Current concepts in CLINICAL NURSING

Volume III

Current concepts in
CLINICAL NURSING

Edited by

MARGERY DUFFEY, R.N., Ph.D.

EDITH H. ANDERSON, R.N., Ph.D.

BETTY S. BERGERSEN, R.N., Ed.D.

MARY LOHR, R.N., Ed.D.

MARION H. ROSE, R.N., M.A.

Volume III

With 22 illustrations

THE C. V. MOSBY COMPANY

Saint Louis   1971

Contributors

Martha Adams, R.N., M.S.
Lecturer in Nursing, School of Nursing, University of California, San Francisco, Calif.

Edith H. Anderson, R.N., Ph.D.
Dean, School of Nursing, University of Hawaii, Honolulu, Hawaii

Margaret Bennett, R.N., M.S.
Instructor, School of Nursing, University of Hawaii, Honolulu, Hawaii

Betty S. Bergersen, R.N., Ed.D.
Visiting Professor, School of Nursing, University of Colorado, Denver, Colo.

Maxine Berlinger, R.N., M.A.
Associate Professor, School of Nursing, University of Colorado, Denver, Colo.

Joy L. Brown, R.N., M.S.N.
Staff Nurse, University of Illinois Medical Center, Chicago, Ill.

Imogene D. Cahill, R.N., Ed.D.
Associate Professor, School of Nursing, University of California, Los Angeles, Calif.

Joyce Cameron, R.N., M.S.
Associate Professor, College of Nursing, University of Utah, Salt Lake City, Utah

Margery Duffey, R.N., Ph.D.
Associate Professor, Department of Nursing Education, University of Kansas, Kansas City, Kan.

Shirley Farrah, R.N., M.S.N.
Instructor in Nursing, Avila College, Kansas City, Mo.

Boonie Ford, R.N., M.A.
Associate Professor, School of Nursing, University of Colorado, Denver, Colo.

Loretta C. Ford, R.N., Ed.D.
Professor and Chairman, Community Health Nursing, School of Nursing, University of Colorado, Denver, Colo.

Nancy Ragsdale Gilien, R.N., M.P.H.
Doctoral Candidate in Anthropology, University of California, Los Angeles, Calif.

†Beulah Gingrich, R.N., B.S.
Instructor, Cook County School of Nursing, Chicago, Ill.

Beatrice Goodwin, R.N., Ph.D.
Associate Professor of Nursing, Herbert H. Lehman College, City University of New York, Bronx, N. Y.

Cheryl Hall Harris, R.N., B.S.
Infant Care Coordinator, Children's Mercy Hospital, Kansas City, Mo.

Doreen M. Harris, R.N., M.S.N.
Instructor, College of Nursing, University of Illinois, Chicago, Ill.

---

†Deceased.

Judy Haselhorst, R.N., M.S.N.
Formerly Instructor, Medical-Surgical Nursing, College of Nursing, University of Illinois, Chicago, Ill.

Mary E. Hazzard, R.N., Ph.D.
Associate Professor of Nursing, University of Virginia School of Nursing, Charlottesville, Va.

Marguerite J. Holmes, R.N., M.N.
Associate Professor, College of Nursing, Arizona State University, Tempe, Ariz.

Shelley Horton, R.N., M.S.
Instructor, School of Nursing, University of Hawaii, Honolulu, Hawaii

Sharon M. Jones, R.N., B.S.
Staff Nurse, Post-partum, Labor and Delivery, University of Kansas Medical Center, Kansas City, Kan.

†Vernita Kay, R.N., D.N.Sc.
Professor, University of Virginia School of Nursing, Charlottesville, Va.

Joan M. King, R.N., D.N.Sc.
Associate Professor, Graduate Program in Psychiatric Nursing, College of Nursing, University of Illinois, Chicago, Ill.

Lily Larson, R.N., M.Ed.
Associate Professor of Nursing, Department of Nursing Education, University of Kansas, Kansas City, Kan.

Mary Lohr, R.N., Ed.D.
Dean, School of Nursing, University of Virginia, Charlottesville, Va.

Mona L. Moughton, R.N., M.A.
Associate Professor of Nursing, University of Virginia School of Nursing, Charlottesville, Va.

Juanita F. Murphy, R.N., Ph.D.
Associate Professor of Nursing, Department of Nursing Education, Associate Professor of Sociology, Department of Sociology, University of Kansas, Kansas City, Kan.

---

†Deceased.

Susan M. Owens, B.S.N.
Public Health Nurse, Albemarle-Charlottesville Health Department, Charlottesville, Va.

Ruth E. Redmann, R.N., M.A.
Assistant Professor, School of Nursing, University of Wisconsin, Madison, Wis.

Olive J. Rich, R.N., Ph.D.
Doctoral Candidate, School of Nursing, University of Pittsburgh, Pittsburgh, Pa.

Hilda Richards, R.N., Ed.M.
Deputy Chief, Division of Rehabilitation Services, Department of Psychiatry, Harlem Hospital Center, New York, N. Y.; Research Assistant, Department of Nursing Education, Teachers College, Columbia University, New York, N. Y.

Marion H. Rose, R.N., M.A.
Professor of Nursing, College of Nursing, Arizona State University, Tempe, Ariz.

Maxine Rubin, R.N., M.A.
Formerly Instructor, Department of Nursing Education, University of Kansas Medical Center, Kansas City, Kan.

Margaret Sagar, B.S.N., R.N.
Lecturer, Preventive Medicine and Public Health, School of Nursing, Queen's University, Kingston, Ontario, Canada

Jurate A. Sakalys, R.N., M.S.N.
Assistant Professor, School of Nursing, University of Colorado, Denver, Colo.

Marie D. Strickland, R.N.
Assistant Professor, Cornell University-New York Hospital School of Nursing, New York, N. Y.

Leonide M. Tanner, R.N., M.S.
Instructor of Maternity Nursing, University of California, Los Angeles, Calif.

Eugenia H. Waechter, R.N., Ph.D.
Assistant Professor, School of Nursing, University of California, San Francisco, Calif.

Lorraine Walker, R.N.
Doctoral Candidate, School of Education, Indiana University, Bloomington, Ind.

Joan E. Zetterlund, R.N., M.S.
Instructor, Department of Nursing, North Park College, Chicago, Ill.

Preface

In 1966 when the idea of a series of books designed to present a broad spectrum of the new or current concerns and functions of nurse practitioners was conceived, there were doubts about the success of such a venture. One of the questions raised was whether every two years the editors could locate thirty to forty contributors with something new and interesting to say regarding patient-care practices.

The three volumes now published represent the contribution of approximately one hundred authors, some of them well known for previous literary works; some venturing to submit their efforts to the scrutiny of their peers for the first time. The variety of ideas put forth by these authors is apparent in the list of chapter titles in these three volumes. Obviously the doubt concerning the adequacy of the source of material for such a series was unfounded.

The reception the members of the profession have given the first two volumes indicates that the series is meeting a need. However, one difficulty that can keep this series from reaching its goal has become apparent. Since the editors cannot know about all of the new and interesting individual things that are happening in nursing today, we take this opportunity to urge all members of the profession who have ideas they wish to share to view this series as one means by which they may communicate with their peers. Also, if you know a colleague, student, or teacher who is doing things in clinical nursing that you think have relevance for nurses in different situations, urge them to contact us. In this time of rapid change, only in this way can this series approach the original goal the editors set for it.

Margery Duffey

Contents

Section III   Maternity nursing
edited by Edith H. Anderson

Psychiatric nursing

With an introduction by
Mary Lohr

This section is dedicated to the memory of Vernita Place Kay, a clinician whose passing has created a loss in all our lives. Some of us grieve the passing of a teacher, others mourn the loss of a perceptive clinician, and many experience the personal bereavement associated with the departure of a friend.

Throughout her life Vernita Place Kay was guided by the central purpose of improving nursing care and strengthening the education of students of professional nursing. From this motivating force she seemed to derive the strength that sustained her frail body years beyond the expectations of her private physicians. Therefore it seems fitting that the objective of this section be to set forth a few ideas that may foster constructive action and may have a favorable impact on nursing care and programs preparing professional nurses.

Contemporary nurses are exploring ways in which they can improve nursing services. The chapters in this section describe a variety of approaches—some are theory guided, others are wholly pragmatic, but each contributor offers some wisdom that may help the reader to use inner resources which will have a favorable influence on patient care and clinical teaching.

A eulogy to Vernita Place Kay written by Mona Moughton follows. The strong friendship bond between these two clinicians was fostered by a mutual interest in psychiatric nursing.

Vernita Mae Place was born in Waterloo, Iowa, on March 18, 1918. She was a middle child, having an older and a younger sister. Her father's work required that the family move quite frequently and the three girls became very close, depending on each other as the constants in an ever-changing environment. Their mother died when Vernita was 15 and her much younger sister said at Vernita's death, 'I haven't just lost a sister, I've lost my sister, my mother, and my friend.'

We have some appreciation of what this means because we have lost not only a valued colleague, but a trusted friend. Vernita was not a letter writer, but one could depend on a telephone call now and then "just to keep in touch" when separated by distance. It still has little meaning, for me at least, that the distance that separates us now is much too great for a telephone call.

Vernita had not always wanted to be a nurse, as with some of us, but she made the decision after several years of college and keeping house for her father and younger sister. She entered Broadlawns General Hospital School of Nursing in Des Moines, Iowa, in 1940 and completed the course in 1943. Her class must hold some kind of record, for they have kept a round-robin letter going without a break since 1943.

During nurses' training, Vernita contracted tuberculosis and after completion of the nursing program she was hospitalized for quite a long time, a period that included surgery for the removal of the greater part of her right lung. She told me one time that her father stayed with her day and night after the surgery and was a source of strength and comfort at times when she felt she could endure no more. Vernita admired her father greatly and particularly appreciated his attempt to be both father and mother after the death of her mother. Vernita and her father shared a passion for baseball, an interest she never lost.

Vernita married James Kay in August of 1946 and he died in 1951. After his death, she returned to nursing, working at the Independence Mental Health Institute in Independence, Iowa. She also decided to further her education and completed the baccalaureate degree with specialization in psychiatric nursing at the University of Iowa College of Nursing in 1955 and completed her master's degree in 1957. Dr. Mary Lohr was chairman of the Psychiatric Nursing Department at that time. In 1958 Vernita left the Mental Health Institute, where she was director of nursing, to teach at the University of Iowa. Although I had known Vernita prior to this, it was at this time that she and I became fellow teachers and friends. Her sincere interest and quiet competence were greatly valued by her students and her colleagues.

However, Iowa did not present the challenge that Vernita needed, so she returned to school in 1961, entering the doctoral program at Boston University. She completed the program and received the degree of Doctor of Nursing Science in 1965. She again turned to teaching, this time at the University of Illinois School of Nursing, in the graduate program in psychiatric nursing. She came to us just one short year ago. She had become quite concerned by our troubled adolescents and the last few years left to her were spent in learning and teaching psychotherapeutic approaches to the treatment of emotionally disturbed adolescents. Through her characteristic intense concentration, within a relatively brief span of time, Vernita became one of the most able and informed clinicians within this highly specialized field. Her loss to this area of concern is incalculable.

Vernita had planned to retire in about two more years and had a number of works outlined to be written when she had the time. She had not yet written much when she died and now we have lost this also. Most of you have heard from her about her lodge in the northern Minnesota woods, a place at which she found much peace. This next summer a tool shed there would have been converted into a study, a quiet place in which to write. She now lies buried one-half mile from her lodge.

Although I had always known that Vernita needed to conserve her energy, I had not known that when surgery was performed in 1943, she was told she had ten good years left. The fact that she extended these ten years to twenty-six attests to her will and determination. One of the topics she frequently mentioned was loss, the personal loss to people when they parted for whatever reason. Apparently she understood that she would leave us first and was trying to prepare us and herself for this parting.

Chapter 1

Rescue fantasy in the nurse—a study of the attitudes of pediatric-psychiatric nurses

Susan M. Owens

The term "rescue fantasy" is widely used to indicate that form of behavior observed in the therapist (nurse, doctor, etc.) in which she appears to hold a persistent, unrealistic fantasy that she can save or in someway meaningfully rescue the child or children with whom she works.[1] It is a construct that cannot be directly observed in most cases, but must instead be inferred from behavior or from active questioning of the therapist involved. The fantasy itself appears to strongly reflect the personality and unconscious motivations of the particular nurse or doctor and does not appear to be an isolated reaction to a specific child or situation.[2]

Many published studies deal with rescue fantasy experience in the physician, but few are reported in the area of nursing. In this chapter, an assessment of the reactions of selected graduate nurses to the care of emotionally disturbed pediatric patients has been made. In particular, the assessment tests the phenomenon of rescue fantasy, which has been used to explain some facets of the nurse-therapist relationship with disturbed children. From a study by Linda Dabritz and associates[1] in which the dynamics of rescue fantasy are discussed in detail, six basic assumptions have been drawn about the nurse's role with emotionally disturbed children. On the basis of these assumptions, a questionnaire was constructed to demonstrate compliance with or rejection of the philosophy and attitudes that may eventually develop into rescue fantasy effect.

Rescue fantasy has been recently proposed as one of the main attitude patterns of nurses entering pediatric-psychiatry, yet it has been minimally explored. It was hoped that this study would lend support to the rescue fantasy theory by providing agreement on the part of respondents about the following six basic assumptions:

1. The nurse has unconscious feelings of omnipotence, and any success she has increases her self-esteem and her feelings of power.

2. The nurse exhibits narcissistic characteristics to a high degree, as shown by her overestimation of her own capabilities.

3. The nurse is overprotective of the child with whom she works.

4. The nurse becomes hostile to the par-

ents, unrealistically excluding them from the therapy program whenever it is possible. She thinks of the staff as a good substitute parent.

5. The nurse identifies with the child.

6. The nurse's feelings are caused by an unconscious attempt to resolve her feelings of debt to her own parents (Freud's parental complex). She considers cure for the child equivalent to a rescue from death.

Methodology

Seven questions were designed for each of the foregoing statements, with the exception of an additional question for assumption 4.

The questionnaire was actually a series of statements arranged on the left-hand side of the page with a Likert-type rating scale on the right-hand side. Respondents were requested to check choices of strong agreement, agreement, indifference, disagreement, or strong disagreement.

Fifty questionnaires were sent out to nurses working in the psychiatric children's units of four different hospitals. Nurses from three hospitals responded (located in New York, Virginia, and Florida).* Sixteen forms, or 32% of the total, were returned.† Personal information about each respondent requested included only age, marital status, number of chil-

---

*Hospitals utilized for this investigation were University of Florida, Inpatient Children's Psychiatric Unit, Gainesville, Fla.; Virginia Treatment Center for Children, Medical College of Virginia, Richmond, Va.; Bellevue Children's Unit, Bellevue Hospital, New York City, N. Y.

†Of the returns, eleven were from the Richmond area, three from Gainesville, and two from New York. The questionnaire forms were distributed through the directors of nursing in each of the hospitals. All of them showed great interest in the study and asked for a copy of the results, and the Virginia Treatment Center for Children asked for permission to use the questionnaire with applicants asking for employment.

dren, education, and length of experience in this type of nursing.

Findings

It was found that eleven of the respondents ($68\frac{3}{4}\%$) were between the ages of 21 and 26, four (25%) were between the ages of 32 and 38, and only one respondent ($6\frac{1}{4}\%$) was above that age group (46 years old).

In regard to length of experience, six persons ($37\frac{1}{2}\%$) had worked with emotionally disturbed children for 5 months or less. Four persons (25%) had worked between 10 and 18 months in this field. Five persons ($31\frac{1}{4}\%$) had worked between $2\frac{1}{2}$ years and 6 years, and the remaining person ($6\frac{1}{4}\%$) had worked 12 years in pediatric-psychiatry.

Nine nurses ($56\frac{1}{4}\%$) were married, whereas seven ($43\frac{3}{4}\%$) were single. Of the married subjects in this study, six ($66\frac{2}{3}\%$) had no children, one ($11\frac{1}{9}\%$) had one child, and two ($22\frac{2}{9}\%$) had two children. The remaining seven nurses, of course, had no children.

One nurse ($6\frac{1}{4}\%$) was a graduate of a program leading to an associate of arts in nursing degree, four were graduates of a baccalaureate nursing program (25%), eight were graduates of a diploma nursing program (50%), and three nurses had attained a master of science or master of arts degree in psychiatric or pediatric-psychiatric nursing ($18\frac{3}{4}\%$).

Fig. 1 was compiled by analyzing the number of "correct" responses each individual made to the questions relating to each individual statement. A response was considered "correct" if it supported one of the six major assumptions previously mentioned. If a person had less than three "incorrect" responses for the seven or eight questions relating to the appropriate statement, it was considered the statement was supported. If there were four or more deviations from the "correct" response, it was considered that the respondent re-

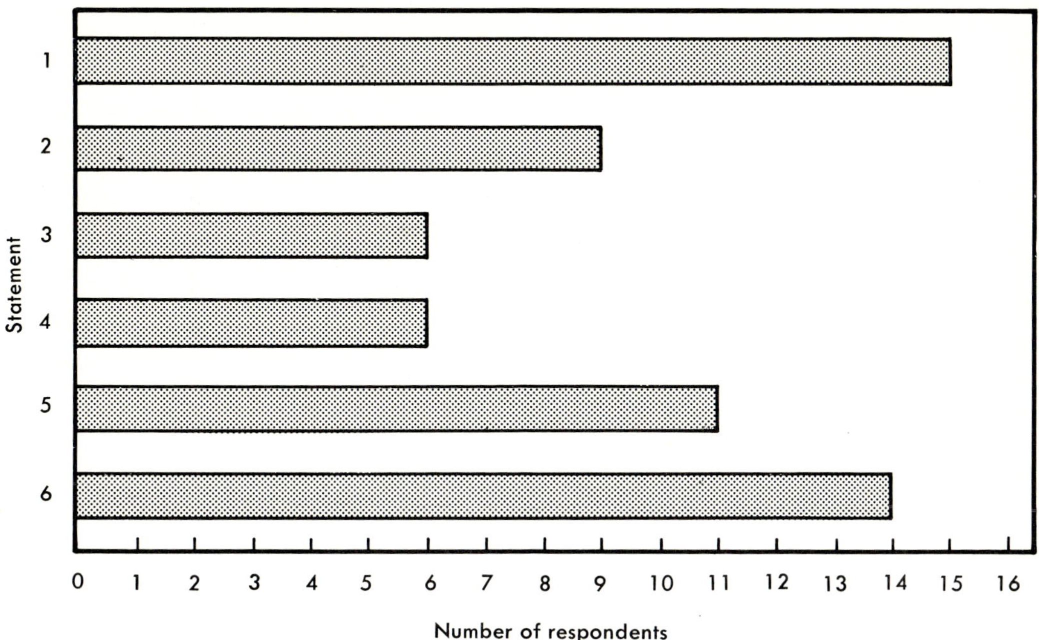

Fig. 1

Number of persons responding in a supportive manner for each of the six major assumptions.

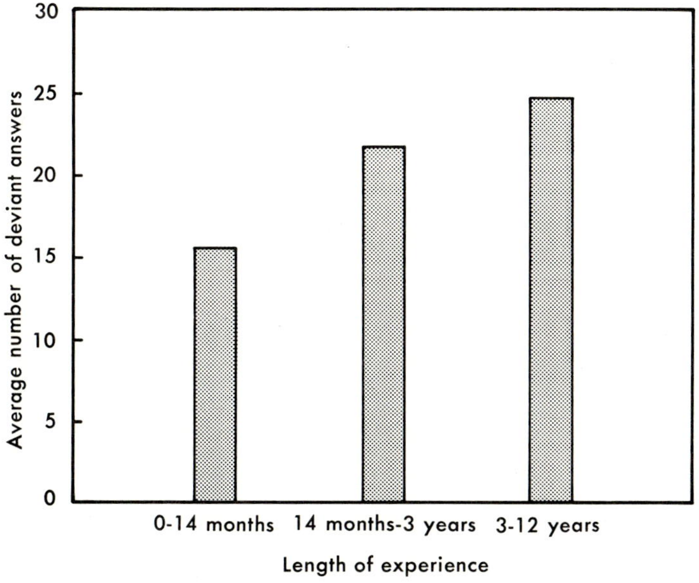

Fig. 2

Length of work experience of respondents and frequency of answers *not* complying with the basic assumptions about rescue fantasy in nurses.

jected the statement and had made a deviant response.

These data clearly demonstrate that the greatest amount of agreement occurred with statements 1 and 6, showing support for the assumptions related to the nurse's unconscious feeling of omnipotence and to her unconscious attempt to resolve her feelings of debt to her own parents by "rescuing" the child. Such dramatic support was not shown for the other four statements. Sixty-two and one-half percent of the respondents showed agreement with questions relating to statement 5, but only 50% sunpported statement 2, which related to the nurse's narcissistic characteristics. Statements 3 and 4 received the least support, when only 31¼% of respondents answered as expected questions designed to indicate hostility to the child's

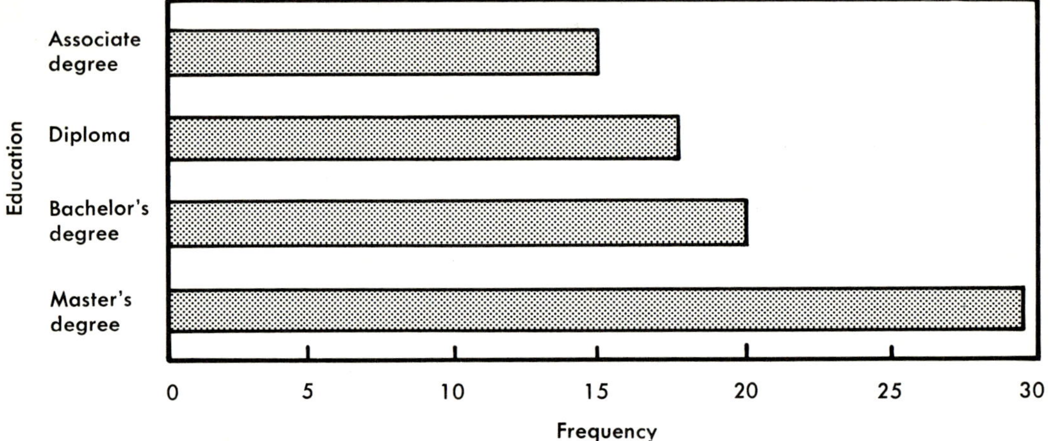

Fig. 3
Education of respondents and frequency of answers *not* complying with the six basic assumptions about rescue fantasy.

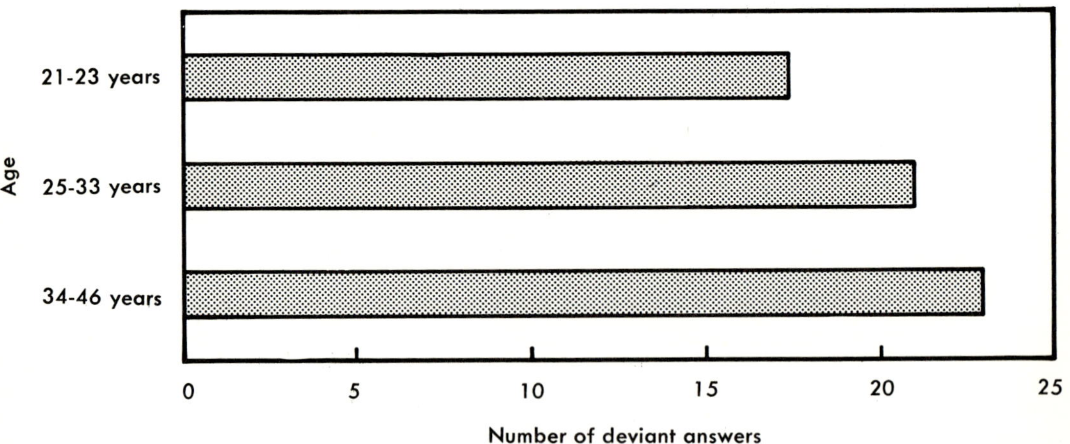

Fig. 4
Frequency of deviant answers according to age of individual respondents.

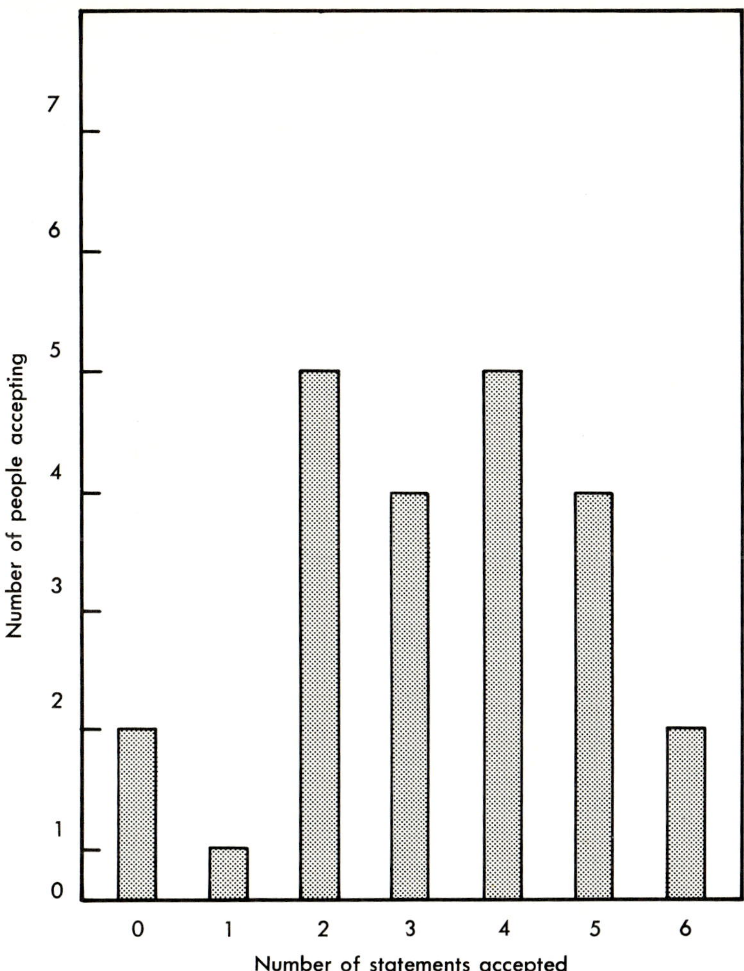

Fig. 5

Tabulation of the number of nurses according to the number of statements accepted by each.

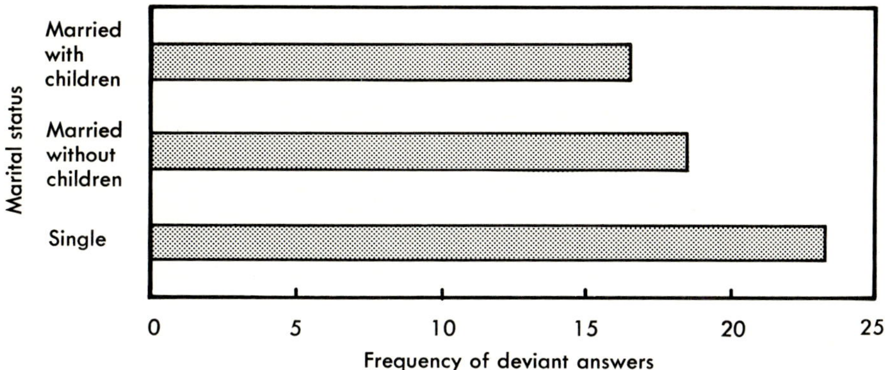

Fig. 6

Frequency distribution of deviant answers according to marital status.

parents and overprotection of the child himself.

In regard to the relationship of the amount of work experience to the amount of rescue fantasy, as can be seen in Fig. 2, those nurses with the least experience appeared to support more strongly the six basic assumptions regarding the rescue fantasy phenomenon. Those with more experience gave a higher average of deviant responses that was directly proportional to the duration of their work experience.

Fig. 3, the next tabulation carried out, was done to demonstrate the relationship of education to the amount of rescue fantasy felt by the nurse. As can be seen, the educational level does appear to have a definite relationship on the number of deviant responses encountered in the questionnaire and, therefore, on the amount of rescue fantasy encountered in the individual. Those respondents with the least education exhibited the greatest amount of rescue fantasy, whereas those with more education exhibited less of this reaction in an amount directly proportional to the amount of education they had received.

The correlation between the number of deviant answers and the age of the individual responding demonstrated a directly proportional relationship. The respondents were divided into three age groups, and the average number of deviant answers was figured for each group. Fig. 4 provides visual representation of the relationship.

After having tabulated group responses in Figs. 1 to 4, it was decided to concentrate on patterns in the individual nurses involved in the study. It soon became evident that few nurses accepted all of the six assumptions related to rescue fantasy and that few rejected all of them. Fig. 5 demonstrates that almost all the nurses accepted between two and five of the six assumptions.

As can be seen from Fig. 6, a definite correlation was found between marital status and frequency of deviant answers in the group tested. The mean number of deviant answers in the single group was higher than either of the other groups. Those nurses who were married and had their own children had a mean number of deviant answers lower than the other two groups.

Discussion

From the preceding results reflecting attitudes, several tentative conclusions may be drawn. It must be kept in mind that data were obtained from sixteen respondents. There are also several other variables that must be taken into account in analyzing these data and considering their validity. It is possible, for instance, that some items on the questionnaire could not be answered truthfully without posing a threat to the individual. From these findings, some observations that may be of use include the following:

1. Pediatric-psychiatric nurses show less tendency to overprotect their patients and to be hostile toward patients' parents than the investigator predicted.

2. Most respondents identify strongly with their patients.

3. Nurses with the least experience seem to have the most rescue fantasy. It is possible that this demonstrates that rescue fantasy is a strong motivation for choosing to work with emotionally disturbed children, but this effect seems not to be sustained in the face of discouraging results and prognosis.

4. Nurses with the least education exhibit the most rescue fantasy. It is possible that this could be explained in part by the fact that formal education leads to a more realistic conception of the persistence of psychopathology. Increased education hopefully also serves to help the individual to edit hostile actions such as those suggested in statement 4 out of her behavior.

5. Younger nurses demonstrate more

rescue fantasy. They are, perhaps, more idealistic and less willing to accept an unfavorable prognosis, and in general they have had less experience and their feelings of omnipotence have therefore been challenged less frequently.

6. Those nurses who are married and have their own children support the rescue fantasy most strongly, whereas those who are single support it least strongly. Most nurses in the field of pediatric-psychiatric nursing are single, and leave the field when they become married; few remain in the field after they have children. Whether this is because they think of their own children when they work with these disturbed youngsters or whether it is because married nurses with children believe more strongly in rescue fantasy and therefore become more easily disturbed and dissatisfied when their expectations are not· met is a point that could be argued and is worthy of study.

Rescue fantasy, if it can be definitely identified as a part of the nurse-child relationship in pediatric psychiatry, is an area in which further research should be devoted. An understanding of this concept could assist in understanding feelings of despondency, frustration, and helplessness that nurses in pediatric-psychiatric nursing often feel. An investigation in this area could assist in clarifying whether rescue fantasy is a saving concept that gives nurses the fortitude to continue working with disturbed children in what is frequently a discouraging atmosphere.

This chapter has only initiated a study of rescue fantasy. Some support for the idea that there is a definite relationship between the concept of rescue fantasy and the nursing care provided pediatric-psychiatric patients has been suggested, but there are many opportunities for further useful inquiry in this area that have not been touched on.

References

1. Dabritz, Linda, Gillis, Sue, and Van Epps, Joan: Rescue fantasy in the nurse therapist relationship with a psychotic child, J. Psychiat. Nurs. Ment. Health Service 6:71-78, 1968.
2. Schneer, Henry: Recent advances in the treatment of childhood schizophrenia, J. Hillside Hospital 10-11:194-204, 1962.

Chapter 2

Role of the nurse with emotionally disturbed adolescents

Vernita Kay

I have been asked to cover the nurse's role in the hospital, the problems of the hospitalized adolescent, and understanding and working with parents and with hospital school teachers. These aspects are rather broad to cover in a short chapter so I have chosen to discuss one or two issues related to each aspect.

In my experience the usual model used to house adolescent patients in hospitals is either to separate them in a ward with their age group or to integrate them throughout the adult wards. It is not always possible, but the latter is preferable in my judgment because (1) it is a more normal arrangement in life to house adults and children together, (2) adult patients provide additional means of impulse control for young persons, and (3) I believe it takes less nursing staff. Adequate staffing in adolescent treatment programs is of primary importance, I believe, to plan corrective experiences that can be carried out, which are useful to the child, and to avoid traumatic end results that call for punitive or unsuccessful outside measures of control. It is useful to house adolescents on adult units, but at the same time, I am not suggesting that they share adult treatment programs, except in carefully structured instances. Adolescent patients have quite different needs than do adult patients. I will cover this point later in the chapter.

Problems that distress adolescents are as broad as within any age grouping and probably greater than most. The child at the beginning of adolescence has no established identity and no certain way of life that would determine his future. There is not yet a capacity to identify with adult figures without loss of personal identity or a sense of personal continuity. In addition, today's teen-agers are the offspring of those persons whom Riesman called "other-directed" a few years ago in *The Lonely Crowd,* which warned of deep uncertainty in a population associated with social and cultural institutional changes. Such uncertainty tends to widen the generation gap even further and to close meaningful comunication between adults and adolescents. In some ways, this state of affairs, if one reads many newspapers carefully, seems to promote tyranny in peer groups that makes young people in a certain sense captives of each other. At least today it often seems so.[1] A main task, then, is for adolescents to establish, from a shifting sense of self, a relatively constant one. Devaluing adults, particularly parents, is part of the growing-up process.

The adolescent who rebels against the dominance of the adult world, its values and its restrictions, needs peer associations as well as associations with meaningful adults. Peers are persons who greatly help him find his own identity. Identification with a structured peer group, such as the Boy Scouts, can provide him some relief from pain and tension by supplying a group code of behavior that wards off overwhelming anxieties involved in making individual decisions because the answers are generalized and stereotyped. In addition to groups structured and led by adults, some clinicians have stressed the need for spontaneous peer group associations by pointing out that gangs may satisfy needs that individuals cannot. In a gang an individual has feedback from the group response to him. The child repeats in a group childhood experiences from his family, and in this situation he does it actively and takes responsibility for it both as leader and as follower, which is something he had experienced previously only in a passive way in his family group. Environmental treatment programs should include opportunity for the patient to participate in both structured and spontaneous groups.

A primary problem at adolescence is further internalization of controls. This is the root of adult conscience. Included are changes from total taboo against sex to integrated total acceptance and from lack of controls in aggressive behavior to more sublimated behavior independent of environment. The norms and values related to internalized controls cover a wide range. However, in our society it is safe to say that the superego in adolescence can be harsh unless it is softened by adult aggression (controls). Depression has been a factor observed in all disturbed adolescents with which my students and I have worked. This is an important understanding for nurses who seem to be constantly struggling with the "contagion" phenomena of behavior, which seems to be either self-destructive or socially destructive and goes from time to time through adolescent populations in hospitals.

The primary source of anxiety at adolescence stems from separation from parents or impending separation from parents. Both parents and child experience a sense of loss and if parents deny felt loss at this time, they are not available to help the child free his energy to seek out mature love objects. Adolescent distress that is experienced may be typical for the age group, but it may be troublesome to the child in a hospital and particularly troublesome to the adults about him. These phenomena include common sexual problems, delinquent acts, rebellion, crushes, asceticism, intellectuality, mood swings, masturbation, shyness, and such transient symptoms as phobias and obsessions. All these symptoms that are observed in disturbed children represent a tremendous effort for control on the part of the adolescent whose fragile ego is simply too weak to handle adolescent conflicts. We often see contradictory traits day to day, hour to hour. During this time it is important that adults do not become confused about their own role with the youngster.

Ego psychology has provided the clinician with tools to assess ego strengths and weaknesses that in turn provide clues to direct relevant nursing intervention.

The nurse's role in treatment programs of adolescents may be as broad as she has the capacity to make it. However, no matter what role a nurse assumes for herself the statements regarding treatment that follow are based on the following assumptions:

1. All persons who are involved in any

way in the treatment program, that is, all levels and all kinds of staff, have common agreement on the norms of acceptable adolescent behavior.

2. All levels and kinds of staff share common goals in the program.

3. All levels and kinds of staff have some basic theoretical understanding of human development, psychodynamics, and psychopathology.

4. Some appropriate supervision is to be attainable.

5. All levels and kinds of staff have the capacity to allow young people to have fun in an adolescent manner, not an adult manner.

With disturbed adolescents the goal of treatment is *not* insight; rather it is to help the adolescent handle the insight he has.

It does not matter what the precipitating factors or the individual psychodynamics are, the child who is hospitalized is first confronted within himself with issues of separation. Initial help must be directed here before anything further can be confronted. The steps as outlined by Grace and Davis[2] that must occur are (1) denial of the unendurable reality, (2) development of awareness of the pain of loss and emptiness, and (3) the restitution phase in which new objects replace lost ones. In my experience, no child is able to engage himself in a therapeutic alliance while denying the immediate and real loss of family and friends.

Second, at no time in the life of individuals is the ego more fragile and battered from increased drives and uncompromising reality than at adolescence. A nurse must therefore make immediate and continual assessments of ego strengths and weaknesses in each child. Primary focus, then, is directed toward ego stability and development. Every emotional disturbance has concomitantly some ego-function damage. Assessment then identifies those ego functions in need of repairs. It is important to use ego strengths as therapeutic allies

to prevent further battering of weakened ego functions. For example, with a child whose thinking process is relatively intact and who is having severe distress with impulse controls, it might be advantageous to encourage intellectualization. In the adult neurotic, one might attempt to cut through the intellectualization. In an adolescent patient, on the other hand, one might helpfully foster it.

In interacting with a disturbed adolescent, the therapist should follow whatever direction the opportunities offer within the situation to promote ego growth and to raise self-esteem and avoid massive assault on the ego as might occur with sarcasm or flippancy. It is terribly important not to back an adolescent in a corner either psychologically or literally so that he has to defend himself maladaptively to save face or to avoid humiliation. He has no controls to save himself or you. Provide him with a real person (as opposed to a transference figure) with whom to form a positive identification. Use yourself to validate reality with the child as he goes through his day-by-day living experiences.

It would follow that it is perhaps also more important to keep track of one's own feelings about patients with a youngster of this age than with any other patient, except perhaps an acute adult schizophrenic. Youngsters are terribly sensitive and perceptive. Evasion, avoidance, and untruths are devastating to a child. And finally, when the task is to help a patient to learn to differentiate and to discriminate, and almost every disturbed adolescent needs help to identify the roles real people have in his life, focus may be helpfully directed to communication habits that tend to foster distortions, misperceptions, unclear referents, and similar problematic speech patterns on the part of the nurse as well as the patient.

I would like to come back briefly now to the point I made earlier—that adolescents need a treatment program which is different from adult programs and which is age appropriate. There will, of course, be some overlapping; but I do not believe that any social institution in our culture makes equal demands, has equal expectations, or has the same rules and regulations for adults and for adolescents. It follows, then, in the real world adolescents need more environmental structure and guidance, school if possible, scheduled study and recreation, and so on than do adults. They need built-in mechanisms to reduce tension and to expend energy. They need opportunity to try on real life roles for size and fit. If the programs are large enough to allow for it, I believe stable permanent staff should be assigned to adolescent programs, so that staff development programs will become more meaningful, delimited, and discriminating.

Certainly a nurse must have the final decision about how many adolescents a ward is able to absorb and which child is to be transferred if one is. Hers is the only discipline that has information about each child, how they relate to the total program as a whole, how much expressed rage a unit can absorb, and whether certain adult patients at all times on the units provide a climate for adolescent growth. It is her responsibility to staff adequately her units and to provide development for her staff. This would be quite impossible if she were often caught off balance with an unrealistic proportion of either adult or adolescent patients. A nurse provides the setting that allows utilization for exploration of life issues on the spot, regardless of scheduled interviews and meetings. She presents rational reality as one choice. Dis-

turbed adolescents need an adequate program to provide structure to their lives, to allow for expression of surplus tension, and to be helped into corrective emotional experiences by a nurse's manipulation of her own role—that of an adult model.

Finally, a few words about the nurse's role with the adolescent's family. The nurse works closely with family members if she is participating in family treatment programs. And some nurses do this—provide family therapy either alone or with others under certain circumstances. Her observations of the visit, for the most part, would center on the adolescent, his reactions, stresses, mood, etc.

These observations would be shared with other levels and kinds of staff working in the program. The school teacher, on the other hand, would be the recipient of the nurse's observations. It would be important for her to have understanding in depth about the adolescent's frustration tolerance, his intellectual interests outside the classroom, the amount and kinds of help he needs with his homework, and obvious distortions in his perception, language, and speech, as well as the mode he is apt to use in communication of frustration and rage. Ideally, the teacher would be an active member in the program for purposes of planning, for carrying out certain program goals, and for evaluation.

References

1. Harris, T. George: The young are captives of each other: a conversation with David Riesman, Psychology Today 3:67, Oct., 1967.
2. Grace, Helen, and Davis, Lucille: Personal communication, 1967.

Chapter 3

Systems theory and the adolescent

Mona L. Moughton and Mary E. Hazzard

If one were to analyze the current notions and catchwords, he would find "systems" high on the list. The concept has pervaded fields of science and penetrated into popular thinking, jargon, mass media, and the nursing literature.[1-3] It is necessary to study not only the parts and processes in isolation but also the order and organization unifying them, which results in a dynamic interaction of parts and which makes the behavior of the parts different when studied in isolation or within the whole. Ludwig von Bertalanffy[4] has postulated the general systems theory, which attempts to apply universal principles to systems or their subclasses irrespective of the particular kind, the nature of the component elements, and the relations or forces between them.

Systems

A system is a set of parts or components together with relationships between the parts and between the properties of the parts.[5] For any given set of parts the relationships to be studied depend on the problem. The interesting or important relationships pertaining to the problem are included and the trivial or unessential relationships are excluded. A system, together with its environment, makes up the totality of all things of interest in a given context. The division into system and environment is arbitrary and ultimately depends on the intention of the one studying the phenomena. The subsystems, components, or parts of a system are themselves concrete systems.

Systems may be open or closed. In a closed system there is no exchange of matter or energy with the environment. This system will eventually run down when maximum entropy is reached. An open system is a system that exchanges matter and energy with the environment. From conception through death the life process continually takes in matter, energy, or information from the environment and releases matter, energy, or information to the environment. The environment does more than affect our well-being in the here and now, for it determines almost irreversibly the future of man and society.

Energy

There are two types of energy. One is negentropy and is ordered, available "free energy," and the other is entropy and is disordered, unavailable "bound energy." Open systems may have irreversible and reversible processes and in order to study these Prigogine[6] extended the second law of thermodynamics. In its simplest form this law states that whenever energy is transformed from one kind into another, only a fraction of the internal energy change is available for doing useful work; the remainder remains as heat energy of the molecules left at the completion of the reaction or entropy.

Information, which is defined as energy by some theorists, is also defined as the degree of freedom that exists in a given situation to choose among symbols, messages, or patterns that have been transmitted. Meaning is therefore the significance of the information to the system processing it. Matter-energy and information always flow together. When information is transferred from one place to another, a channel for transmission of the information is necessary. If a message is put in at one end, that is, the mouthpiece of the telephone, another message comes out the other end, that is, through the telephone receiver. Under ideal circumstances these messages are closely related, but if there is interference or "noise," the output is altered. The information available in a message as it is received depends on the meaning of the message and the distorting effects that occur between input and output.

In an open system there are states of nonequilibrium, or the steady state, where variables tend to remain within a predetermined range of system parameters, but a process or processes may lead to change or changes in the value of the system variables. The living organism is thus able to dispense existing potentials or tensions in spontaneous activity or in response to relieving stimuli and can advance toward higher order and organization. Even under constant external conditions and in the absence of external stimuli the organism is an active and not a passive system. It appears, therefore, that internal activity rather than reaction to stimuli is the fundamental issue. Stimuli do not cause reactions in an otherwise inert system; it only modifies reactions in an autonomously active system. In a steady state environment the processes are irreversible and the system does not return to its original state after the process has been completed. An analogy that might be used is that one cannot step into the same river twice. The molecules of the river are different and changes have taken place in the foot.

The life process

The life process in man has been identified as (1) an open system, (2) manifesting pattern and organization amid constant change, (3) a self-regulating system, (4) a dynamic system, and (5) subject to the universal laws governing all living systems.

As frequently noted in the literature,[10-12] the study of man encompasses the multiplicity of events that take place as man moves along the continuum from conception through death. Time and rate are involved in the system processes and the progression is from initial to final state. Equifinality is the tendency toward a characteristic final state from different initial states and in different ways based on the dynamic interaction in the open system as it attempts to attain a steady state.[4] Growth is equifinal; the same species' characteristic final state, death, can be reached from different initial states, size at birth. Some achieve the final state rapidly; others take a longer period of time. The rate of entropy increase influences the length of the life-span of the individual.

The living system can maintain itself in a steady state by the importation of material rich in free energy and through exchange can avoid an increase of entropy,

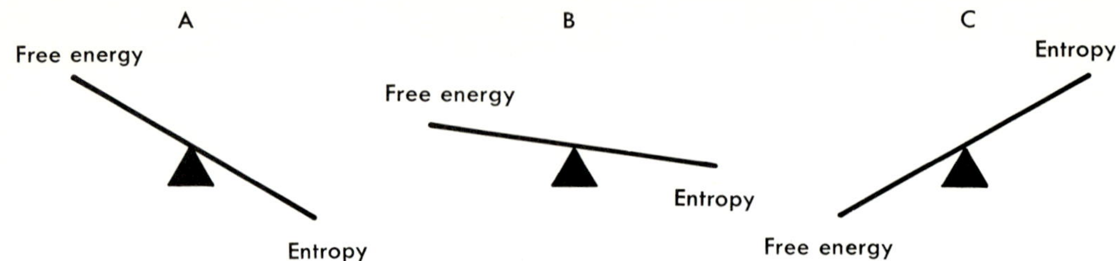

Fig. 7
A, Childhood. **B,** Adulthood. **C,** Aging.

which cannot be avoided in a closed system. This control of entropy allows the organism to develop toward states of increased order and organization. Growth is based on a balance of anabolic and catabolic processes, and when the building up surpasses the breaking down, the individual grows. Growth becomes stationary when both processes are equal and aging occurs when breaking down, entropy, surpasses the building up, negentropy. A set of balances may be used to demonstrate these phenomena (Fig. 7).

In Fig. 7, *A*, childhood, there is more free energy than entropy within the system. As the person grows and develops, a quasi-steady entropy or free energy state exists as demonstrated in Fig. 7, *B*. As the person approaches the death dimension of the life process, there is a reversal of the levels of entropy and free energy. In the elderly, Fig. 7, *C*, there is a high incidence of entropy or "bound energy" and a low incidence of negentropy.

The use of models

A model is a symbolic assertion in logical terms of an idealized, relatively simple situation showing the structural properties of the original factual system. Our thoughts are a progression of symbols that we put in relations and sequences according to established rules. No part of the universe is so simple that it can be grasped and controlled without abstraction. An incongruence between a model and reality often exists, but this does not hinder the use of such models. Models may show an array of approaches to investigate systems that had otherwise been considered beyond the scope of exploration. There are advantages in the use of mathematical models—unambiguity, possibility of strict deduction, verifiability by observed data—but this does not preclude models formulated in ordinary language. One assumption with the use of models is that order can be imposed on the phenomena under study.[13]

For purposes of this discussion a model of living systems is diagramed in Fig. 8. In this model the center box represents the system under consideration—the individual, the family, or the hospital. The input into the system, interacting with previously acquired information through an internal feedback loop, will result in decisions and actions, output, which through an external feedback loop further affects the input.

The individual

A biological system is characterized by its ability to be self-regulating for the purpose of survival, given optimum conditions. The human organism is just such a system. It can regulate the input of energy, matter, or information, transform this matter or information by checking it against previously stored data, and, acting through feedback controls, produce an output related to the need to survive. The

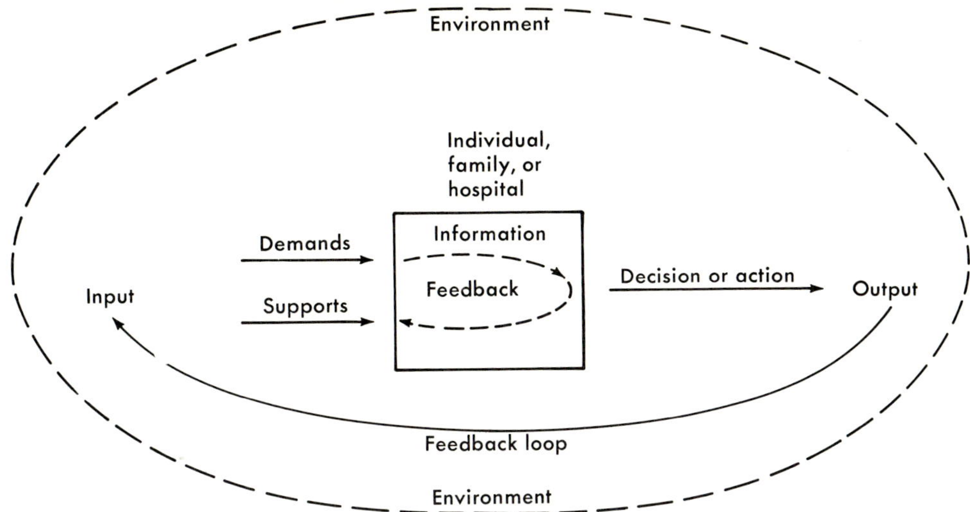

Fig. 8
A model of living systems.

output consists of matter, energy, or information.

The family

In the same way that a person may be described as an integration of subsystems, groups of persons may be seen as systems that create new and larger systems for ensuring survival of group members.

The family also can be viewed as just such a system. The basic family system is a young couple who, to ensure survival of the newly created system, relinquish some individual needs while together resisting possible outside influences that might separate them. This system will function as long as the common goal, the family system, takes precedence over the need to function as independent persons.

With the addition of children this family system enlarges and the original system, now the parent system, has greatly increased responsibilities. During the growing-up process much information passes from the adults to the children in the system, the intent being to ensure the ability of each child to function increasingly as an independent system.

The hospital

The hospital may be thought of as one of the social institutions that has risen in the course of social evolution. As a system the hospital tends to have a life of its own and has emerged to fill the needs of the community that would have been impossible to achieve otherwise.

Interacting subsystems within the hospital are tightly coupled and this closeness of coupling may be either an advantage or a disadvantage. The conscious intentions of the participants (nurses, doctors, patients, administrators, ancillary personnel) are important factors. The existence of a stable organization implies a degree of harmony and coordination, or a sharing of intentions. To do this, the participants must communicate with each other to formulate common goals and the means for attaining such goals. It is possible to measure such communication.

In the hospital system the input consists

of sick people and their relationships, transformation is constituted of the therapeutic interaction taking place, and the output is healthier and better functioning individuals or groups. A good therapeutic system will achieve these goals in a reasonable time and with a high incidence of good and lasting results.

The family

Individuals are born into a family, and every family is a component part of a society or a culture. The individual, the family, and the society are each a system, yet the individual can be viewed as a subsystem of the family, and the family as a subsystem of the culture. The model of input, feedback processing, and output with external feedback affecting further input can be seen to operate at each level. However, these systems do not operate independently, since they are in constant contact with each other. Thus the output from the individual as a system will affect further input into that same system, but the output will also affect the input into the family system and the system of the larger society. If there are more than two family members, each of the additional persons will affect and be affected by the output of one individual system. It can readily be seen that there is rarely a single cause for a specific event, and that studying or explaining behavior out of its wider context will be valid more often than not by chance only.

To understand why the family is what it is, it must be considered as a part of the total culture within which it exists. The family and the child-rearing that is a part of it are the earliest influences that surround the infant and the child. The child grows up in the family system that provides for his survival and is responsible for his personality development and enculturation. The foundation established by the family will provide the model for all future responses made by the child to the

experiences he encounters; later experiences will influence and modify these responses but never really change them wholly. It is through the family system that society has provided for the transmission of culture to ensure the ability of the next generation to fit into the cultural pattern. However, the personalities of the parents and that part of the social pattern they have internalized will affect what they teach their children, and at the same time will influence the culture, resulting in a slow but constant cultural evolution. Except for small isolated cultural groups that have tended to behave as closed systems, such as some African tribes, cultural groups behave as open systems and are subject to constant change.

As noted by Ackerman,[14] the task of the family is to socialize the child and foster the development of his identity. The child becomes a microcosm of his family group: the image of self and the image of the family are reciprocally interdependent.

Information processing in the child

Arbib and Kahn[15] postulated an interesting model for information processing in the child. The large time-sharing computers have a monitor permanently programed into them when they are first installed. After the monitor is found to function properly, it will schedule and control the various programs as they are run through. The monitor itself never changes and is good for the life of the computer. These authors suggest that the period of interpersonal contact with the mother and then the family is equivalent to writing a monitor. This process yields such affectual qualities as "basic trust" and such informational qualities as "learning to learn."[15] Faulty responses at this stage would result in a defective monitor. Later programs are run by this monitor and it does not matter how good the new programs are, for there will be malfunction if the monitor is faulty. Some system would be needed to modify the monitor before programs could begin to run more appropriately.

The infant is dependent on activity about him for normal development to occur. "It is the input and state (memory) of the system which together yield the output . . . (so that) the system actively seeks information to update its internal model of the environment . . . (and thus) the system uses its output as a stimulus to the environment to elicit a meaningful response to serve as its input."* So, if the mothering one consistently receives relieves tension in the infant, "basic trust" develops, or a model of the external world develops that helps the infant internalize adaptive actions which lead to tension relief. Environmental cues come to be recognized as information rather than as vague feelings, and information and feelings become mutually self-modifying while "inside" and "outside" are gradually becoming differentiated.[15] Interaction with the outside world is a central factor in determining if certain processes will develop at all, the age at which they will evolve, and the intensity with which they will feed back to help the inner system modify itself.[15] This process would be repeated, with increasing sophistication, while the infant and child work through the developmental tasks at the appropriate stages. If this developmental process breaks down, fragmented inconsistent behavior results, with rituals developed earlier being run through inappropriately.

The adolescent

After the major changes in growth and development that occur prior to 6 years of age, a somewhat quasi-steady situation arises between 6 and 12 years of age during which mostly minor crises occur. Rela-

*From Arbib, Michael, and Kahn, Roy M.: A developmental model of information processing in the child, Perspect. Biol. Med. 12:397-416, 1969.

tively speaking, the quieter this latter period has been and the more rapid the rate of change at the onset of adolescence, the greater will be the problems of the individual in coping with change.

A systems approach to growth and development should recognize decision procedures and attitudes that will maximize the growth and development not only of a particular system of interest, but also of relevant ecological systems. The problem is not to argue whether adolescence is a biological or psychological effect or to try to describe on a statistical basis to what degree the problem *is* biological or psychological in nature. The problem is to gain insight into the ways that the whole functions and the parts interact and work together or against each other.

The period of adolescence has been referred to as a period of transition—transition from childhood to adulthood. The input into the adolescent system is great and quite varied. One area of concern for any individual is his own body. Generally, one knows what he can expect from his body and how it will react under given circumstances. In adolescence more or less new and strange bodily experiences arise and what was known and reliable becomes unreliable. An awareness of the anatomical and physiological changes confronting the adolescent is essential to understanding this concern.

Under the influence of the central nervous system, especially the hypothalamus and the pituitary gland, the onset of hormonal activity begins. The major consequences are an increased elaboration of the adrenocortical and gonadal hormones and the production of mature ova and spermatozoa. Broad-spectrum changes that occur include the development of primary and secondary sex characteristics; changes in size, weight, body proportions, and muscular development; and related changes in strength, coordination, and skill. The length of time over which these changes occur varies; in some adolescents it is five to six years and in others one to two years. The person experiencing the changes over a short period of time is more likely to have troublesome problems, since he has difficulty coping with so much change in so short a period of time.

During the first five years of life, the child begins to define his self-concept. The healthy child begins to clarify the distinctions between himself and other people in the environment. From this time until adolescence the child is relatively stable in this definition of himself. Changes in personality occur, but the self in relation to others has been defined. When the individual reaches the period of adolescence, he has established some working relationship with himself and others based on a more or less healthy concept of himself. Adolescence upsets the even tenor of the days. The child develops toward adulthood beset by conflicting emotions and struggling to maintain self-control and to achieve self-expression under the impact of sensations and impulses that are scarcely understood but insistently demand attention. The youth feels estranged from the self the child had known. For some the emotional stability achieved in childhood and the security of family relationships permit a fairly steady direction; others are not so fortunate.

During adolescence the perception of the world changes, and the adolescent begins to think beyond the present and forms theories about everything including that which is not, the stage Piaget refers to as formal thought.[16] Reflective thinking is characteristic of the adolescent, and formal thought consists in reflecting on the operations or in thinking about thinking. Adolescent thought is directed toward the utopian, and the imaginal standards of what life and society might be supply the standards that motivate the adolescent toward reforming the world that exists. Yet some adolescents of today are said to be

uncommitted and to feel helpless in doing much about any large problem. Everything seems impossibly large and insoluble.

The passage through adolescence is a critical period. The period leading up to the closure of adolescence is particularly important for this personality must become something workable. A useful personality results from the successful completion of tasks specific to adolescence that lead to reintegration and reorganization of the personality structure and permit functioning as a reasonably self-sufficient adult.

The sum of the experiences of one person from conception through death can be seen to form a system. The various experiences as they occur can be seen as subsystems, or as the components for interaction that build up over a period of time and are stored in the personal memory bank. Each new experience provides input which, through processing in the internal feedback system, changes and is changed by the already stored data. The outcome of one experience will affect the way in which an individual enters into the next experience and result in an ongoing dynamic equilibrium between the parts of the organism and its total functioning. The individual is continually being influenced in the present by what his memory tells him of the past.

Adolescent task: identity

The chief task of adolescence is to establish a sense of identity, or a sense of who he is and how he fits into the world. This task is greatly helped or hindered by the past experiences that each adolescent has had to process while accomplishing the infancy and childhood stages of growth and development. Adolescence represents the end of dependency and the beginning of a long period of increased responsibility. Behavior during this time can be expected to be a mixture of new, relatively untried responses and the old familiar responses of childhood with which he is comfortable. As noted by Ackerman,[14] the adolescent does not mature in a consistent forward movement because anxiety induces a backward and forward irregularity. The fear of being a child pushes the adolescent forward yet the fear of being an adult pushes him backward.

The behavior of adolescents is understood only superficially if it is viewed out of context of the family and the culture. The input into the adolescent system must be taken into consideration before an evaluation of the output is made. However, when the adolescent is attempting to detach himself from the family in preparation for establishing his separateness as a person in the world, the effect of the behavior of the parents on the adolescent is often overlooked. Separation anxiety can be acute in adolescence and the mourning which accompanies the struggle of the adolescent to disengage himself from his parents can be too painful to bear at times, as evidenced by the vacillating behavior that seems to say "I hate you—no, I love you." The adolescent does not suffer alone, however, because the parents must bear this parting also. Both parents and child need to have practiced the letting go in small ways so that the affectional bonds that hold them together can be more gently stretched, although this does not mean there will be no pain. This can prevent the massive wrenching apart that sometimes occurs and that requires much repair before the systems can again effectively interact. In *My Language is Me,* David says, "Someone was telling me that the only way some people can leave home is to get mad and stomp out."[17] When this happens the prior preparation for the experience of separation has not been made.

One of the needs of the adolescent is the reassurance that his parents believe he is capable of functioning independently and will stand by while he tries. This can be very difficult, since devaluing adults, and particularly parents, is part of the growing-up process. The hostility directed toward the parents and their values and standards must make them sometimes wonder what happened to their lovely child. Yet if the devaluing did not take place, probably no one would ever leave home. It would be too painful.

Parents, then, also need to be committed to the goal of independence for the adolescent. However, the ability to take independent action is the goal and the markers along the adolescent route lead to this end. In the meantime he is discovering various life-styles, testing them to see what they feel like to him and checking what reactions he gets from others (feedback). He must get some sort of response from his environment before he can begin to crystallize the kind of person he wants to be or to establish his identity. Feedback is particularly important on those occasions when he has responded in an adult manner. This affords him the opportunity to learn what it feels like to be treated as an adult and hopefully will help to increase his ability to act the adult role acceptable in his culture.

One of the pressing problems for the adolescent is impulse control. The wish of the young child to express aggression is followed by the fear of retaliation, which he anticipates will be some form of bodily mutilation. These aggressive urges have been controlled through the internalization of parental values and standards. This serves him well until adolescence when things change, controls are relaxed, and one must become aggressive to make one's mark in the world, to be recognized as a person with tasks to be accomplished. Without the childhood controls, the adolescent has a difficult time organizing both his aggressive and sexual impulses and in deciding when to be assertive and when to be yielding. If he is assertive at the wrong time his childhood fears of bodily damage are reactivated yet, if he is yielding he fears being dominated and engulfed, of losing his identity. It is in this setting that all the unsolved problems of the earlier stages of growth and development are reactivated, and at a time when the adolescent, whose personality changes almost from day to day, is most vulnerable. If the input during these earlier stages was flawed, the adolescent may have failed to develop adequate basic trust or personal autonomy or may have developed an expectation of rejection. This further complicates internal feedback processing and, with a personality in a very fluid state, may have widespread deleterious effects on the adult who finally emerges from adolescence.

Adolescent peer groups

The adolescent period presents the individual with the problem of reformulating his concepts of himself as different from those of childhood. To do this, he must have some social group that will reflect to him how his "new identity" is accepted as it grows. The family cannot be of much help to him during this period because relating closely to them would keep him feeling dependent, and besides he is inevitably disillusioned by the values and standards of his parents and their society. The search for new and more satisfying standards leads him to join forces with his peers, who are also making the same search. They create within their own group a small world with unique standards and values suited to their particular needs. Adolescent groups tend to cushion the demands of the expectations facing group members and prevent them from being overwhelmed by the decisions that will affect them the remainder of their lives—how will they earn a living, will they find someone with whom to share the future, what will it be like to have children to raise? In addition, group codes provide badly needed impulse controls while the adolescent learns to internalize

aggression control in terms acceptable for adults in his culture, as well as helping him learn to adapt to a wide variety of behaviors.

Adolescent situations in systems terms

The events peculiar to the adolescent era lend themselves easily to systems theory explanation. The use of the model previously outlined and an elementary knowledge of systems theory principles make it easier to predict the outcome in each instance.

If the parents of the adolescent are able to decrease their demands but maintain support (input), the adolescent can gradually become increasingly responsible for his own behavior, processing each response against previously stored data and feeling secure enough to try new actions that affect the environment, getting further feedback to process and on around again. If as each new action is extended to be tested it is realistically assessed and reacted to, the adolescent has new raw data for processing against previously stored data, and the reaction received may, and probably will, change the stored data so that the information storage center is constantly being updated.

Feedback mechanisms are closed loop systems, but they need an energy supply to keep going. If the power supply balances the energy loss in the loops, the system will work at a steady state. The adolescent whose communication with his parents is faulty or nonexistent may set in motion a positive feedback system. In positive feedback the activity increases with each turn of the loop until the limits are reached. The system may then oscillate between an upper and a lower limit. The adolescent and his parents may find themselves in an intensely emotional situation that builds to the point at which both seek escape from the relationship (upper limit of the oscillation). They withdraw from the relationship and after respite (lower limit of the oscillation) may try again to communicate with each other. The intensity of the emotion will provide the needed power supply to keep the reaction going. This situation may also become a vicious circle if an energy loss balances the power supply, thus creating a situation in which no one can win but no one can withdraw. Energy in this situation could be drained off if the participants in the relationship can take the problem to someone else for a sympathetic ear. The adolescent may use his peer group and his mother may use her mother in just this way. If the energy loss does not occur and the system continues to increase its own output, it may stop or burst. This would be the kind of setting in which delinquency could occur.

A negative feedback situation may result from interpersonal family discord. In negative feedback the activity is damped at each turn of the loop until standstill is achieved. This system cuts down its own input, always tending to stop at zero resting level. If disturbed, it tries to return to the reference value. The mechanism continuously compares the reference value with the actual output and aims at zeroing the difference. If the parents of an adolescent are unable to decrease their demands (input) and the adolescent is prevented from seeking to function independently through threat of disapproval or of loss of love and support, negative feedback results with dampened oscillations that prevent the system from being disturbed (output), the adolescent usually keeping a zero balance through avoidance behavior (low amplification). However, the internal information processing center is at the same time producing lowered self-confidence and reduced self-esteem because the need for autonomy is being denied.

The period of devaluing parents, better known as adolescent rebellion, is a difficult time for those who experience it. However, systems theory principles may

be used to explore the concept. When the system tries to return to the reference value after a change, there is some inertia in the system and an overshot may occur. This produces instability through time lag, high gain, or resistance. Time lag refers to time delay or the correction if an overshot comes late. High gain refers to feedback that is too strong and there is a heavy overshot. Resistance in the system will tend to correct overshot by dampening the oscillations. The parents of the adolescent who have standards and values to which they rigidly adhere are causing high gain in the system, which results in a situation that may cause an adolescent to rebel in kind. This could result in acting-out behavior of various kinds. Those parents who vacillate, sometimes changing their standards and values in attempting to seek the approval of an adolescent, may produce time lag in the system and thus be one step behind the demands. Those parents who have a set of values and standards to which they adhere with some flexibility are putting resistance into the system, thus preventing the problem presented by time lag and high gain.

The hospitalized adolescent

In the hospital the adolescent may have similar problems. If housed with other adolescents only, there is the security of the peer group but he is denied the opportunity of testing behavior against adult standards that will give him further experience with what is acceptable in the adult world for which he strives. Conversely, if housed with adult patients, the need for activity to reduce tension in coping with anxiety and uncertainty would probably be frowned upon. It would seem, then, that adolescents should, in the hospital, be housed according to need rather than age, thus keeping the feedback systems functioning as nearly as possible in a steady state with the power supply and the energy loss in balance.

Summary

Adolescence is life between childhood and adulthood during which the individual bids farewell to the self and the objects of the past and gradually, with much hope and anxiety, approaches adult responsibilities and prerogatives. The adolescent must free himself from his attachments to persons who were all important during childhood. How this separation is accomplished will have implications for the future because learning to deal with one loss in a mature fashion will facilitate coping with other losses. The adolescent preparing to leave home must reach out for adult sex, love, and responsibility, for a new and different type of social relationship, new interests and sublimations, and new values, standards, and goals. A complete reorientation to life is required.

Maturity is the goal of the life process. It implies that the individual is able to differentiate the inner and outer worlds of his life and to accept and assess feedback from other people. The maturing individual can accept the gradual loosening of affectional bonds in his nuclear family while gradually developing relationships outside the family to substitute for the loss. Selecting a mate, establishing a new nuclear family, and achieving mastery at an occupation will indicate that the family system is functioning optimally to meet its goal.

Adolescence has been utilized to demonstrate the application of principles of systems theory. Given input from the environment into the adolescent system and internal feedback processing, the output from the system (decision or action) can be predicted. With a means of predicting the decision or action, appropriate nursing intervention can be instituted.

References

1. Finch, Joyce: Systems analysis: a logical approach to professional nursing care, Nurs. Forum **8**:177-190, Nov., 1969.
2. McKay, Rose: Theories, models and systems for nursing, Nurs. Res. **18**:393-400, Sept.-Oct., 1969.
3. Smoyak, Shirley: Toward understanding nursing situations: a transaction paradigm, Nurs. Res. **18**:405-411, Sept.-Oct., 1969.
4. Bertalanffy, Ludwig von: General systems theory, New York, 1968, George Braziller, Inc.
5. Hall, A. D., and Fagen, R. E.: Definition of a system. In Buckley, Walter, editor: Modern systems research for the behavioral scientist, Chicago, 1968, Aldine Publishing Co.
6. Prigogine, I.: Introduction to thermodynamics of irreversible reactions, Springfield, Ill., 1955, Charles C Thomas, Publisher.
7. Miller, James G.: Living systems: basic concepts, Behav. Sci. **10**:193-237, July 1965.
8. Miller, George A.: What is information measurement? In Buckley, Walter, editor: Modern systems research for the behavioral scientist, Chicago, 1968, Aldine Publishing Co.
9. Weiner, Norbert: The human use of human beings, New York, 1954, Doubleday & Co., Inc.
10. Herrick, C. Judson: The evolution of human nature, New York, 1961, Harper & Row, Publishers.
11. Dubos, Rene: Man adapting, New Haven, 1965, Yale University Press.
12. Rogers, Martha E.: An introduction to the theoretical basis of nursing, Philadelphia, 1970, F. A. Davis Co.
13. Rosenbleuth, Arturo, and Weiner, Norbert: The role of models in science, Philosophy Sci. **12**:316-321, 1945.
14. Ackerman, Nathan: The psychodynamics of family life, New York, 1958, Basic Books, Inc., Publishers.
15. Arbib, Michael, and Kahn, Roy M.: A developmental model of information processing in the child, Perspect. Bio. Med. **12**:397-416, 1969.
16. Piaget, I.: Psychology of intelligence, Totowa, N. J., 1966, Littlefield, Adams & Co.
17. Parker, Beulah: My language is me, New York, 1962, Basic Books, Inc., Publishers.

Bibliography

Brodbeck, May: Models, meaning and theories. In Gross, Llewellyn, editor. Symposium on sociological theory, Evanston, Ill., 1959, Row, Peterson & Co.
Group for the Advancement of Psychiatry: Normal adolescence, New York, 1968, Charles Scribner's Sons.

Haberstrok, Chadwick J.: Control as an organizational process. In Buckley, Walter, editor: Modern systems research for the behavioral scientist, Chicago, 1968, Aldine Publishing Co.

Josselyn, Irene M.: The adolescent and his world, New York, 1952, Family Service Association of America.

Laqueur, Peter H.: General systems theory and multiple family therapy. In Gray, William, editor: General systems theory and psychiatry, Boston, 1969, Little, Brown & Co.

Lewin, Kurt: The field theory approach to adolescence. In Seidman, Jerome M., editor: The adolescent—a book of readings, New York, 1960, Holt, Rinehart & Winston, Inc.

Rizzo, Nicholas D., Gray, William, and Kaiser, Julian: A general systems approach to problems in growth and development. In Gray, William, editor: General systems theory and psychiatry, Boston, 1969, Little, Brown & Co.

Winnicott, D. W.: The family and individual development, London, 1965, Tavistock Publications, Ltd.

Chapter 4

Systems theory and the aged

Mona L. Moughton and Mary E. Hazzard

Senescence is a decline in the ability of an organism to produce free energy and this follows a definite pattern. Only energy systems senesce. The decline of functional efficiency occurs with time even without interference from the environment. The onset of senescence has been identified as beginning at or near the onset of conception, since fertilization of the ovum takes place when two cells that have some type of past history and age unite. These gametes carry the genetic pattern and calendar for the organism. The processes that produce enlargement and differentiation cannot be distinguished from those that produce senescence or the slowing down of the organism. These processes are more rapid in the early years of the life process than they are in the later years. The living system tends to delay senescence by three fundamental processes: elimination of system products, replication of essential components, and control of aberrant or side reactions.[1]

Old age is considered somewhat arbitrarily to start at 65, the traditional retirement age for man. The person who reaches 65 still has a life expectancy of over twelve years and must plan accordingly. When a person reaches 80, as many will, he will still have an expectation of another ten years. For some reason with advancing age the decline of the body seems to slow down.

The aged population is a social problem and its ever-increasing size must be faced. In 1963 over 18 million people, about one tenth of the population, were over 65 years of age. Responsibility for those persons under 16 years of age and over 65 years of age falls on about the equivalent number between these ages. The population rise has developed more rapidly than have measures designed to meet the ensuing problems. In 1840 the life expectancy of an infant was forty years and in 1950 it was sixty-eight years. In 1950 there were 10 million people over 65 and by 1980 this figure is expected to be 25 million.[2] The problem has been created almost entirely by medicine. Medical science has changed the structure of society, yet medicine has dragged its heels and been reluctant to attend to the problem it has created. One of the most pressing problems is still medical care, despite Medicare and related programs.

The life-span

Man is the longest living mammal and his life-span has been estimated at about 150 years. Each species and all organisms of that species have a fixed life-span that can only be realized in a perfectly optimal environment, which is rarely realized.

The living system, man, regardless of the initial status and efficiency, finally becomes senescent and dies because he cannot perfectly replicate, eliminate, and control disproportion that arises within the system. The processes within the living system are not perfect and some cells do not divide and regenerate after birth. One example of this is the brain cell that when it dies is never replaced. There is a constant tendency toward equilibrium in the life process, and this enables free energy to be transferred within the system. Reactions must constantly take place for free energy to be transferred. Senescence occurs with time and varies with the genetic makeup of the organism. The decline in biological efficiency may be explained by the decrease in the individual's ability to produce or utilize free energy.[3]

Entropy and aging

Entropy, which can be expressed mathematically, is currently being studied in relation to the aging process. If the reaction is reversible, then the entropy is reversible; this is particularly true in open systems. The equation can be shown to represent how energy is lost to the system, or how it becomes "bound" and therefore is not available to the system. Entropy is involved in every energy transfer in the universe; it is not limited to chemical, mechanical, or physical processes and it may be positive or negative. The sequence, order, timing, and nature may be altered in the living system, making it impossible for the system to produce the necessary free energy at the time, place, and velocity necessary for the system to function.[3, 4] Order within the orga-

nism and within the cell is relative and related to the eye of the beholder. All of the matter and substance remains after the individual dies, and although the individual can no longer function as a person, many reactions are still going on. The synchronous behavior of the system has been disturbed, but the parts remain.

Cellular senescence

At least three mechanisms of cellular senescence have been identified by Calloway.[5] The first mechanism involves the normal processes of the organism. The rate at which the steady state is approached may be altered by rate changes or by slight changes in the steady state. Normal processes that decline in rate, increase in rate, or change their relationship to other processes may alter the energy system. The second mechanism involves the appearance of new processes in the cell or in the system. The immunological theory states that with time, mutated cells may stimulate development of proteins that results in the useless production of an amyloid-type obstructing material which is then laid down. This immunological reaction leads to the degradation and eventual death of the organism.[6] The third mechanism involves imperfect repair. Theories have been developed about the repair of proteins, connective tissue, or replicating tissue. Monotonic cross-linkage of proteins and nucleic acid molecules may account for changes in the nucleus of a cell or in the chromosomes themselves.[6] Cross-linkage of all types of molecules is proportional to the metabolic rate and is dependent on the density of chemical free radicals within the system. Increased stress on the person as input results in biochemical changes that enhance the rate of cross-linkage. Changes in one part of the system affect the whole system; for example, collagen formation leads to shrinkage of tissue about the capillaries, decreasing the supply of chemicals to a localized area leading to increased deposition of collagen. Another example is that immunological reactions change the chemical environment and therefore change the rate of cross-linkage, dissociation, and waste product production.

Transition

The period of senescence can be referred to as a period of transition—transition from greater independence to greater dependence—even though the input into the system may be as great and varied as in the adolescent period. One area of concern, as in the adolescent, is the body. In the adolescent there was greater differentiation and increase in size, coordination, and strength, but now dedifferentiation and decrease in size, coordination, and strength occurs. An awareness of the anatomical and physiological changes confronting the aging individual is essential to understanding his concerns.

Under the influence of ribonucleic acid, deoxyribonucleic acid, and related metabolites,[7] broad-spectrum changes occur in the living system during the senescent period of the life-span. Component parts of organs may be replaced by malfunctioning fibrous tissue due to degeneration of cells through accumulation of pigment, formation of vacuoles, or hyaline changes in the cell. Some cells may proliferate rather than degenerate and produce a benign or malignant growth. Changes that occur in the connective tissue consist of an increase in the amount of fibrous connective tissue, less contractility and more rigid and thickened collagen as well as end fragmentation, and sometimes splitting or aggregation of elastic fibers into irregular masses. There is wrinkling of the skin due to a loss of elasticity, fat, and water. The epidermis becomes thinner and its cellular components at the basal layer undergo changes in shape and organization. Well-known lines and wrinkles become more prominent in the hands and feet because

of deposition of glycogen that was not there previously. Atrophy of the sweat glands occurs. As the testosterone and estrogen decrease, the hyaluronic acid and water in the skin decrease, resulting in dry, scaly skin. In males there is an increase in connective tissue surrounding the sperm-producing tubules and in some there is cessation of spermatogenic function. Pigmentation occurs in the interstitial cells where testosterone is produced, causing a decrease in this hormone. In females many of the ova degenerate, the uterus atrophies, and estrogen production decreases. Changes occur in the thyroid, thymus, adrenals, pancreas, and pituitary, with resultant decrease in hormones or secretions. Changes take place in cardiac tissue leading to conduction abnormalities and decreased output. A decreased conduction velocity in the central nervous system leads to changes in reaction time. The shorter the period of time in which changes occur, the greater will be the difficulty of the individual in coping with these changes.

Lidz[8] has defined three possible phases of the later years of the life-span, but they do not necessarily happen to all people. The first phase is "the elderly." The person at retirement is essentially unchanged from middle age except for work and is capable and competent to take care of his needs and affairs. The second phase is that of the "senescent." If changes occur in the life of the individual, the person may be forced to rely upon others. The person who has been able to provide for and guide his children now may become dependent on them. Self-esteem is undermined and the dependency commonly provokes anxiety and friction that occur at a time when the capacity for ego control is lessened. The third phase is "the senile." In this situation the brain no longer serves in its essential function as an organ of adaptation and the person enters his "second childhood," requiring someone to be responsible for his complete care. All persons do not become senile even at advanced years. The failing intellectual abilities may also become manifest in diminished control over impulses and emotion. Frequent displays of anger or distrust may make it difficult for others to get along with the aged person. Sexual drives or sensations may no longer be properly controlled, and masturbatory activities may cause embarrassment to the family or to the persons caring for him.

The mandatory retirement age is a mixed blessing, since it assures that the incompetent will not stay on the job; but sudden complete retirement appears to be a problem for many and some institutions favor gradual transition. Many people have been impressed by the frequency with which sudden death occurs soon after retirement; the pattern of gradual retirement has been one attempt to answer this phenomenon.

The systems model and aging

Through the use of a systems model (Fig. 9), the expected reactions (output) can be demonstrated given a specific input in a stated context. By using this model the response of the individual to acute physiological changes within the system and to the introduction of a drug into the system as well as the response within the system to an acute emotional crisis can be demonstrated.

Acute physiological change within the system

The ability of the body to cope with infection decreases with age. Fever is a natural weapon against disease but the elderly often have severe infections without a fever or even a subclinical temperature.[9] Available information suggests a decline in the immunological system with age, resulting in a reduction of lymphoid tissue due to nodules of fat that replace the majority of tissue and leave only a rim of lymphoid tissue in the lymph node. Symptoms of hayfever in women are reported to abate or disappear at the menopause and to become less severe in middle-aged men. Although the ability to form antibodies seems to decline, studies with

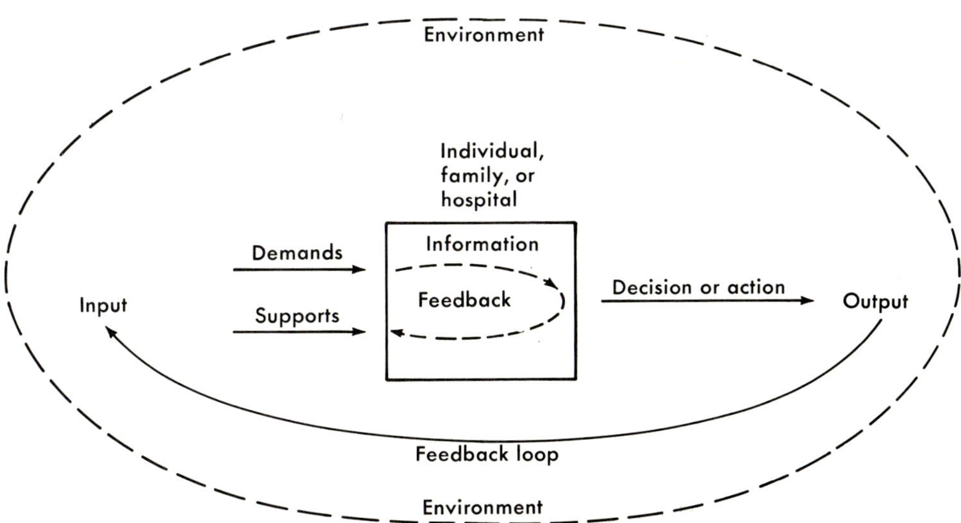

Fig. 9
A model of living systems.

mice indicate that homograft reactions do not decline with age; hence, tissue transplantation is not likely to be easier in the elderly.[10]

During an acute illness, such as pneumonia or heart failure, the diminished oxygen supply to the brain may be too great for the degenerating brain cells. The input of oxygen into the system is too small, and through a feedback mechanism, respiration and heart action decrease further. The output of the system will be decreased activity and independence that feeds back as input into the system and leads to continued degeneration of the functioning whole. For this reason the sooner the elderly person with an acute illness in a general hospital can be gotten out of bed and rehabilitation started (increased input), the less will be the debility, and the sooner the individual can go home.

When the aged person becomes bedridden, the demands on the system are great and pressure on the skin at bony prominences can lead to decubiti. The trophic changes that occur in the skin, as well as related changes in blood vessels, can constitute an input too great for the system to process, and preventive measures that include frequent turning and attention to skin care are essential. In this instance the output, the condition of the skin, will demonstrate the quality of nursing care given.

A related situation involves the elderly person who must have a series of tests extending over several days. Because of the loss of physiological flexibility, decreased metabolism, and slowed adaptive responses, the elderly person is not able to tolerate a three-day regimen of tests. This is too much input in too short a period of time, and the output will often be irritability, hostility, refusal to cooperate, and even transient confusion. If the tests are done over a longer period of time, the individual can usually cope.

Introduction of a drug into the system

The input into the aging system may be a drug or other substance that causes a toxic dysfunction. The energy within the system becomes bound and cannot be utilized by the system. Those medications not tolerated well are steroids, barbiturates, potent hypotensives, oral hypoglycemic agents, and even aspirin, and the thiazide diuretics can produce serious complications.[11]

Response to an acute emotional crisis

A senile break may be brought on by the input of an overwhelming emotional crisis, such as the death of a spouse, or a change that requires adjustment beyond the capacity of the individual, such as moving to a new home with a son or daughter. Conflict and turmoil may result and the person cannot cope. The output may be confusion that tends to become a disability and may through feedback gradually spread.

Theories of aging

There are a number of theories about aging, but two among them are interesting to consider when viewed in relation to systems theory. These are the two contrasting theories called the activity theory and the disengagement theory.

Activity theory

The activity theory[12] holds that except for the inevitable changes in biology and health (entropic changes) older people are essentially the same as middle-aged people. The decreased social interaction that characterizes old age (output from the system) results from the withdrawal by society (decreased input) from the aging person, and the decrease in social interaction proceeds against the desires of most aging men and women. The person maintains activities of middle age as long as possible and finds substitutes for work when he is forced to retire and substitutes for friends and loved ones whom he loses by death. The older person who ages optimally is the person who stays active and manages to resist having his social world shrink.

Disengagement theory

In the disengagement theory[13] the decreased social interaction is interpreted as a process characterized by mutuality in which both society and the aging person withdraw, with the aging person accepting and perhaps desiring decreased interaction because of decreased energy levels. There is increased preoccupation with the self and decreased emotional investment in persons and objects in the environment. Disengagement, then, is a natural rather than an imposed process. This older person reaches a new equilibrium characterized by greater social distance, altered types of relationships, and decreased social interaction.

According to systems theory, however, if the input is decreased, then the output must be decreased because there is less to be processed by the individual. With an increase in physical deterioration, death of peers, the stigma associated with aging in our society, enforced retirement, and the preponderance of a mobile nuclear

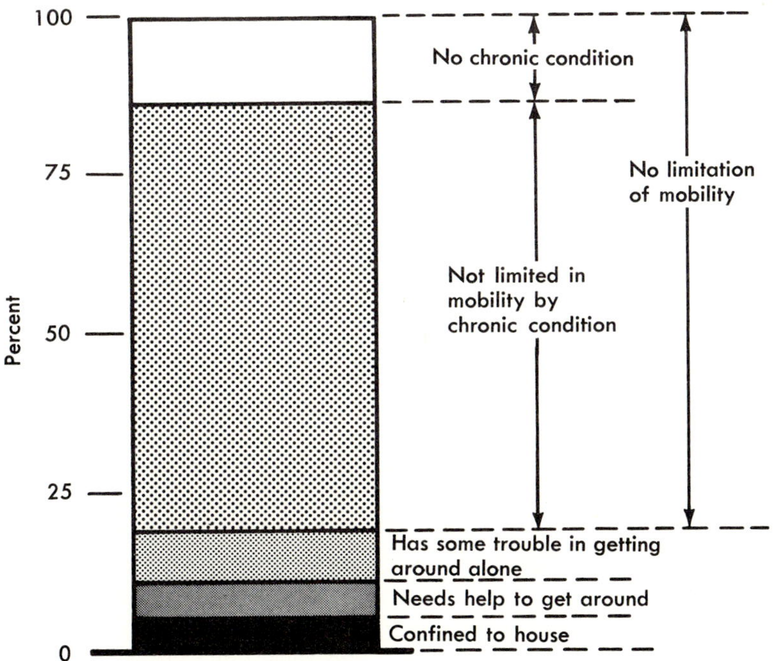

Fig. 10
Effect of chronic conditions* on mobility of noninstitutionalized older people, July, 1965 to June, 1967. (From Brotman, H. B.: Older Americans speak to the nation, 1970 Senior Citizens Prologue to 1971 White House Conference on Aging, Aging, No. 187, May, 1970.)

---

*Chronic conditions are conditions or impairments that have lasted for more than three months or those with an onset more recent that appear on lists of medically determined long-lasting conditions. They range from visual impairments corrected by eyeglasses to a completely disabling stroke.

family, there is not only less support for the individual but greater demands on the system. Input transformation within the system leads, through the feedback loops, to greater social withdrawal as the output.

It would seem then that if the disengagement theory is valid, it should be interrupted, rather than accepted. By intervening to increase the supports and simplify the demands, the aging individual can more successfully process and transform the information input, resulting in increased ability to care for himself and increased interest in his environment.

The elderly and the community

The community and the family both function as open systems. Input, internal feedback processing, output with external feedback affecting further input as well as affecting the environment can be understood readily in this context.

According to the latest available data there are, in 1970, 19 million people over 65 years of age or older.[2] By 1980 it is expected that this number will be 25 million. The majority of the elderly are not ill and less than 5% are in institutions.[14] However, most of those who remain in the community have some condition that is disabling to a degree (Fig. 10).

The information on this graph represents a great deal of input not only for the community, but also for the family if there is one. The elderly and their families need positive supports (input) to help them learn best how to live together, to accept each other, to understand each other, and to communicate. This is a difficult task. Elderly persons have had many years to become differentiated, and since they are not all alike, mass solutions to the problems are not the answer.

Psychiatric therapy

Psychiatric therapy can be useful with the elderly by providing support for the person. It is not directed at making pro-

found personality changes, thus increasing the demands on the system, but is directed at providing comfort for the person.[15] The consistent, supporting attitude tends to increase self-esteem, which is quite low in many of the elderly. Sessions may be 15 to 50 minutes and the individual is encouraged to ventilate (output). Frequently, particularly in the elderly person who is having increasing interpersonal conflict, anxiety "binds" the energy so that entropy builds up and the output is disordered, as would be expected of the process of entropy. Psychotherapy helps to clarify the meaning of events so that the input, when processed by the individual, becomes increasingly ordered and therefore more understandable. Through feedback the output affects the input, further clarifying meaning.

Many of the elderly have been sent to mental hospitals because they were seriously depressed and disorganized. In large part this was probably because they lacked suitable places to live and inadequate financial and emotional support. Unless they are suffering from chronic brain syndrome, much of the effect of the inadequacies is reversible.

Once the person is hospitalized, the input is minimal because of a lack of personal attention, barren surroundings, and depressing atmosphere. With less information being processed, the feedback decreases and input is further limited. Transformation of limited input leads to apathy and progressive deterioration. It is therefore easy to understand why a person entering a long-term care institution at the present time tends to stay there.

A study carried out at Langley Porter Neuropsychiatric Institute has shown that this need not be the case. This study was based on the principles of systems theory, although the investigators did not apparently use systems theory in the study design. The study showed that careful placement of the elderly mentally ill person in a setting suited to his needs or the provision of supportive services to allow him to live independently in the community is a much more satisfactory solution from the point of view of the person and is more likely to result in an efficient use of community resources than routine commitment of these patients to state hospitals. This was true even though the person suffered from the "typical" conditions for the age group. The patients in the study were considered to be older, financially poorer, physically sicker, and more socially isolated than their peers in the community. Their admission diagnoses fell into at least one of three categories: chronic brain syndrome, acute brain syndrome, or psychogenic disorder. A three-month sample of 99 patients in 1965 showed that 48% had been referred to a general hospital psychiatric ward or medical ward for treatment from which they went directly to nursing or boarding homes; 11% were left where they were and 11% were referred to outpatient departments of other hospitals. After one year, 47% of these persons were in nursing or boarding homes, 25% had died, 20% were in the community, and only 2% were in state hospitals.[16] A boarding-out program at an English mental hospital was equally successful.[17]

In reading these studies it is apparent that the investigators were most concerned with the input into the aging human system. Demands were made but supports were given that allowed the individual to live out his life in a more normal manner rather than in deteriorating behind locked doors. This quality care requires much more from the care-taking persons in the environment.

In an open system, matter and energy are exchanged freely with the environment. Some reactions within the system are reversible up to a specific point, beyond which they are irreversible. Thus apathy and confused, disordered behavior

in the elderly can be halted. This is done by simplifying the environment and the tasks demanded of the person. For the elderly person, who has a tendency toward greater entropy, there is a need for a relatively stable environment to minimize the demands on the system and increase the support for the system. If the individual feels secure, enjoys good health, companionship, a sense of dignity in daily living, finds meaning and purposefulness in life, and has sufficient funds and appropriate housing, there will be fewer demands on him. These factors will act as supports entering the system. As the individual grows older, there is a slowing down of the internal feedback mechanism with a delay in output or action; hence, greater calm, simplicity, and familiarity become more essential.

Input into the system of self-esteem and a purpose that provides meaning beyond tomorrow interact within the system and provide a look toward the future for others, if not for the self. This helps to counteract apathy and leads to an output of increased alertness or maintenance of alertness. Religion has often been an input giving support to the system and aiding the individual in his search for a purpose in living. This is particularly true when religion continues to be a way of life rather than a way of dying.

Death may not be feared by the very old, who may regard it as a relief from the effort required to continue living. As they lose close relationships, their feelings of being needed and wanted lessen. Those who look forward to death are not necessarily depressed.

The elderly, their families, and the nurse

The family functions as a system and as a subsystem of society, as well as having subsystems itself composed of the individual family members. Numerous interactions are possible among the people involved in these systems. With the possible input so varied, it is readily understood that error occurs and results in maladaption at some level. Systems theory can be quite useful to those providing psychiatric therapy where it is indicated because it allows for analysis of where the maladaptation is occurring and for better understanding of how this system affects and is affected by its environment.

There are myriad ways for the aging and their families to disagree. The young are impatient with the slow, cautious responses of their elders and are probably somewhat threatened also by this evidence of what the future holds for them. Their elders are made anxious by the seeming haste with which the young family members make moves that are vital to the family, and they are probably somewhat envious of this ability to move confidently ahead. The young have busy lives occupied with work, children and their activities, entertaining, and much more, and there is never quite enough time to complete all that one intended to do. For the elderly, who tire more quickly, have fewer demands on their time, and are more urgently aware that the number of days left to them are preciously few, the busyness of their young compared to the time spent with elders may become a point for covert or overt dissention. If the elderly person lives with the younger family, the contrast between activity and attention may be more acute, and certainly the possibility for dissention is greater.

The number of people who live to be 65 years of age and more grows steadily; therefore the problem of difficult relations between the generations is quite likely to keep pace. The elderly and their families need positive supports as input to help them learn to live together, to accept and understand each other, and to communicate with each other. This is a difficult task, yet it must be accomplished in some way to prevent ever increasing numbers of the aging from finding their way behind locked doors in our long-term care institutions.

It has been estimated that there will be 25 million people 65 years of age and older by 1980. It is also estimated[2] that about 80% of these people will have a chronic medical condition that will be delimiting to some extent. It seems quite likely that the nurses of the immediate future will be having much contact with the elderly in their homes, in clinics, or in hospitals. It would seem, therefore, that one focus in nursing should be the aging individual in the community. This would include health supervision counseling, direct nursing services when indicated, and preventive services such as diabetic detection and remedial services in such areas as hearing and visual deficiencies. In all these services a knowledge of systems theory would enable the nurse to assist the person in ordering and organizing thought processes. This can be done by providing support and helping the person to decrease the demands made on him (input) and by offering feedback (external), thus helping him to know that he is understood or helping him to understand how his communication is faulty. This increases the accuracy of the input, which increases the probability that decisions or actions which follow will be appropriate, resulting in approval from those in the environment and in an increase in self-esteem for the elderly person. Whenever possible the nurse may provide the same service for family members when she meets them. A focused conversation, which can be very meaningful to both the elderly person and his family, need not take a long time, may be of greater value than medication, does not require a medical order, and may be repeated as necessary.

Because of repeated contacts with the elderly, the nurse also is in a position to be useful to community groups when they begin to plan programs for the elderly of the community, such as Meals on Wheels. The nurse could be quite helpful in reviewing the problems of the elderly in a specific community and helping get action to solve such problems. One problem about which little has really been done is the waste of time and talent among the elderly who could contribute much more to each other than they currently do. This would require the talents of an organizer, but even that may be found among the elderly. Group discussion procedures are badly needed to find out who has what to offer, to sort out the activities in which group members would be interested, or just to talk and to be heard. Although the nurse may not wish to take on the task, and indeed may not have the talent, this is another activity to bring to the attention of those who are concerned.

There are groups of elderly, retired persons who are organized for personal pleasure, such as travel, or to help others, such as the grandparents clubs, but these are far too few to make much of an impression on the immensity of the problem which is rapidly approaching.

Summary

"The life process, the living person, is an open system. It is self-regulating and self-repairing up to a point if there is the proper input of food and other forms of information. However, entropy eventually overtakes energy, and the living system dies. We live with this certain knowledge of death. Our comfort comes from the use we put to our days before they are ended, or the manner in which we spend our time."[18]

With the expectation of 25 million people over the age of 65 by 1980, and estimating that 80% of these people will have a chronic medical condition that will be debilitating to some extent, it seems likely that the nurse will become more involved in the care of the elderly. As the person grows older, there is a slowing down of the internal feedback mechanism with a delay in output or action. Probably the current major focus for intervention should be on the secondary prevention level, for example, early case finding and treatment. The tertiary level, rehabilitation, is also of prime importance. The nurse will be involved in health supervision counseling, direct nursing services when indicated, remedial services, preventive or detection services, and general community planning. As studies continue and more and more data are gathered, the prevention of the more disastrous effects of aging can be initiated.

If the aging individual is to realize his full potential, an optimum environment providing adequate supports and limiting the demands (input) is essential for proper internal feedback processing of the input and hence result in appropriate decisions or actions (output) which will in turn feed back as input into the system. For the elderly person who has a tendency toward greater entropy, there is a definite need for a relatively stable environment to minimize the demands on the system and allow for an increase in the supports for the system.

References

1. Calloway, N. O.: The onset of senescence, J. Amer. Geriat. Soc. 14:1134-1137, Nov., 1966.
2. Aging: older Americans speak to the nation: Prologue to the 1971 White House Conference on Aging, Washington, D. C., 1970, U. S. Department of Health, Education & Welfare.
3. Strechler, Bernard L.: Time, cells, and aging, New York, 1962, Academic Press, Inc.
4. Calloway, N. O.: The role of entrophy in biologic senescence, J. Amer. Geriat. Soc. 14:342-349, April, 1966.
5. Calloway, N. O.: The factors of senescence, J. Amer. Geriat. Soc. 14:826-833, Aug., 1966.
6. Carpenter, Donald G., and Logod, James:

An integrated theory of aging, J. Amer. Geriat. Soc. **16:**1307-1322, 1968.

7. Frank, Benjamin S.: Nucleic acid therapy in aging and degenerative disease, New York, 1969, Psychological Library Publishers.

8. Lidz, Theodore: The person: his development throughout the life cycle, New York, 1968, Basic Books, Inc., Publishers.

9. Thau, Marcel: Fever as a defense against disease, J. Amer. Geriat. Soc. **12:**366-367, April, 1964.

10. Williamson, J., and Johnson, D. B.: Ageing. In Passmore, R., and Robson, J. S., editors: A companion to medical studies, vol. 2, Philadelphia, 1970, F. A. Davis Co.

11. Ford, Amasa B.: Distinguishing characteristics of the aging from a clinical viewpoint, J. Amer. Geriat. Soc. **16:**142-148, 1968.

12. Havinghurst, Robert J.: Personality and patterns of aging, part 2, Gerontologist **8:**20-23, Spring, 1968.

13. Cumming, E., and Henry, W. E.: Growing old; the process of disengagement, New York, 1961, Basic Books, Inc., Publishers.

14. Smith, Eleanor: Distinguishing characteristics of the aging from a medical care administration viewpoint, J. Amer. Geriat. Soc. **16:**136-141, 1968.

15. Wolff, Kurt: Comparison of group and individual psychotherapy with geriatric patients, Dis. Nerv. Syst. **28:**384-386, June, 1967.

16. Simon, A.: The geriatric mentally ill, part 2, Gerontologist **8:**7-15, 1968.

17. Whitehead, J. A., and Graham, J. V.: Boarding out elderly psychiatric patients, Geriatrics **23:**164-168, 1968.

18. Moughton, Mona: Perspectives on aging and time. In Bergersen, Betty S., et al., editors: Current concepts in clinical nursing, vol. 2, St. Louis, 1969, The C. V. Mosby Co.

Bibliography

Ackerman, Nathan W.: The psychodynamics of family life, New York, 1958, Basic Books, Inc., Publishers.

Amburgey, Pauline I.: Environmental aids for the aged patient, Amer. J. Nurs. **66:**2017-2018, Sept., 1966.

Birren, J. E.: Handbook of aging and the individual, Chicago, 1959, University of Chicago Press.

Bortz, Edward L.: Retirement and the individual, J. Amer. Geriat. Soc. **16:**1-15, Jan., 1968.

Comfort, A.: The biology of senescence, New York, 1956, Holt, Rinehart & Winston, Inc.

Gray, William, editor: General systems theory and psychiatry, Boston, 1969, Little, Brown & Co.

Kutner, Bernard: Socio-economic impact of aging, J. Amer. Geriat. Soc. **14:**33-40, Jan., 1966.

Warner, B. A.: The process of aging, Nurs. Clin. N. Amer. **1:**407-415, Sept., 1966.

Chapter 5

Nursing intervention with a dying patient

Marguerite J. Holmes

In recent years considerable interest in the process of dying and the care of the dying patient has been stirred. Caring for the dying is an important part of nursing. Probably it has always been a difficult task to care for the person who is dying because death reminds us of the fragility of our own lives. It is difficult, too, because we must share the pain and suffering of the person who is dying and of the family and friends he leaves behind.

Recent work by such authors as Kübler-Ross,[1] Glaser and Strauss,[2] and Quint[3] has contributed greatly to our understanding of some of the problems faced by the person who is dying. Kübler-Ross has provided us with some valuable insights into what the person goes through as he faces his own death. We have long been aware of the meaning of grief as it is experienced by the living, and we understand something about the pain and anguish of the bereaved as they mourn the loss of a loved one. Kübler-Ross has helped us also to understand that the terminally ill person experiences a similar process of grieving as he suffers more and more losses. These may include the loss of body parts and the loss of ability to function in normal ways.

If surgery and repeated or prolonged hospitalizations are required, the financial burden becomes enormous. Added to this may be the loss of a job due to absences or the inability to function. All these losses add to the sadness and depression of the person suffering them.

We can only begin to imagine the grief experienced by the one who is losing not one person, but everybody; not one relationship, but all relationships; all functioning, all abilities, all activities, all possessions; even his own body, his consciousness, his very being. It is no wonder his grief is so immense, his anger so great, his envy of the living so painful.

Dying is made even more difficult by some of the cultural changes that have occurred. Death is often viewed not as the natural conclusion of a life, but as the enemy of life.[4] Modern medicine wages a hard fought battle against the enemy, death. Many times the final battle between medicine and death is waged in a hospital where it is fought in a fierce but impersonal way. The patient becomes not a man who is dying, but a "case"—an object of medical and nursing interventions. Hospitalization usually means incurring enormous expense, being subjected to strange and painful procedures, and being separated from familiar surroundings and, for the most part, from familiar people.

For many people, talking about dying is both a painful and difficult task. The person who is dying frequently becomes alienated from those he loves the most, with the tragic result that he and his loved ones are unable to talk together about the meaning of their lives and about the impending death that will separate them forever.

The patient who is experiencing all of this may behave in ways that are difficult for the nursing staff to comprehend and to cope with. The patient's behavior may reflect his own reactions to the multiple losses he is incurring; to illness, incapacitation, and pain; to separation from familiar people and places; and to the many unpleasantries of hospitalization. To the nursing staff, reasons for the patient's behavior may not always be as obvious as it would seem. Their reactions to the patient are likely to reflect their feeling of adequacy about themselves as helping people, the nursing unit at that moment, their expectations of the patient (based perhaps on previous experience with the patient or with others they perceive to be like him), as well as their interpretation of the meaning of the patient's behavior.

Talking with a dying patient is difficult for many people. Many of the ordinary topics of conversation seem inappropriate, particularly future-oriented topics. A nurse may feel awkward about asking a patient how he is feeling for fear of upsetting him. On the other hand, she may be distressed by his depressed, angry, or critical remarks and wonder if they are directed at her personally, when most often they are not.

Many nurses have told me that they are reticent to engage in conversation with dying patients because they fear that the patient will ask them, "Am I dying?" They are unsure of how to deal with this ques-

tion so rather than facing having to give a "yes" or "no" answer they avoid getting into any serious discussion with the patient. However, one interpretation of the meaning of the question, "Am I dying?," is that the patient who asks it is aware of his state and is seeking an opportunity to talk with someone about what he perceives to be happening to him and how he feels about it. Thus the helpful role is not to say "yes" or "no" to the question, but to give the patient an opening to express his thoughts and feelings about what is happening to him. This is difficult to do because it requires that the nurse then be able to listen to his expression without cutting him off, without trying to cheer him up with false platitudes, and without withdrawing from his anger and grief.

How can we best provide nursing care for the patient with a fatal illness? Ujhely sees the main focus of the nurse with any patient as ". . . sustaining the patient through the experience which has brought him into contact with her in the first place."* "Sustaining" is defined as ". . . an overall term that covers all of the nurse's interventions that are designed to help the patient cope with or profit from his experience. . . ."* Ujhely clarifies that the nurse's concern with the patient's subjective state does not imply a lack of concern for the objective world (the more technical aspects of his care), but quite the opposite. "If the patient's experience is important to her, she will also attach importance to well-cared for instruments and well-executed procedures."* Ujhely's meaning is clear—that nurses should concern themselves with the experiences of the patient and the reality of the situation for the patient—and not merely with the overt behavior of the patient and their own reactions to this behavior.

---

*From Ujhely, G. B.: Determinants of the nurse-patient relationship, New York, 1968, Springer Publishing Co., Inc.

During the course of some recent work as a consultant to a group of coordinators at a large, modern, general hospital, I have had the opportunity to become involved in the nursing care of patients with fatal illnesses. The work to be reported below was begun in an attempt to better understand not only the problems faced by a patient who is dying, but also the problems that confront nursing staff as they attempt to provide nursing care for the patient. During the course of the work we learned, too, that working with a dying patient can be a rewarding experience for the staff.

The situation was one that could easily have developed into a disaster for both the patient and the staff. Fortunately for all concerned, the coordinator was a nurse who was sensitive to the experiences of both the patient and the nursing staff.*

In the following section of the report the data about the patient and the related nursing carse are presented in summarized form. The final section is an analysis of the situation and reiteration of what seemed to be the most significant learnings about the patient and the process of nursing intervention.

This is in no way intended to be a comprehensive study of the nursing care of the dying patient, for it is a detailed study of only one situation. It is hoped that such a study will increase our understanding of some aspects of the experiences of a dying patient and of some of the problems and satisfactions in the process of nursing intervention. It is further hoped that knowledge of the method of exploration and intervention in this situation will be useful to others who wish to increase

their effectiveness in working with dying patients.

The story of Mrs. X
The staff's experience with the patient

The setting was a medical-surgical unit with about 30 very sick patients. It was 3 P.M. on a busy day when both shifts of nursing personnel were on the floor, and report time was drawing near. The phone rang. After requesting to speak to the charge nurse, a man on the line (without identifying himself) curtly asked the coordinator if she had a certain kind of narcotic on the unit. Mrs. D, the coordinator, asked why he wanted to know. The man then explained that his wife, who was being admitted to the unit, needed that specific medication for pain.

This phone call was the initial contact between the nursing staff and the X family. It was not a good beginning for a new relationship. Mrs. D was irritated by the question and by the man's curt manner. She felt his request to be an implication that he thought the staff would not be ready for the patient, and she wondered if the man felt that they should give their entire attention to his wife—as if she were the *only* patient being admitted that day.

The scene that followed was unforgettable. In rapid succession, 6 new patients arrived on the floor, and Mrs. X was among them. She arrived on a stretcher moaning loudly and requesting not to be moved too rapidly because of pathological fractures in her chest and pelvis. She also had tremendous lymphedema of her left arm and was wearing a neck brace. Transferring her to her bed and positioning comfortably was a tedious and time-consuming task. It seemed impossible to do anything to Mrs. X's satisfaction. Within minutes of Mrs. X's arrival on the unit, one of the licensed practical nurses (LPN) appeared at the nurses' station, irately demanding a transfer or threatening to re-

---

*Special thanks is given to Mrs. Ruth Davenport, R.N., who was at the time of this study the coordinator of the unit involved. She was most instrumental in planning for and providing the nursing care and was very helpful to me in providing information for this report.

sign if the coordinator did not reassign her from Mrs. X.

Shortly after this a student nurse who had recently been assigned to the unit came to the nurses' station and said, "I understand you have my mother on the unit." Six new patients had been admitted that afternoon, so Mrs. D did not associate the student with Mrs. X. Mrs. D reported later to me, "I almost had a stroke when I found out that she was Mrs. X's daughter! They seemed to me to be complete opposites. The daughter was very quiet, never complained, took everything in stride, was always supernice to everybody. She's the kind of person who goes out of her way to make everybody else comfortable, and there was her mother—just the complete opposite!"

Mrs. X's doctor arrived in the unit later and added more negative impressions to the staff's already grim perception of her. First he told Mrs. D that no other floor would take Mrs. X, so he had sent her to "nice little" Mrs. D's floor. Then, before entering the patient's room to see her, he groaned, "Oh, God—give me strength." After seeing Mrs. X he told the staff about her condition and previous hospital reputation. Her illness was cancer that was now in an advanced state (she had had a radical mastectomy about three years previously). More recently, she had been hospitalized on another unit in the same hospital on which the nursing staff had threatened to walk off their jobs if Mrs. X ever returned to their unit. Furthermore, shortly before she was brought to Mrs. D's unit she had first been admitted to another unit. Because of a minor conflict between Mrs. X and her roommate, the staff quickly shuffled Mrs. X off to another unit rather than make any adjustments within their own unit.

Mrs. D thought the whole situation to be unfortunate for and unfair to Mrs. X and decided to try to find a more positive approach to her care. With a nursing care-plan form in hand, she went to Mrs. X's room and asked for her help in planning for her own care. She told Mrs. X that she would record all the information on the nursing care plan so that it would be available to all the staff to read. Mrs. X then began to dictate her entire schedule, detailing exactly what procedures to follow. This dictation lasted for an hour, after which Mrs. D again assured her that the information would be shared, and then bade her good night. Mrs. D returned to the nursing station and shared the information with the nursing staff, including the LPN who had threatened to quit. This LPN then accepted her assignment of caring for Mrs. X.

Request for consultation

Two days later at a group meeting of several coordinators who had been meeting weekly with me, Mrs. D brought up her problem with Mrs. X and asked that the group try to help her find some solutions to the problems which this patient was presenting. Mrs. D described Mrs. X and the nursing situation to us. It was evident that she was interested in trying to understand this patient and offer her the kind of nursing care that would make her hospital stay as agreeable as possible. She was quite aware that some of her staff were responding to Mrs. X's demands with anger and might even resign unless they could be helped in some way to accept this patient better. Mrs. D also shared with us some of Mrs. X's background and history, so we knew about Mrs. X's condition and about her previous hospital stays. During this discussion it became apparent that we had little information about Mrs. X as a person, about how she might be feeling, and about how she viewed her illness and her hospitalization. At the end of this conference I went to the unit with Mrs. D to interview Mrs. X in an effort to obtain some more information about her experience. Hopefully, as a result of this interview, we would both understand Mrs. X better and Mrs. D then would be able to help her staff work with her more effectively.

Interview: the patient's experience

Mrs. D and I went in together to Mrs. X's room, and Mrs. D introduced me to the patient. A woman who had been taking care of Mrs. X at home prior to her hospitalization was sitting quietly at the bedside (she sat beside the bed in such a way that her back was turned to Mrs. X so that they could not even exchange glances). I further introduced myself to Mrs. X by telling her that I was a nurse and that I worked one day a week as a consultant at the hospital. I explained that Mrs. D was concerned about her and her care, and that she had asked me to see if there was any way in which we could plan together for the best possible nursing care for her. I told Mrs. X that I thought we might best be able to do that if I knew her a little better, and I wondered if she would be willing to talk with me for awhile about herself and her difficulties. She said that she would be quite willing to do that. I indicated that I would like to have Mrs. D stay with us while we talked, since she was coordinator on the floor and she would be involved in any planning that went on; then I asked her whether she would like to have her "sitter" stay also, thinking that she probably would. To my surprise, Mrs. X said no, she would prefer that the sitter did not stay for this conversation. She then asked the sitter to leave the room. Mrs. D sat on the edge of the overstuffed chair where the sitter had been so that she faced both me and Mrs. X. Since there was no other place to sit in the area, I asked Mrs. X if it would be all right with her if I sat on the foot of her bed so that I could face her while we talked. She said that was fine with her.

Let me describe Mrs. X's appearance briefly before going on. She was a middle-aged woman who seemed to be quite large and heavyset. She wore heavy glasses, was clean and neat with her hair combed, but she definitely looked sick and in pain. Her left arm was tremendously swollen and was lying across the covers with the hand resting near her abdomen. The arm looked like it was quite useless. I was not sure whether she was able to move it at all, and I assumed that it had very little function. The head of the bed was in an upright position. She wore a neck brace with her head cushioned against some pillows. Her mouth was visibly dry. Periodically, throughout the interview, she would ask for sips of water to moisten her mouth.

To begin the interview, after the introductory remarks, I asked her first of all how sick she was. Her answer was, "Well, I am not exactly sick." That surprised me. I asked her what she meant by that statement. She explained that she had a "problem" that kept recurring and that bothered her quite a lot, but it was not exactly what she would call being sick. I then asked her how she was feeling and she said that she had a lot of pain. I asked where the pain was. She indicated that she had a lot of pain in her pelvis. When I asked her what that was about she said that there were some broken bones there. Then she further described her problems and gave me some of the history of her illness. She said she had had a breast removed three years ago. The tumor, which of course was cancer, had recurred in other parts of her body. She was in the hospital now because her pelvic bones had broken so that she could not walk any more. In fact, she could barely sit up.

The manner in which Mrs. X described her illness was an interesting progression of expression, for she gradually moved from seeming denial of the problem to speaking quite freely and openly about the nature of her illness and her approaching death. In the beginning she said she was not "exactly sick" (she just had this problem that kept recurring), and then as she began to talk more and to give the details and history of her illness, she began gradually to use words such as malignancy and cancer. She talked about the cancer spreading to other parts of her body and before long she was mentioning death and the fact that she knew she had not much longer to live. Although I asked for more details about how she felt and about what was happening to her, in *no instance did I introduce any of the emotionally laden terms such as malignancy, cancer, or death.*

I asked her what she expected from this hospitalization and how long she thought she would be there. She told me she was there to have cobalt treatments, and that she expected that after the treatments were finished she would then be able to go home again for awhile.

As she described herself it became quite easy to picture the extreme discomfort she was in with her body riddled with cancer to the extent that bones in the pelvis and in the chest were fracturing spontaneously. She could no longer bear weight on them and could scarcely ever get in a position, even in bed, that was comfortable for her. She was also uncomfortable because of the dryness of her mouth, which she thought was due to some of the medications she was taking, presumably tranquilizers. She did not seem particularly anxious, but she did seem depressed, despairing, and pained. She was, however, freely willing to discuss her feelings and her experiences.

I asked her if she had been able to talk with anyone before about what was happening to her. In answer to my question she described a situation in which she and her family had been mutually avoiding the subject, each for fear of upsetting the other. She said she would like to talk with her husband about what she was experiencing but that she did not want to make him cry, and she was sure that he avoided saying anything to her about her illness or her death for the same reason. She cried quietly during part of the interview and seemed to feel relieved to be able to do so.

Mrs. X talked about herself as always having been a dominant person. In her family she made all the pertinent decisions and, for the most part, ran the affairs of the family. She said she was finding it difficult, now that she knew she was dying, to transfer the control of the family to her husband. It was not only difficult for her to give up the control, but it was also difficult for her husband to begin to take over.

Then she told me about her daughters, about whom she was quite concerned. The older daughter was a student at a nearby university and the younger one was a senior nursing student. She was very concerned about these two daughters and wished to be able to say certain things to them, to impart some of her values to them, she said, before she died. This emerged quite clearly as one matter that she was greatly concerned about and hoping that someone would be able to help her with.

Mrs. X was also concerned about the mounting cost of her care and hospitalization. She realized that she would die soon anyway, and she regretted leaving such a large financial burden for her husband to bear after her death.

(Following the conference I located Mr. X in the lounge and talked with him briefly about his wife and about who I was and why I was seeing her.)

Nursing care: sustaining the patient

If in nursing we take as our focus "sustaining the patient in his subjective experience," then we must know something of what that experience is. It is not enough to know facts about the patient, we must know how he feels and what he thinks about himself and his situation.

The interview with Mrs. X provided us with considerable appreciation of her experience. Mrs. D was able to share this information with the nursing staff so that they too could understand something of what Mrs. X's life was like for her at the present time. The staff then began to be able to view Mrs. X as a *person* who was experiencing the greatest difficulty of her life, rather than as a *patient* who was trying to make life difficult for the staff. As they began to appreciate her experience, they were able to understand her behavior in new ways. They began to think of her as a dying, needful patient, rather than as a demanding, irritable patient.

With Mrs. D's leadership, the staff was able to revise the nursing care plan in many small ways which contributed to Mrs. X's comfort. Interestingly, but not so surprising, as the staff became more interested in meeting her needs, Mrs. X's demands lessened. Her call light was no longer turned on every 10 minutes or so. The staff began relating to Mrs. D some of the positive things that were happening with Mrs. X, rather than only negative incidents.

Mrs. D spent a period of time each day talking with Mrs. X. She found that as Mrs. X became more relaxed, and as the staff became more interested in working with her, the period of time that Mrs. X needed with her gradually lessened.

A week later, when I was again at the hospital, Mrs. D and I went in together to see Mrs. X for about 15 minutes. She seemed much more relaxed than she had the week before. She said she had been anticipating this visit and the chance to talk. She had obviously given considerable thought to our original interview and had some things on her mind that she wished to discuss with us. She knew that Mrs. D knew her daughter, Andi, who was a

senior student nurse at the hospital. She asked Mrs. D if she would be willing to talk with Andi about her future in nursing (Andi was nearing graduation and was undecided about what field of nursing to go into). Mrs. D said that she would be willing to talk with her about nursing and the various fields in it in order to help her make that decision. Mrs. X's concern with her older daughter was of a different nature. She felt quite close to Andi and could talk with her about many things, but there seemed to be a serious communication barrier between her and her older daughter. Mrs. X wondered if I would be willing to talk with her sometime. I was not sure what she thought I could do to help the situation, but I told her I would be happy to talk with her daughter any time if she wanted to.

During this brief discussion Mrs. X also told me that she had learned this week that the cancer had now spread to her brain. She seemed to be accepting of this additional information and fully aware of the implication. In fact, her concern seemed to be more with the additional cost of the x-ray examinations.

The next time I saw Mrs. X was the day she was leaving the hospital to go home. She talked further this time about her daughters, again asking us to talk with them. Mrs. D and I restated our willingness to talk with them if they wished to. Mrs. X also said that she was able to talk with her family more now. In fact, she had decided to get the daughters together for a family conference. I was not sure what she intended to say to them; the implications seemed to be that she wanted to talk with them about her impending death and some of the things she wanted them to know and consider for the future. During this discussion her husband came in and joined us. I suggested to Mrs. X that she include him in the family conference. She readily agreed to this.

Mrs. X told me about the plans for her

care at home. She asked me to help her think about what she might be able to do at home. We talked about what capabilities she had left that would determine what she could do. Her vision was fairly good so she could read and watch television. She could not walk, nor could she sit up unassisted. Her right arm was functional, but her left was not. She was having progressively worsening headaches. The pain from the bone tumors and fractures had abated somewhat, but even so she required narcotics regularly to keep her (even remotely) comfortable. I felt quite helpless during this discussion and wished that I could come up with something creative and satisfying for her to do, but I could not.

In parting I told Mrs. X that it had meant very much to me to get to know her as well as I had. I told her she could contact me at the university any time if she wished to talk with me again. She thanked me profusely for talking with her and was genuinely appreciative of my interest in her.

This was the last time I saw Mrs. X. Mrs. D saw her later that day, shortly before she was discharged home. She thanked Mrs. D and the staff and requested to come back to that unit if she returned to the hospital again.

One week after the discharge Andi came to the unit to see Mrs. D, saying that her mother had asked that she come to talk with her. Mrs. D explained to Andi her mother's concern about her future in nursing. Andi, instead of speaking about her future in nursing, spoke about her mother's condition and how it was becoming increasingly worse, with ever-increasing pain, and increasing demands. (Andi was temporarily living at home to be with her mother from 4 A.M., at which time Mr. X went to work, until 7 A.M. when another caretaker, employed by the family, arrived.)

Mrs. D expressed to Andi her concern for her. She asked Andi if she were extremely tired, taking care of her mother, going to school, and then returning home to take care of her mother. Mrs. D then shared some of her own feelings of becoming supersaturated at times with the many complaints of patients, and then becoming angry at herself because she was less patient at home than she thought she should be. Andi agreed to having all these types of feelings, and went on to say that because she was "the nurse" in the family she felt a responsibility to each one of the family members. She realized that she was not only physically tired, but that she needed someone else to talk with about her own problems. She said that she did not have anybody to talk to at the school; she felt that the other students did not really want to be burdened with her problems. She then began to discuss her future in nursing and some of the clinical areas she was interested in. At that time Mrs. D just listened, and Andi came up with the suggestion that she thought a general nursing care unit, rather than a specialized unit, would be better for her to begin employment. After she reached this decision she thanked Mrs. D and told her that she would see her again for it was helpful for her to be able to share her feelings with an interested and an understanding person.

Two weeks later Mrs. D saw Andi in the hallway. Andi said that her mother's condition was very critical. Andi did not know what to do—one doctor had said "keep her out of pain" and another doctor had said "keep her awake as much as possible." She was giving injections to her mother at home and Mrs. X was taking narcotics frequently. However, if she had enough narcotics to be relieved of pain, Andi reported her mother slept most of the time. Andi was in a quandary about what to do. Mrs. D asked her, "What do you think, and what does your father think?" Andi thought it would be best to keep her mother out of pain, since she did not have much longer to live. She said then, "That's what I'll do. I'll just keep her as comfortable as possible because when she is awake all she does is ramble on without making much sense." Mrs. D asked if Mrs. X had recognized that Andi was there at her bedside. Andi replied that her mother had intermittent periods when she was lucid. She also said at this time that the care, she realized, was only custodial. She felt the situation was very traumatic to her father and she was concerned about him. Her father wondered if perhaps they should consider taking Mrs. X to a nursing home. Andi felt that this would be very difficult, especially since she was in nursing, but she realized that this might be the best thing to do.

The family never had to make the decision about taking Mrs. X to a nursing home because she expired within three days after Andi spoke to Mrs. D. Andi had asked one of her fellow students to call Mrs. D and let her know about the death.

Conclusion and review

This section of the report presents a brief analysis of some of the problems the nursing staff experienced in working with this dying patient, some of the problems the patient was experiencing, and the method and effect of the nursing intervention. Of the many things we might learn from such a situation, I have selected for discussion only those few which seemed most meaningful to us who were in the situation. Unquestionably, other conclusions could be drawn and other ideas could be generated than those that I am presenting here.

The nursing staff's problems with the patient

Prior to Mrs. X's admission the scene was already set for the nursing staff to develop negative feelings about her. The husband's phone call, which was undoubtedly an anxious attempt on his part to ensure comfort for his wife, was felt by the staff as an affront to their competence. Mrs. X's reputation as an impossible, demanding patient reached the unit almost as soon as she did. It would have been difficult for the staff, even under the best of circumstances, to resist being influenced by the many negative feelings of other nursing and medical personnel toward Mrs. X, since their own experiences with her began on a hectic note.

Unfortunately for all concerned, Mrs. X's anxiety about herself was expressed as a barrage of demands on the nursing staff. Given the situation as it was, the staff reacted to these endless complaints and demands as an implication that they were not adequate to the task of providing her nursing care. The staff felt Mrs. X's behavior a threat to their sense of competence or adequacy, rather than seeing it as an expression of her inner experiences —her anxiety, pain, depression, and anger, which was *not* directed at the staff personally although they reacted to it as if it were.

I think the perception of her as a "dying" and painfully needful patient was new to the staff and helpful to them in their understanding of her. According to Sudnow,[5] members of the staff reserve "dying" for those patients who are likely to die during their current hospital admission, rather than thinking of persons who are on a steady downward course as dying. Thus "dying" has a very different meaning for the staff than it does for the patient. Mrs. X was well aware that she was dying, but to the staff she was not a "dying" patient (meaning generally comatose or nearly so), but a "demanding" patient.

The staff's attitude and feelings about Mrs. X changed when they were helped to understand how she was experiencing the situation. As they began to know what she was going through, they could understand her behavior as an expression of her own needs and not feel it as a hostile attack on them.

In this situation the information given the staff about what Mrs. X was experiencing as she faced her own death was sufficient to help them to shift their focus from their *own* subjective experience to *her* experience. This relationship with Mrs. X was new, and although there had been much input of negative feelings about Mrs. X from other people, this staff had not had a long-term negative relationship with her. Had this situation been allowed to develop into a bitter, deadlocked experience of long standing for the staff, changing the staff's attitudes would have been much more difficult. In such an instance it would be important to deal first with the *staff's* feelings about the patient, and only then begin to interest them in learning about how the patient is feeling in this situation.

The patient's problems

Mrs. X willingly told us a great deal about what she was going through. Her pain and discomfort were great; she was anxious about her care and handling. She recognized herself as a woman who characteristically controlled and dominated things. It was important that she be allowed to retain as much control as possible of her nursing care. She was concerned with how to occupy her time and her mind. Realistically, however, there was little left that she could do because of her failing physical abilities.

She was well aware that she was facing death within a short while. Both pain and grief were clearly lined in her face. She was concerned about the mounting expenses of her treatment and care and regretted leaving such a burden for her husband to bear.

Like so many dying patients, Mrs. X was surrounded by silence. She and her husband were both afraid to talk about her death, each for fear of upsetting the other. Our discussions with Mrs. X helped with this, and both she and her family were able to talk, at least a little, about her approaching death.

Mrs. X was "putting her house in order." It was important to her to express certain ideas and values to her daughters before leaving them forever. She was concerned about the problems they were facing in their lives and wished to be of help to them. She was able to make some progress with these concerns, partially by being better able to talk with them herself, and partially by using Mrs. D and myself to communicate with her daughters.

Intervention: the interview

The one-hour interview provided us with considerable information about Mrs. X's thoughts and feelings as she courageously faced her own progressive disability and approaching death. I think it was important that the interview focused not on death *per se,* but on *whatever* Mrs. X was feeling and was concerned about.

Having the coordinator present during the interview was important for at least two reasons:

1. The coordinator had the opportunity to learn directly from Mrs. X what she was experiencing, rather than having the information reported to her by the consultant.

2. The interviewing style was important as a role model for Mrs. D. She expressed her feelings about the interview as follows: "You can read many books on interviewing technique and have many classes on interviewing, but you have to experience an interview like this one to really appreciate what has been done and what you yourself could do with a patient." Mrs. D further stated that the interview had improved her relationship with the patient by opening up the communication between them. She felt more comfortable

in asking Mrs. X how she felt about things and in telling her more directly her own thoughts and feelings. The communication became more direct, open, and more realistic.

Nursing care: sustaining the patient

If we want to sustain the patient in his experience of struggle, we must be able to inquire as to what he is experiencing, what the struggle is all about. Mrs. X was relieved to be able to talk about what she was going through. All patients need this opportunity, although a few may choose not to use it, and most will not want to talk about their experiences all of the time. Nurses must be sensitive to the patient's need to talk seriously about his situation and receptive to his communications about himself.

Nursing care can be more specific to the needs of the patient when it is based on detailed information about the patient's condition and physical and emotional needs. Such care helps relieve the patient's anxiety about what is happening to him. Many patients, like Mrs. X, need to control their environment as much as possible. It is important to respect this need and plan care *with* rather than *for* the patient.

Relatively brief but regular opportunities for a patient to talk with someone about what he is experiencing may be felt as supportive by the patient. Mrs. X anticipated our brief sessions, planned what she wanted to discuss, and used the talks to help her clarify her thinking and work on her "unfinished business."

Nursing care extends beyond the hospital and beyond the patient. Mrs. D's talks with Andi were helpful, not only for Mrs. X's peace of mind, but even more importantly, they were supportive of Andi as she struggled through what surely must have been the most excruciating experience of her young life. The opportunity to talk with the older daughter never arose. It is regrettable that we were able to have only minimal contact with the husband. The nursing care would surely have been even more meaningful if we had been able to include him in it more completely.

References

1. Kübler-Ross, E.: On death and dying, New York, 1969, The Macmillan Co.
2. Glaser, B., and Strauss, A.: Time for dying, Chicago, 1968, Aldine Publishing Co.
3. Quint, J. C.: The nurse and the dying patient, New York, 1967, The Macmillan Co.
4. Schneidman, E. S.: The enemy, Psychology Today 4:37-41, Aug., 1970.
5. Sudnow, D.: Passing on, Englewood Cliffs, N. J., 1967, Prentice-Hall, Inc.

Bibliography

Anonymous: Death in the first person, Amer. J. Nurs. 70:336, Feb., 1970.
Ujhely, G. B.: Determinants of the nurse-patient relationship, New York, 1968, Springer Publishing Co., Inc.

Chapter 6

A therapeutic approach to acting out and its ramifications

Joan M. King

Acting out in its many forms is a frequently encountered experience. Yet, strangely, it is one of the most problematic situations encountered by nurses and other health professionals. The problems inherent in acting-out behavior manifest themselves in diverse ways. What, then, are the issues involved in acting out for the patient and for the nurse? In what manner are these issues illustrated in patient and nurse behavior? In what fashion do these issues influence experiential learning and hamper or encourage successful resolution of acting-out behavior? What intervention facilitates reduction of acting out and of the many problems associated with this behavior? These questions will be explored in this chapter.

Phenomenon of acting out

Maloney[1] describes the lack of precise meaning inherent in many terms common to psychiatric nursing. She identifies the tendency to attach personal meaning to common terminology. The private connotations ascribed to a term may be shared to some extent with others in a specific environment. However, the meaning is not universal; the definition of the same term by "outsiders" would be at variance with the meaning ascribed to that term by "insiders." Although this situation has some functional value within the context of a specific social system, it is limiting in both theoretical and practical spheres. Critical aspects of a concept must be identified to devise appropriate nursing intervention. Explicit universal definition of a specific term is basic to reducing confusion and misinterpretation in the intraprofessional and interprofessional communication required to plan and implement therapeutic endeavors.

The term acting out has acquired a multitude of meanings. In loose, but common usage, it applies to behavior that is in some manner repugnant to the individual applying the term. Repugnance may stem from transgression of social norms, role assignments, or values held by the observer. In a theoretical framework, acting out refers to ego syntonic behavior that involves "partial discharge of instinctual tension . . . achieved by responding to the present situation as if it were the situation that originally gave rise to the instinctual demand."[2] Bellak[3] and Ekstein[4] further clarify this definition by viewing acting out as an unconscious statement, which may be a stereotyped behavioral pattern or circumscribed and episodic in nature. An example of circumscribed episodic acting out can be seen in the frequently encountered unwarranted negative response to figures in authority positions. Arguing, accusation, firm resistance, suspiciousness, and expectation of exploitation are common expressions of this pattern.

As implied in the definition, acting out represents a displacement from the original to the existing situation. Something within present experience is associated with repressed memories and acts as a stimulus for action. Acting out may also be stimulated by guilt. Under these circumstances the behavior is unwittingly designed to bring forth external punishment or failure that functions to absolve guilt from instinctual demands unacceptable to the individual.

Acting-out behavior represents an inability to tolerate frustration. Detour behavior is not used. Impulses are translated into immediate action that prevents the experiencing of frustration and anxiety. The action relieves inner tension through allowing partial expression of impulses. Thus acting out also involves either a reduced ability or an inability to control impulses.

Furthermore, the rapidity of the push for behavioral expression prevents or limits ability to contemplate and to assess the appropriateness and consequences of specific action in terms of the situation in which the individual is presently involved. This lack interferes with inhibiting or altering behavior into actions congruent with the situation and personal needs. Thus acting out involves a disturbance in functions of self-observation and self-criticism. These functions are prerequisites for internal behavioral mastery and control.

Specific disturbances in reality assessment are inherent in acting out. Elements of present reality are distorted in terms of past experience. The individual acts in accord with his view of the situation without recognizing the distortion. This misinterpretation of reality may prevent the individual from recognizing the inappropriateness of his actions in relation to present reality. Also, the individual may not be able to identify the cause-effect relationship that exists between his actions and their consequences. He may ascribe effects to fate or to chance. When this situation prevails, there is little incentive for change.

Shapiro[5] discusses the cognitive style of the psychopath. Although acting out is not synonymous with psychopathy nor limited to a single diagnostic category, certain elements of this style are relevant to this discussion of acting out. Of prime interest is the emphasis these individuals place on immediate concerns and pleasures. Lacks exist in objectivity, in self-criticism, in active searching for and organizing information, and in planning. Shapiro believes this cognitive style supports whim behavior; individuals do know the consequences of their actions, but do not think before acting.

The following example of acting-out behavior illustrates not only distortion of present reality in terms of prior experiences, but also coping functions of the behavior.

An adolescent, acting-out boy was hospitalized at a considerable distance from his home. When his parents wrote they would visit him at a specific time and requested he obtain a pass, he consistently complied. However, several hours prior to the designated time of his parents' arrival, the adolescent would act out to such an extent that his pass would be revoked. After several such incidents, it became apparent that this was a pattern and, further, that his parents frequently did not come to visit.

It was learned that as a child he frequently returned from school to find his parents had left home for several days without telling him in advance. While adequate provisions had been made for his care during these periods, there existed a question in the child's mind about the whereabouts of his parents and the possibility of their not returning.

His actions prior to the arranged time of his parents' visits to the hospital managed to reduce his uncertainty and frustration about whether or not they would actually come, to express his anger toward them, and to alleviate disappointment if they did not arrive.

Issues involved in acting-out behavior
Patient issues

The many problems involved in acting out for the performer can be identified readily from the prior discussion. This behavior, whether limited to a single sphere or more encompassing, is self-destructive in terms of continued growth. It inhibits control over behavior and planning for the future course of life either minimally or, in some instances, extensively. Actions are not based on choices resulting from information held and from hypotheses about the situation, other persons, and results accruing from a specific course of action. The repetitious, impetuous nature of the behavior is not based on an inability to learn, but rather an inability to effectively use learning. There is insufficient time between impulse stimulation and action on that impulse for intellectual processes to alter or deter behavioral expression. Thus, initially, acting-out behavior cannot be controlled without external assistance, and self-defeating actions will continue until the individual learns to delay action, to tolerate frustration, to increase his capacity for tension, and to develop internal restraints.

In addition to the limiting effects of acting out, the behavior may have more concretely punitive effects on the individual and his family. The acting-out pattern may involve behavior that is illegal, threatening, or harmful to others and may result in involvement with the legal or penal system.

Staff issues

Acting-out behavior tends to bring about a strong emotional response in others. These responses are particularly problematic for those involved in patient care, since the emotional response may find expression in behavior that either inhibits a therapeutic approach to acting out or actually encourages further acting out. Countertransference is the term applied to staff's strong emotional responses to patient behavior when responses are based on a staff member's own unresolved conflicts. The term implies the patient has been invested with certain characteristics relative to the staff member's past experience. Not all responses to patient behavior are countertransference phenomena; some responses are reality based and unrelated to prior conflicts. When emotional responses occur, it is essential that each individual staff member scrutinize his own response to determine whether it is related to past or present reality. It is not always possible to make this determination, since conflicts are frequently out of awareness, but it is necessary to make the attempt.

One of the most common responses to acting out is a feeling of helplessness and hopelessness. Personnel feel unable to control or to reduce frequency or intensity of patient behavior. This feeling may be expressed directly through ignoring the behavior, failure to establish limits, or assigning responsibility for behavioral control to others. Such responses allow continuation of acting out by omission. An unwarranted magical belief in the capability of drugs, physical treatments, or physicians to interrupt behavior and control the patient is another expression of helplessness embodying the hope of rescue from highly unpleasant feelings. Magical solutions such as these are generally not accompanied by actions toward the behavior itself but toward the individual who controls the magical solution. Therefore the desired outcome does not materialize and strife between various professionals frequently results. Staff strife presents the patient a rich opportunity to play staff members against each other, creating further chaos and lessening the opportunity of developing a rational and effective approach to acting out. All involved in the patient's care must be able to freely and openly discuss the behavior and their response to it, and arrive at a mutually agreeable plan of action if the behavioral approach is to be implemented with the degree of consistency required for effective intervention. When strife exists between staff members, it is extremely difficult to undertake such joint action based on cooperation and compromise until the strife itself is resolved. It might be said that at the point staff strife develops, personnel are indeed helpless to effectively approach patient behavior directly. However, this "helplessness" is not due to patient behavior but to staff response to patient behavior, which inhibits effective planning and action.

Overindulgence, which again encourages maintenance of acting-out behavior, is a response that may be encountered. This response pattern may arise from various motivations. It may express a desire to be liked by the patient or a belief that "love" will bring about a cessation of acting out. Overindulgence may also be a defense against feelings of anger or helplessness generated by patient behavior.

Anger is one of the most common responses to acting-out behavior and may be directly related to an initial response of helplessness; anger may be easier for the individual to tolerate than a feeling of being overwhelmed. Or, anger may be experienced because the staff perceives the patient as "getting away" with behavior that they will not permit themselves to express. In either instance, anger experienced by personnel may lead them to be overrestrictive and punitive toward the acting-out patient. This course of action may be seen as necessarily protective to others and preventative in nature; it may involve limits in unneeded areas and unwarranted restrictions for minor infractions of ward rules. However, undue and punitive restrictions encourage further acting out.

Anger toward the patient or toward staff members with divergent views about this behavior may lead a staff member to unwittingly encourage further acting out. The following is an example of this phenomenon.

Morning report was attended by a staff nurse who repeatedly expressed anger toward an 18-year-old boy who had demonstrated an acting-out pattern of eloping and smuggling alcohol into the ward. She also expressed anger toward his psychiatrist for "letting him get away with murder." At morning report, it was mentioned another patient had overheard the adolescent bragging about arson and stealing cars.

Later that day, the nurse told the patient in a loud accusing tone that he was not sick, but enjoyed getting away with being a no good delinquent. The adolescent ran out of the ward. The nurse made no effort to physically or verbally stop him. During this absence from the hospital, the adolescent wrecked a stolen car. As a result of this action, charges were brought against the adolescent and he was removed from the hospital.

The nurse's accusation was demeaning and undercut security. It also suggested a course of action—delinquent behavior. Although the nurse may not have been able to stop the adolescent nor predict his subsequent action with full accuracy, sufficient information was available to anticipate acting out of a serious nature. Her inaction permitted successful elopement and provided an opportunity to act out in a way that was self-punitive; it also prevented the psychiatrist from further action and removed the adolescent from the ward.

Staff members may encourage acting-out behavior because of their own wish to undertake a specific action that is unacceptable to them. Through identification with the patient, the staff member can obtain some gratification of this wish when this act is performed by the patient. The specific act may be unwittingly suggested to the patient, and staff activity that would prevent occurrence of the act is omitted. After patient acting out, the staff member frequently rebukes the patient for his behavior. This action is based on denial of participation in encouraging the behavior.

Staff may also respond to acting-out behavior with hopelessness, anger, or overconcern because it does not rapidly diminish or disappear. Main,[7] in discussing patient improvement, states "When a patient gets better it is a most reassuring event for his doctor or nurse." Conversely, a lack of improvement or slowness to respond to expectations can be disappointing. The patient's response may become intertwined with the staff's view of themselves as helping persons. Limited therapeutic response then becomes threatening to the individual's professional image. This state might be described in this manner, "I am a poor nurse because he is not getting better."

Group issues

Individuals, both patients and staff, on psychiatric wards become involved in group experiences. These experiences may be formalized in such activities as group therapy, patient-staff community meetings, or treatment-planning sessions. Informal talking with friends or co-workers is another form of group activity encountered in a ward setting.

One might think of the overall group on a psychiatric ward as being composed of all patients and staff who have sustained contact with patients. This large group encompasses many subgroups; staff members and patients may be seen as two of these subgroups.

Group experiences hold the potential of providing members with valuable opportunities to develop satisfying relationships, validate ideas, and obtain information about their behavior from others. This potential may be nullified if the group develops an intense response to the acting-out patient or his behavior.

Polarization is a group phenomenon that may be one response to acting-out behavior. This phenomenon may be displayed in both patient and staff groups. It involves group members assuming opposing stands on some issue, the pro and con factions. These stands may be highly emotional and result in group splintering and bickering. The group's purpose may be forgotten and goal-directed action set aside. This situation does not facilitate the open sharing of views and opinions necessary for operation of an effective therapeutic milieu. Energy and emotion that could be used more productively are tied up in circular arguments. No one benefits; successful experiences in modifying behavior, in changing one's environment, and in expressing opinions are not available to group members under these conditions.

A second group response to acting-out behavior is pervasive anger or disgust. These emotions may be expressed directly or indirectly through demeaning comments to the individual or in side comments to other group members. The acting-out patient may become a ward scapegoat. He may be ostracized from the group. This pervasive response is not directly related to specific instances of acting out but to group members' projected anxiety, fear, and anger. Such scapegoating can produce a cohesive group but one that is not beneficial, since growth of members and opportunities for trying out "new behaviors" are not fostered.

Group polarization and group anger have been discussed in terms of the total group, but what effect do these situations have on the individual who acts out?

Every group has devised what has been

termed "group values." These values are guides to acceptable and nonacceptable behavior within the group. They have been developed by the group and have group support. Transgression of these implicit or explicit operating rules brings forth group responses directed toward stopping errant action or, occasionally, the behavior may be accepted, which requires altering existing values. Only rarely are group values in opposition to society's norms governing acceptable human behavior. However, therapeutic groups offer an important divergence from social values, which holds particular opportunity for modifying acting-out behavior. Group members are expected to express directly and honestly opinions about their own and others' behavior. A related value is that these expressions may result in disagreement, but not retribution.

Polarization and group anger prevent utilization of one of the most effective tools in limiting acting-out behavior. Group opinion and pressure are powerful forces in molding human behavior. In terms of altering acting out, they are far more effective than individual opinion and limit setting. However, to be successful, group pressure, just as individual action, cannot be motivated by anger or the wish to punish. Group and individual actions that are so motivated will be resisted and the frequency or intensity of acting out may increase.

Intervention
Team issues

The diverse issues relating to acting-out behavior mentioned in the previous section indicate that sole reliance on a diadic relationship is inadequate during hospitalization. In addition to individual therapeutic endeavors, group effort, including all staff who have contact with the patient, is required. Individual and staff actions should augment one another to achieve therapeutic goals. Group staff meetings are needed to identify and work out divergent responses to the patient, to set goals, to plan realistic approaches to patient behavior, and to obtain consistency in limit setting and other therapeutic actions. In general, the goals of these meetings are to reduce manipulation and to provide a predictable environment in which the patient can learn to alter his behavior.

Staff care-planning conferences are not meant to be therapeutic vehicles for staff. However, meetings can be helpful in identifying and resolving some emotional responses to acting out that interfere with therapeutic activity. Mature open communication between co-workers can be beneficial in establishing realistic expectations for oneself and for others. Staff members may be of aid to each other in identifying feelings that were not in awareness or whose expression in action had evaded recognition. Also, awareness that other staff members respond to acting out with anger or helplessness can reduce denial and feelings of guilt. This recognition assists each individual to identify specific actions that bring forth the emotional response and to deal with their own responses more appropriately. Open discussion of such emotional response to patient behavior as anger do not eliminate the anger, but can alleviate the expression of anger in action.

Staff members rarely respond to patient behavior in a similar manner if planning meetings are initiated shortly after admission. This diversity of response provides an opportunity to direct group attention toward possible means of intervention, thus preventing or alleviating anger, helplessness, or other inhibiting responses.

Staff care-planning conferences can provide an additional function in moving members toward a realistic therapeutic approach. A frequent response to countertransference involvement in acting-out behavior is the development of a pseudorationale to explain and to justify one's own behavior. Such explanations serve to maintain existing action with the patient and to inhibit development of therapeutic strategies. Staff may be helpful in identifying, exploring, and altering these pseudorationales.

Limit setting

Planning realistic approaches to acting out requires cooperation and compromise if these plans are to be translated into consistent activity carried out by all personnel. To develop a unified approach, it may be necessary to specify the boundaries of acceptable behavior. This involves verbal identification and agreement on what behavior is and is not acceptable. In this manner, behavior that requires limitation can be agreed upon, reducing the possibility of inconsistent limit setting. Consequences to the patient of violating these limits must also be discussed and agreed upon. Again, the aim is to reduce the possibility that overrestrictive or underrestrictive action will be applied should the patient not abide by the limits set for his behavior. Consequences that are not, or cannot be, enforced simply become idle threats that permit continuation of the behavior.

Perhaps of even greater importance is the understanding that each staff member has of limit setting. This is not a punitive action taken when a patient is disobedient, rather it is a means of helping him to clearly delineate unacceptable behavior, to understand why the behavior is unacceptable, and to develop awareness of the relationship between his actions and the consequences of those actions. Staff must understand and apply limit setting with this connotation to achieve the desired results. At the time limits are set, the patient must be clearly told exactly what behavior is unacceptable, given specific concrete reasons for its unacceptability, and informed of the consequences of transgression. When feasible, seeking patient participation in establishing limits is the most effective approach to self-control. Limits

that are nonpunitive, clearly applied, and consistently carried out will teach the patient to delay acting out on impulse, to predict behavioral consequences, and to control his behavior. Singer[8] speaks of rational limits as being devoid of arbitrariness. They are established solely for the benefit of the patient and those around him.

Behavioral control and limit setting are not the only therapeutic issues and actions that will need discussion at staff meetings; effective intervention also requires consideration of the specific elements of acting out. Behavioral control and limit setting were selected for group attention because both involve all staff members and require some degree of consensus for appropriate application.

Specific therapeutic considerations

A basic tenet of this chapter is that nursing intervention is based on the interaction of theoretical considerations and clinical data. Five major aspects of acting-out behavior have been identified as a basis for intervention as follows:

1. An unconscious behavioral statement
2. Action that reduces tension and prevents experiencing anxiety
3. Inability to tolerate frustration
4. Inability to delay action
5. Disturbances in reality testing and self-criticism

Hospital admission may remove a patient from those individuals and circumstances that have become involved in behavioral expression of his adaptive difficulties. However, similar patterns are rapidly reactivated within the ward setting. The patient responds to various staff as he has to significant individuals from his past and present extrahospital living situations. The conflicts reside within the individual and he responds with coping patterns used previously.

Ekstein's reference to acting out as a communication of unconscious conflicts in action can be used as a guiding principle in planning and implementing a therapeutic regimen. Observations of specific instances of acting-out behavior offer clues to underlying conflicts and aid in developing therapeutic strategies. Since acting out is a rapid response to some element in present experience representing prior conflictual situations, thought should be directed toward the situation immediately preceding the acting out. A pattern or theme may begin to emerge as a series of these observations are gathered. For example, a patient may repeatedly act out in those situations in which he is ordered to do something. These patterns and themes must be validated by further observations and exploration with the patient before they are used as a basis for planning care.

Themes not only offer guides to possible conflicts and the adaptive function of the behavior, but also can be helpful in predicting potential acting-out situations. This predictive information is useful in a variety of ways. If patient behavior is destructive to self or others, efforts may be directed toward reducing frequency or intensity of those situations and messages within the patient's encounters that are likely to stimulate acting out. Frequently this approach is not feasible, and effort may be directed toward maintaining the patient's anxiety at a level he can tolerate. In this situation the need to act out is reduced because an anxiety level sufficient to stimulate acting out occurs less often. Predictive information may also be useful to personnel in anticipating potential acting-out responses and used to alleviate the intensity of their own response should it actually materialize. Predictions of acting out may also be used in therapy sessions to abort behavior. In the latter instance, predictions must be used with caution, since the goal is to underscore and alter behavior with a series of accurate forecasts.

It is important to observe the nature of acting-out behavior as a basis for planning

therapeutic intervention. Anticipated consequences of the specific behavior most frequently used should be considered fully. Certain behaviors have serious results for the patient or others. Actions that bring about physical or psychological harm and have legal or serious financial consequences require more direct and immediate effort in behavioral control than do trying but "nonharmful" behaviors. Short-term intervention may be of use in effecting behavioral change. Overall treatment goals may or may not require prolonged therapy and consequent use of long-term techniques.

Short-term techniques

The principle basic to all short-term therapeutic strategies is establishing external ego and superego controls while attempting to strengthen internal prohibitions. Three means of applying this principle have already been discussed: removing the individual from the situation, reducing stresses that potentially activate the behavior, and limit setting.

Physical and chemical restraints may be useful at times to alleviate or prevent acting out. These means may be seen by the patient as punitive rather than as protective measures. This interpretation is particularly likely to occur when seclusion or cuffs are used to constrain behavior. This viewpoint is often shared by staff and other patients and may reinforce the acting-out patient's beliefs. While the notion that restraints are punishment for infraction of "rules" may be a misinterpretation, in some instances it may be a valid interpretation of the situation. The staff has the responsibility of critically assessing the purpose behind use of these measures. Restraints, when used judiciously, represent concern for the well-being of the restrained individual and others on the ward. Restraints are of service when other control methods are ineffective.

It was mentioned earlier that acting-out

behavior is ego syntonic. One of the most useful approaches is an attempt to make behavior ego alien. This involves helping the patient to develop distance or some discomfort about the behavior so that it no longer occurs "naturally." Bellak[3] suggests the harmful aspects of the action and its repetitive nature be clearly pointed out to the patient. Patient recognition of his actual role as victim of his own impulses rather than master of self and situations will help him obtain distance from behavior that, with this understanding, becomes less desirable.

Emphasis on harmful aspects and consequences of acting out can also be used to strengthen the superego. This approach reinforces internal prohibitions and uses healthy aspects of patient personality. It may also help develop awareness of the relationship between behavior and its consequences for those individuals who have difficulty with this concept.

Two other elements of acting out present useful guides to intervention: acting out involves immediate action and action reduces tension. Initiating a period of delay will help abort acting out, particularly when a substitute action can be undertaken during the delay period. Ideally, the substitute action would involve discussion of what the patient wishes to do and related feelings and thoughts. Talking in this manner not only furthers patient and therapist understanding, but alleviates some tension through allowing verbal expression of wishes. However, this course involves considerable control and may be beyond patient abilities. In such instances, physical action may be a useful tension reducing mechanism; pacing, ping pong, sanding, or other available activities can be used. Patient involvement in the delay process should be sought whenever feasible. Mutual agreement on the length of delay is one approach to increasing frustration tolerance that is not limited to potential acting-out situations, but can be used in a wide variety of daily living experiences.

Long-term techniques

The objectives underlying long-term treatment strategies are development of self-awareness and internalization of behavioral control. These goals are implemented through verbal exploration. Instances of acting-out behavior are repeatedly discussed in specific detail so that the patient may gradually recognize that anxiety leads to acting out. Experiential awareness of anxiety permits other avenues of expression, avenues that are less problematic to the patient and his associates. Verbalization and physical activity are two possible substitute behaviors. Recognition of anxiety is also the first step toward understanding the cause of that anxiety.

The anxiety generating acting out cannot be experienced unless the behavior ceases or there is a period of time between development of anxiety and action. Patient group meetings or group therapy can be an important support system to help the patient delay or prevent acting out.

Assessment of intervention

Perhaps one of the most inhibiting factors in implementing a therapeutic approach to acting out is the conviction that nothing can be done to alter this behavior pattern. In some instances this is true. We do not have sufficient understanding of the phenomenon of acting out, nor has successful intervention been fully identified. However, acceptance of inevitable failure promotes failure, since it interferes with judicious therapeutic action. An attitude that holds prejudgment in abeyance is needed. This attitude will facilitate thoughtful consideration of issues relevant to acting out with consequent development and implementation of therapeutic strategies directed toward behavioral alteration. Whether treatment plans culminate in success or failure, it is essential that all aspects of therapy be scrutinized. Assessment may yield valuable clues to guide future therapeutic efforts to similar situations. Critical evaluation can identify both successful and unsuccessful intervention patterns and may further our understanding of the phenomenon of acting out.

Summary

Acting-out behavior presents a host of problems to health personnel who have assumed responsibility to therapeutically intervene in this self-defeating pattern. The behavior frequently stimulates strong emotional response in other patients and personnel. The nature of these responses is such that continuing or escalating acting out may be unwittingly encouraged. Thus an individual approach to the problem behavior is inadequate if not accompanied by group planning and consistent group action. It is hoped this exploration of the concept of acting out and related intervention will be helpful in reducing the dilemma and emotional turmoil related toward management of patients demonstrating this behavior.

References

1. Maloney, E.: Regression as a conceptual tool. In Bergersen, B., et al., editors: Current concepts in clinical nursing, vol. 1, St. Louis, 1967, The C. V. Mosby Co.
2. Hinsie, L. E., and Campbell, R. J.: Psychiatric dictionary, ed. 3, New York, 1960, Oxford University Press, Inc.
3. Bellak, L.: The concept of acting out: theoretical considerations. In Abt, L. E., and Weissman, S. L., editors: Acting out, New York, 1965, Grune & Stratton, Inc.
4. Ekstein, R.: General treatment philosophy of acting out. In Abt, L. E., and Weissman, S. L., editors: Acting out, New York, 1965, Grune & Stratton, Inc.
5. Shapiro, D.: Neurotic styles, New York, 1965, Basic Books, Inc., Publishers.
6. Wolberg, L. R.: The techniques of psychotherapy, New York, 1969, Grune & Stratton, Inc.
7. Main, T. F.: The ailment, An address to the Medical Section, British Psychological Society, March 20, 1957 (mimeographed).
8. Singer, E.: Key concepts in psychotherapy, New York, 1965, Random House, Inc.
9. Rome, H. P., and Barry, M. J.: Problems of therapeutic management of acting out with hospitalized patients. In Abt, L. E., and Weissman, S. L., editors: Acting out, New York, 1965, Grune & Stratton, Inc.

Chapter 7

Hopefulness in the face of crisis: can nurses participate in community action?

Hilda Richards

Man needs myths to survive, to block out the realities of the insensitivity, stupidity, and inhumanity he sees about him. He needs the illusion that there will be a better tomorrow to calm the mixture of rage and disbelief within, while hearing fantastic justifications given for spending millions to kill millions. Presently, I am reacting to two myths: (1) that there is "community mental health" and (2) that professional groups really are interested in or wish to participate in the development of mental health services that address themselves to critical social issues. The relative inadequacy of services for those whose lives are scarred not only by poverty, deprivation, and a devalued, restricted, imposed social position, but also by mental illness as well is all too clear once attention is turned from concentration on the perfection of technical skills to the application of knowledge to man's needs.[1]

Poverty and racial discrimination, according to one sociologist,[2] are the major mental health concerns facing our society. This position seems to parallel the findings of a study done to explore needs as viewed by clients. The major needs identified were those of finance, basic necessities, isolation, physical problems, psychological symptoms, problems in dealing with the "system," employment, and housing.[3] All of these factors are interrelated, and focusing on one without regard for the total seems senseless.

"To varying degrees, the worlds of disadvantaged persons demonstrate some of the features characteristic of the society: the unequal distribution of goods, urbanization, the expendability of groups of people, dispersion of social responsibility, automation, the uncertainty of life. Men are affected in many ways. They are deprived of goods and services, crowded in slums and ghettos, beset with a sense of marginality and treated as marginal. They are powerless, dehumanized and hopeless."* Little has changed since this quote was written four years ago on completion of a study concerning the utilization of

---

*From Christmas, J. J., and Richards, H.: An overview of group psychotherapy with socially disadvantaged adults in an urban area. Paper presented at 24th Annual Conference American Group Psychotherapy Association, 1967.

group approaches with socially disadvantaged adults in an urban area. Too often it was found that mental health workers attempted to shape the client to meet the needs of the therapists. A remark such as "disadvantaged persons have too many reality problems and must have them resolved before they will be good candidates for group therapy" was not uncommon among therapists of various disciplines in the more traditional treatment institutions, and was reflective of their personal and professional philosophies.

Yet each treatment approach should be questioned as to whether the intervention will facilitate the articulation of the individual within the society.[4] Educators tell us that the extent to which an individual feels some control over his destiny is a crucial condition of learning.[5]

The dependency brought about by the stagnation and strangulation of institutions produces a loss of self-responsibility and an erosion of self-realization, and is thus a measure of personality inadequacy. We like to think of nursing as an educative process and of illness as a potentially useful and usable experience.[6] We like to fantasy that we are advocates for the patient, guiding him through the labyrinth of agencies and caretakers and coordinating his service.[8] Yet are we fulfilling our roles as therapeutic agents by helping him adapt to archaic systems? Are we not saying to him "your self-responsible choices are few, you must remain in a subordinate position, and your possibilities of moving toward independency and maturity are minuscule"? Have we as nurses related ourselves to client needs; or have we, along with other professionals, participated in the game playing, the navel musing, the irrelevancies kept alive by the argument of role and role definitions?

If service effectiveness is defined as assisting the opening up of the total opportunity structure, then social change becomes an integral part of service. Nursing's preoccupation with individual and small group behavior, although good (as motherhood and brotherhood are good), has limited relevance to client need. Instead of focusing on nursing in isolation, it might be of more benefit to see how this profession along with other human service workers might analyze the ingredients necessary for planning appropriate service. How might we use such concepts as hopefulness, community control, advocacy planning citizen participation, and accountability? What tools have we to bring about a working coalition between consumer and giver of services? A case study analysis of a client-staff organization faced with a struggle for survival might assist with the identification of factors that help groups maintain hope and move forward to improved functioning.

The setting

The Harlem Rehabilitation Center, a community-based facility, is a division of the Department of Psychiatry of Harlem Hospital Center. It has developed an organized system of interdisciplinary, multi-focused rehabilitation services. These approaches are modified to meet the needs of clients with social and physical disabilities. A social system model that includes group and individual approaches, as well as clearly defined vocational and community action approaches was chosen. By doing this the multiple leadership of professional-paraprofessional teams, with paraprofessional staff working with experienced professionals, serve as the primary rehabilitative agents.[8] The service goals are as follows:

1. To develop and utilize sociopsychiatric group rehabilitation approaches to provide social, psychiatric, educational, vocational, and community services to persons in need of rehabilitation because of mental disorders, medical handicaps, and social disability.

2. To provide related rehabilitation ser-

vices and assistance to family and community individuals and groups to aid, directly or indirectly, in the rehabilitative process.

3. To serve as a force for individual, group, and social changes through the operation of preventive, habilitative, and rehabilitative systems and their transactions with other social systems, directed toward altering psychological or social disorder or both.

4. To develop and implement relevant and effective systems of human service, participating in the development with other members of the professional, paraprofessional, and lay communities, including recipients of service.[9]

These goals are incorporated in two service programs: The Psychiatric Program and the Vocational Rehabilitation Program. Other types of programs incorporate these goals, such as research and evaluation programs and training and education programs. Multiple approaches are central to service; thus, automatically provided are social, community, medical, and psychiatric services.

Since 1967 when the small staff attached to a pilot project moved into its present facility, the Harlem Rehabilitation Center has grown from a staff of 7 to 63; a sound training program for the 35 professional workers has been developed, with a beginning career ladder. Throughout its life it has been viewed as unique for its philosophy, its services' model in a black community, and its accomplishment in new careers for the health service field. Its reputation and that of the center's chief (Dr. June Jackson Christmas) draw visitors internationally.

Despite this, most of the center's funding came from project grants of various types (National Institute of Mental Health, State Department of Mental Health, Rehabilitation Services Administration of the Department of Health, Education and Welfare). Although this was prestigious,

the lack of permanent money, particularly for paraprofessional staff, precipitated major crises. The financial problems were brought to a head when staff and clients were confronted with the possibility of the center's closing on July 1, 1970, if permanent funds were not appropriated by city officials. This crisis had been precipitated by the termination of a major grant and a cut in the hospital budget.

Additionally the group was placed in the ironic position of knowing that if the essential operating funds were received, additional money was assured for improvement and expansion of vocational services, the incorporation for specialized services to addicts, and the development of a Public Service Careers Program Training Center. All of these had been long-term dreams of staff and community residents. Yet dreams are irrelevant when survival is at stake!

The integrity of an institution

Philip Selznick, in his book *Leadership in Administration*, points out that the key problems of institutional leadership are related to the persistence of an organization's distinctive values, competence, and roles—in other words, the defense of institutional integrity. His analysis of the relationship among what he refers to as the elite, social values, and autonomy comes alive when applied to the center. These three concepts are defined as follows:

> Elite—any group that is responsible for the protection of a social value
>
> Social values—objects of desire that are capable of sustaining group identity
>
> Autonomy—a condition of independence sufficient to permit a group to work out and maintain a distinctive identity[10]

Selznick[10] states, "The maintenance of social values depends on the autonomy of elites." The therapeutic community of staff and clients constituted an elite, and they maintained values as related to mental health services that were in contradiction to the traditional psychoanalytic-medical model held by the remainder of the Department of Psychiatry. Three major themes in the center's philosophy of mental health services were as follows:

1. It is not the individual who has faltered, but rather the system in which he is embedded that has failed to sustain him and maximize his potential functioning.

2. The paraprofessional worker, who has less formalized and much more specific training than that of the traditional professional and who comes with life experience, has the skill both to help the client and to help the professional to create a more pragmatic service model.

3. Social change is essential, since present rigidity of organizations and institutions is frequently destructive to the obtainment of human freedom and effective functioning.

A high degree of self-selectivity among the twelve or so professional staff who work in this system was apparent, since all at least partially supported the philosophy —a philosophy alien to the majority of professionals. The close relationships among all staff had helped all incorporate these values. The fact that the center was located at least ten blocks from the hospital itself had given a realistic (and oftentimes unrealistic) feeling of autonomy. The training program that included sensitivity training for all staff (including clerical) and the therapeutic community–systems approach to service "strengthened the isolations of the elite, [and] its capacity to shape its own identity free of external pressures."[10]

Although the center met Etzioni's criteria for normative organization,[11] commitment of paraprofessional workers was maintained by the fact that their salaries were higher than most nonprofessional salaries, and there was apparent possibility for advancement within the system. For many this is the first time that their job

combined respect for the person and respect for his background—where having a prison record, being an ex-addict or ex-alcoholic, or having been on welfare was an asset rather than a liability.

Much of the commitment was also due to the leadership. Dr. J. J. Christmas agreed that leadership is "the art of coordinating and motivating individuals and groups to achieve desired ends."[12] She played what could be classified as a charismatic role in the agency.[13] Her strong convictions, persuasiveness, and ability to surround herself with creative people (who could work to implement her ideas), the recognition she received within her profession, and the fact that she has been the most influential person in the hospital in acquiring continuing grant money had been relevant factors in the maintenance of the center's life.

Other persons performing leadership roles in the agency had been with the group since its days as a pilot project in 1964. The assistant chief's actions generally complemented those of the chief, playing either the instrumental or expressive role[14] as group and individual needs varied. The senior psychiatric rehabilitation technician was frequently the spokesman for the worker group.

The concepts of shared power and citizen participation had been incorporated into the organization. This had resulted in inclusion of both clients and paraprofessional staff on the administrative committee and in the formation of a client-staff advisory council. With this fuller participation in the therapeutic community of the center, vocalness and commitment increased in various subparts.

Throughout the incubation and maturation period of the agency's growth, the members were faced with many external factors that have assisted in the maintenance of the system:

1. Positive publicity and recognition was given to individuals and the total system.

The staff at various levels had given papers and talks at professional conferences, engaged in consultation, and were offered and sometimes moved into more prestigious positions.

2. The larger system (the Department of Psychiatry) viewed the staff group of the center as mavericks and as a group to admire. High morale had been maintained in the face of crisis, when the rest of the department had low morale and high turnover. The commitment of the staff was exemplified when as a total group they asked to have their salaries lowered for a period of time to save the center.

3. Even though financial worries had been present, expansion had also been progressing at a consistent rate, new staff had been added, services were revised, and planning continued.

4. The group had a common "enemy"— the affiliating university and frequently the administration of the Department of Psychiatry or the hospital system. When all else fails, get an outside scapegoat! This had been used to cope with internal power struggles, role conflicts, and anxiety produced by a shifting environment.

All the factors of leadership, power relations with other organizations, communication with the surrounding community, and communication patterns and social interactions within the group were important in sustaining hopefulness within the system when confronted with potentially threatening events.

The stages of crisis

Within the 5 months that the community of the Harlem Rehabilitation Center was in its most precarious financial state, the group experienced identifiable stages of crisis similar to those described by Caplan[15] and Lindemann.[16]

The initial blow was dealt at the beginning of the year. With the realization that one of the center's major grants would not be renewed for six months, the departmental director insisted that all paraprofessionals on that payroll (sixteen persons) be terminated and rehired when grant funds were renewed. All were stunned! Until this time budget details were withheld from staff. Thus they had not taken seriously the various warnings expressed by the assistant chief over the previous year. Even then, with sixteen people holding termination slips, there was the assumption that "the chief will pull us through." And, in fact, she did; but only partially. She used her contacts to solicit foundation money and obtained an advancement on other grant funds. It was obvious to the center administrators that this was not enough for continual survival.

The assistant chief presented the budgeting facts to the total staff. With repeated confrontation their immobilization and passivity were penetrated. The message conveyed was that they, the staff, *must* do something to assist in the struggle for survival.

Slowly the paraprofessional workers began to mobilize their internal forces. The group's approach was to see how they, by themselves, might help stretch the center's budget. This resulted in the development of a committee that looked at the situation and as a group prepared a proposal to lower their own salaries in an effort to save the center. During this period the focus of staff anger was transferred from the departmental director to the center's chief and assistant chief. Tension among the staff ran high with the feeling that the administration was using staff, forcing them to fight a battle that was not theirs. With the budgetary changes that took place over the two months that followed no one knew which "sixteen persons" might lose their jobs, since criteria shifted from those last hired to those with the poorest work evaluations. Subgrouping was constant and shifting, backbiting ran nonstop, and rumors oozed from the woodwork. After putting their salaries on the line, with little guarantee that this would bring the center stability, their gesture was frustrated by the labor union to which they belonged, who refused to allow the proposed salary readjustment. Increased frustration and depression resulted.

A new crisis peak was reached mid-May, when it was announced that the center's doors would be closed on July 1, if budgetary problems were not resolved. This "reality" was shared with the total community of staff and clients by the chief who stated that she could no longer carry the weight of struggle with the establishment by herself. The budget allocation for the center that had been built into the overall hospital budgetary request had been cut by the city officials. The threat of death produced a new struggle for life! The focus of anger again became those persons in power outside the center system; the clients who had attempted valiantly to assist in the struggle were finally welcomed as full participants. These two elements allowed for group cohesion.

What followed was a series of activities geared toward crisis resolution. The major steps that took place were as follows:

Monday: The possibility of closure was announced.

Tuesday: It was decided to attend an already scheduled community meeting that had been called by one of the local organizations. Several members of the staff were there, but it was the assistant chief who presented the center's plight. This drew community support and gave officials notice that a fight was on.

Wednesday: The problems of the center were presented to the entire Department of Psychiatry. This was done in a scheduled staff meeting by a group of ten, which included clients, paraprofessional workers, and professional staff. Thus support within the hospital was obtained from staff-level persons and heads of divisions. A spontaneous steering committee was formed.

Friday: A community meeting was held at the center. Many grassroot persons and organizations concerned about the Center were present. The chief presented budgetary problems. A struggle

became apparent after the chief's seemingly insistence that "community" proceed in what seemed a conservative manner, that of sending telegrams and letters to key officials, while community members were stating their wish for more active behaviors and more autonomy from hospital. The staff seemed to be caught between two positions; much anger and anxiety were evident. A meeting was planned for the following Monday morning between the borough president and Harlem and Center community people.

Monday: Approximately 100 persons met with the borough president who gave support, explained political budgetary maneuvering, and suggested strategy. Fliers were prepared for distribution. Committees were gelling, but many persons were still functioning in isolated pockets. Cross messages were given, with little validation before reactions took place.

Tuesday: Committees had been formed the previous week and the overall chairman had been appointed by the chief. Internal struggles became obvious; much nonfunctional behavior was apparent. Radio stations were contacted; interviews were taped.

Wednesday: The chief talked on an evening radio program with the sanction of the hospital administration. A community meeting was held; a large group of staff attended and presented the problem, but they disrupted the meeting at times.

Thursday: A scheduled meeting of the total center was held. The assistant chief presented concerns about leadership. The staff-client group expressed anger because they did not have sufficient authority; yet they were asking what the assistant chief wanted them to do. Feelings were ventilated while group behavior was examined; a new co-chairman of steering committee was elected. The feeling that administration and rest of agency were in different camps was discussed. What emerged more clearly were conflictual views concerning advocacy. The two positions were (1) poor communities get governmental response only through disruption and (2) planned advocacy, pulling in and developing community support but still not severing ties with establishment, is necessary. All staff and clients decided to pull together. The group felt a need to confront the chief so as to move her from what they viewed as a conservative position. (This is ironic, of course, since most persons outside the center hold an opposite view of her.) Anxiety about performing unfamiliar behavior was expressed.

Monday: The staff confronted the chief, who also saw herself as receiving much group support. More leadership behavior was to be shared among staff and clients. Plans were finalized for a group to appear before the city Board of Estimate on the next day and for a press conference on Thursday. There was insistance that all staff be on some functioning committee, while clients could make a choice of community action work or following a usual daily routine. *Letter writing* to city officials began with gusto. This activity was seen as low pressured, yet it allowed for all to feel a part. It continued all week. Telegrams and letters were sent to persons asking them to write letters. Community people began spreading the word and making themselves heard. In a meeting with the mayor's assistant in charge of hospital affairs, the case was presented by committee of staff and clients.

Tuesday: Large groups of clients, community persons, and professional and paraprofessional staff testified before Board of Estimate of the city. Much support was received from officials who seemed to be impressed. Some assurance of understanding financial needs was given, but the group was warned to keep pushing. Other contacts were made by the administration, while staff and clients contacted councilmen and community persons.

Wednesday: Dr. Christmas approached the mayor in an open meeting, presented the state of financial problems, and pressed him for support. An important official testified before the Board of Estimate in the center's behalf.

Thursday: A press conference was held. Official and grassroots leaders in all areas participated. Clients themselves gave strong verbal support; strengths were brought out in the client group that had not been apparent three weeks earlier. The mayor's budget staff called the chief for information, and expressed the mayor's wish to give support.

Friday: A representative of the comptroller's office (person in charge of the city budget) appeared at center unannounced asking for more budgetary information. A news team from a local television station came to cover the center for a presentation on news special for following day. Press releases were sent out.

Monday: A meeting between center administration and paraprofessional representation and city officials in charge of health and hospitals was held. By this time a shift in discussion with officials was apparent. Conversations moved from there is no money to money will be found somehow, but do you need all you have requested. This shift was attributed to community support.

Tuesday: A telephone call from the mayor's office informed us that over a thousand letters and telegrams had been received supporting the center. This did not include mail sent to other officials. By this time the center had received ample coverage from mass media, and telephone calls offering help were coming in from all sides. There was nothing more to do but wait for the vote by the city council.

Friday: The center group had a party!

Monday: Word was received that the total amount of money requested was appropriated by the council and that the job positions of all but two paraprofessional workers were made permanent. Success!

The above outline does not give justice to the group process that took place. Contagion was used to advantage. Movement forward emerged out of what appeared to be confusion and inefficient behavior. The varieties of activities allowed for enough latitude for all to participate at different levels. By the middle phase, strong staff and client leadership emerged that allowed professional staff to fill the roles of consultants and team members. Although the roles played were new to many professionals, causing discomfort, they were essential. Examples of this were helping committees plan for a press conference, writing and sending out press releases, obtaining names and addresses of public officials, pulling together effective material for distribution, and helping to think through what were useful group alliances. Confrontations with leadership helped the group to accept the reality that there would always be an internal conflict concerning advocacy roles, since both positions were necessary for system maintenance.

Inclusion of community persons on the center's advisory committee was one of the many positive outcomes of the crisis resolution. Thus the group was propelled toward its ultimate goal of true community control.

Analysis of factors affecting hopefulness

What are the factors that maintain or destroy hopefulness for staff members?

How can hope be sustained when the events of everyday life do not support it? The problem of potential conflict between hopefulness and realism is a general concern for all groups and individuals. Writers such as Bales[17] and Homans[18] regard the development of the social processes among members of groups as a derivative or function of the environmental pressures of the group. In these terms the internal structure of a group, the pattern and content of interactions, is heavily influenced by the external system or by the way the group relates to its environment. The way the group functions is assumed to be a function of "facts." Yet the perceptions of the group, the way in which it sees or interprets the environment, are the decisive elements in the decision of how "facts" are seen. Frustration with the environment can lead to hopefulness instead of hopelessness.[19]

The facts that social change is slow, that job permanency is uncertain, that the parent institutions do not give the support "that they should," and that professional groups put blocks in the way of new careers development can be withstood when the "group" assumes these facts to be reality and when their ideology lets them know that the right is on their side.

According to March and Simon[20] there is little question that the goals of mental health institutions lack "operationability," that is, one cannot ascertain empirically how well the organization is attaining its goals. The goals are too diverse, too diffuse, and too potentially contradictory to be easily operationable. Thus the fact that mental health workers encounter frustration regularly can easily be interpreted in a negative fashion, yet a positive interpretation is necessary for their effective functioning.

Hopefulness in this case was maintained through the ideological system. Some of these sources can be listed.[19]

1. The relationship of the values concerning mental health as listed earlier and the struggles of people who are black and poor.

2. The support given the agency from other institutions, groups, and persons who are not expected to participate in its function. This has come nationally, internationally, and from the local black community.

3. Support from experts outside the institutions; recognition from many professional groups and funding groups.

4. Data collected by the research unit in the center that support our contention that our approach to service has value.

5. The growth of the center over the years, adding staff and service programs.

6. The perception by the group that the center was new, innovative, and different. It was considered the first in the nation to use its service model and has a reputation for giving the best training in the country to paraprofessional staff.

7. The communication and socialization and education process within the agency. In addition to the formal-training system already mentioned and the informal systems always operating, all staff and clients grew in knowledge and closeness with the live-learning experience of crisis resolution.

8. The commitment of the leadership. The fact that the leadership has much personal confidence allows it to also have much confidence in the functioning of the group. Thus high expectations of performance are maintained.

9. The philosophy itself required commitment. The leadership required by the normative nature of the setting was consistent with agency needs: the chief and assistant chief play the expression and task roles necessary for leadership balance.

10. Hope encouraged by ultimate success and sustained by continual positive feedback.

Implications for nursing

"It is part of the wonder of man that even the state of hopelessness can be used to generate hope."[21] The human personality matures by utilizing the process of problem solving in moving toward greater self-responsible behavior. This we say is the goal of psychiatric nursing and community mental health. The challenge to nurses, then, is how to capitalize on the group experience just described by using it to meet the professional goals of appropriate and effective health services for all.

This is not to say that old knowledge is not incorporated into a new approach to service. As we look at the case study we are actually reading a description of how a group of human service staff, clients, and community participants are working toward a viable therapeutic community, one that allows all to be involved in decision-making. The group phenomenon portrayed a living example of putting a theoretical framework to use, that of a social systems approach to group behavior. The task-oriented groups pursued therapeutic goals, focusing on real problems around authority and peer relations. The role of the leader or therapist was to act as regulator of the group and at times to shift his regulatory behavior in response to a reevaluation of group needs and aims. Crisis resolution resulted through the use of both the psychoanalytic and social-psychological models of group therapy.[1]

If, then, the concepts of advocacy, agitation, and the sharing of power are instruments to be used in the forwarding of therapeutic goals, why the professional anxiety and concerns of self-worth and self-maintenance? Social change is painful, and requires "an exertion of all man's will and strength in the face of hopelessness."[22] And professional strivings become weighty, frequently limiting sight and creativity. The professional, we say, is generally the supervisor; but what does it do to one's image as a supervisor when the supervisee is performing functions with which the professional himself would have difficulty. It is not always easy, even in traditional settings, to see your student go beyond you.

Teaching, for roles that we as nurses have had no preparation, is one of many concerns. As the nurse's vista broadens, she will see need for more knowledge of community organization, change theory, administration, the politics of interrelated institutional structure, the manipulations of budget, people, and systems, the principles underlying community control, and the complexity of urban problems. Psychiatric nurse-clinicians traditionally have seen these knowledges as beneath them; yet these seem to be crucial to the existence, if not the success, of service. Are we as professionals able to make the necessary role shifts? What does this mean in terms of our educational preparation? How do we, ourselves, keep a sense of sanity and a center of gravity amid ambiguity and change? Can we teach for this?

The new professional, according to Matthew P. Dumont, is responsive to citizens, is indifferent to credentials, has a sense of superordinate purpose, is critical of current health practice, is impatient with the rate of change, and is driven by compassion for his fellowman.[23] What does this mean to us as nurses attempting to find ourselves in the frothy sea of turmoil in community mental health centers? How can we both learn from and contribute to the growth of the paraprofessional mental health worker who has already proved himself to be indispensable for the development of a pragmatic service model?[7, 24-26] How do we build in agency and professional flexibility that allows for necessary organizational change? Do we wish to absorb these workers into established professions or to allow them to emerge as a group with a separate identity? The absorption of paraprofessionals into subprofessional roles has been shown to cut down their effectiveness as change agents. Indeed, the anticipation of change from within, through cooperative and collaborative[27] effort, seems counter to many of the models of community action.[28-30]

We are in a struggle that involves the utilization of a manpower group previously labeled dispensable in our society, which may allow for the development of relevant human services, and which will include the disenfranchised in meaningful decision-making with control over their destiny. Movement is slow, lonely, and discouraging, particularly when viewing the futility about us. Remember that the "radical, chaotic, unpredictable, and perhaps inefficient behavior, [that is part of the] process of community involvement is also therapeutic, rehabilitative and healthy."[31] It is good to be a participant in man's movement toward self-fulfillment. For, as the fox said to the Little Prince, "It is only with the heart that one can see rightly; what is essential is invisible to the eye. . . . It is the time you have wasted for your rose that makes your rose so important."*

---

*From De Saint-Exupery, Antoine: The little prince, New York, 1943, Harcourt, Brace & World.

References

1. Astrachan, B. M.: Toward a social systems model of the therapeutic group, unpublished paper, 1969.
2. Rainwater, L.: Mental health and social action. Presented at dedication ceremony of Department of Psychiatry, Mental Health Center, Division of the University of Rochester, Rochester, New York, 1969.
3. Campbell, P.: What are the expressed needs of aftercare clients? unpublished, 1970. Prepared for completion of M.Ed. requirement in Psychiatric Nursing-Mental Health, Department of Nursing Education, Teachers College, Columbia University.
4. Levine, L. S.: The racial crisis suggestions for a national program, Santa Barbara, 1966, Center for the Study of Democratic Institutions.
5. Riessman, F., and Gartner, A.: Community control and radical change, Social Policy 1: 52-55, 1970.
6. Fagin, C.: Psychotherapeutic nursing, Amer. J. Nurs. 67:2, 1967.
7. Richards, H.: The relationship between group approaches and social action in community mental health settings. In Bergersen, B., et al., editors: Current concepts in clinical nursing, vol. 2, St. Louis, 1969, The C. V. Mosby Co.
8. Christmas, J. J.: Socio-psychiatric rehabilitation: principles and practices, 1969 (mimeographed).
9. Christmas, J. J.: Socio-psychiatric rehabilitation in a black urban ghetto: conflicts, issues and directions, Amer. J. Orthopsychiat. 39: 651-661, 1969.
10. Selznick, P.: Leadership in administration, New York, 1967, Harper & Row, Publishers, Inc.
11. Etzioni, A.: Modern organizations, Englewood Cliffs, N. J., 1964, Prentice-Hall, Inc.
12. Bennis, W. G.: Leadership theory and administrative behavior, Administrative Sci. Quart. 4:12-15, 1959.
13. Weber, M.: A theory of social and economic organization, New York, 1947, Oxford University Press, Inc.
14. Parsons, T.: Family, socialization and interaction process, New York, 1955, The Free Press.
15. Caplan, G., and Parad, H.: A framework for studying families in crisis. In Parad, H. J., editor: Crisis intervention: selected readings, New York, 1965, Family Service Association of America.
16. Lindemann, E.: Symptomatology and management of acute grief. In Parad, H. J., editor: Crisis intervention: selected readings, New York, 1965, Family Service Association of America.
17. Bales, R. F.: Interaction process analysis: a method for the study of small groups, Cambridge, Mass., 1950 Addison-Wesley Publishing Co., Inc.
18. Homans, G. C.: The human group, New York, 1950, Harcourt, Brace & Co., Inc.
19. Stotland, E., and Kobler, A. L.: The life and death of a mental hospital, Seattle, 1965, University of Washington Press.
20. March, J. G., and Simon, H. A.: Organizations, New York, 1958, John Wiley & Sons, Inc.
21. Gaylin, W.: The meaning of despair, New York, 1958, Science House, Inc.
22. Dumont, M.: The absurd healer, New York, 1968, Science House, Inc.
23. Dumont, M. P.: The changing face of professionalism, Social Policy 1:26-31, 1970.
24. Richards, H.: Implications for nursing in the training of paraprofessional workers in the community mental health setting. Presented

at American Nurses' Association, Conference on Community Mental Health Nursing, New York, February, 1970.

25. Richards, H.: Opportunities for new careerists in the community mental health field. Presented at American Nurses' Association Convention, Miami, Florida, May, 1970.

26. Richards, H., and Daniels, M. S.: Sociopsychiatric rehabilitation in the black ghetto. II. Innovative treatment roles and approaches. Amer. J. Orthopsychiat. 39:662-676, 1969.

27. Ross, M. G.: Community organization: theory and principles, New York, 1955, Harper & Row, Publishers.

28. Brager, G. A.: Advocacy and political behavior, Social Work 13:5-15, 1968.

29. Grosser, C.: Neighborhood community development programs serving the urban poor, Social Work 10:15-21, 1965.

30. Kurzman, P. A.: The new careers movement and social changes, Social Casework 51:22-27, 1970.

31. Prigoff, A.: Concepts and techniques of community control. Presented at the 49th Annual Meeting, American Orthopsychiatric Association, March, 1970.

Pediatric nursing

With an introduction by
Marion H. Rose

In an emergency room a father stands by his listless, feverish child who is lying on an examining table. A box on the wall says, "Mr. Jones, come to the desk, come to the desk."

Mr. Jones, looking bewildered, voices his concern, "Who will stay with my child?" He continues to stand, gently touching his child.

The box bleats impatiently, "Mr. Jones, come to the desk. There are papers to be signed."

Mr. Jones says with despair, "My child."

An aide, busily cleaning thermometers across the room, intones, "She won't fall off."

Mr. Jones walks hesitantly from the room, glancing back with a look that says, "She won't fall off? Does anyone care?"

None of the following chapters are directly concerned with this incident, one small episode in a busy urban hospital. Indirectly they are all concerned with it, since the authors, by presenting new ideas and information, are challenging nurses to give thoughtful consideration to nursing as it is practiced today.

It is evident from the following chapters that a sound knowledge of the behavioral, physical, and biological sciences is indeed necessary in nursing today. The authors provide data and illustrative case material or present a theoretical basis for their ideas. Thus the reader has information that she may thoughtfully consider before accepting, rejecting, or modifying the ideas as presented. However, the presenting of one or two "cases" to support a point does not mean that *truth* has been achieved. It is only by comparing and contrasting information and ideas with others that we may move toward a sound basis for giving nursing care. The authors of these chapters are helping nursing move toward this goal by submitting their ideas to the scrutiny of their peers.

Chapter *8*

Nursing care of high-risk infants

Cheryl Hall Harris

Birth is a stressful period for the healthy infant; for the abnormal one, it may be overwhelming. Although his parents expected a normal child, they must cope with one who may die or have extensive and continuing health problems. The nursing care of a high-risk infant requires a nurse who observes carefully, acts when necessary, and communicates well with physicians and parents.

This chapter will present some of the types of infant problems found in high-risk nurseries. At any given time in such a nursery, there will be infants in a critical state, infants who are dying, and infants who are convalescing in preparation for discharge. These infants will have different health problems from a variety of causes. The nursing care of these infants is the subject of this chapter.

High-risk centers

One of the trends in medicine today is toward regionalization of medical care, that is, the development of major centers that can provide the most complete care for each patient. This is the most practical and economical means of providing the patient with the highly specialized services he needs. One such trend is to develop high-risk maternal and infant centers to provide care to high-risk mothers and their infants.

High-risk delivery centers are hospital areas where mothers with known problems may be referred prenatally. In these centers, equipment and personnel are prepared to give optimal care to the mother during her prenatal course and labor and delivery and to give the same optimal care to her infant as well. The two main categories of high-risk mothers are (1) mothers who have a previous history of abortions or infants with unusual problems and (2) mothers who have experienced difficulty during their current pregnancy or labor and delivery. These two categories of mothers produce infants who (1) are premature, (2) are hypoglycemic, (3) have respiratory distress syndrome, or (4) have some other type of problem. Infants with these abnormalities are commonly found in intensive care nurseries.

An intensive care nursery center will have both infants born within the high-risk maternity center and infants who were transferred from surrounding hospitals. All of the infants will demonstrate some type of problem, and they will be at various levels of illness. Some problems such as temperature regulation, fluid and electrolyte balance, and maintenance of adequate ventilation are common to all of the infants in the center. Other problems such as congenital anomalies and neonatal sepsis are not common to all infants at the center.

Problems common to all intensive care infants
Environmental regulation

Infants with all types of distress should be placed in an area that provides necessary warmth, humidity, oxygen, and infection control. Isolettes can provide the proper environment; however, other infant incubators are now available. There are also prototypes of intensive care infant beds currently being developed that allow for improved patient access, while maintaining current features of temperature regulation and cleanliness of the infant's environment.

Temperature and humidity control of the infant's air mixture can be accomplished by passing the infant's breathing gas through a humidifier with a heating device (such as a nebulizer). If additional oxygen is required, it should be introduced into the air source before the breathing mixture enters the humidifier.

The primary means of infection control is meticulous handwashing by personnel before handling each infant. Bathing the infants with hexachlorophene has also been proved beneficial in reducing infection rates. Many different state regulations control such procedures as gowning, formula preparation, and construction of nurseries, which are designed to assist in the prevention of infection as well as to provide environmental control.

Fluid, electrolyte, and glucose control

Infants have a delicate electrolyte balance that may be quite difficult to main-

tain. If the infant is unable to eat normally, infusions must be utilized either by peripheral intravenous sites or through umbilical catheters inserted by the physician. Small infants have frequently changing fluid requirements. Therefore blood samples for electrolyte levels should be obtained often, and corrective measures begun when necessary by administering sodium or potassium salts in appropriate proportions with fluids.

Hypocalcemia exists when the level of serum calcium is below 8 mg./100 ml. of serum.[1] Infants of low birth weight and prematures seem especially prone to this condition. Symptoms include muscular hyperirritability manifested as twitching, tremors, and frank seizures. It is treated by giving 10% calcium gluconate or calcium chloride intravenously. Whenever calcium is administered, careful monitoring of the heart rate is essential, since increasing bradycardia is common during such administrations.

Hypoglycemia is a below normal level of glucose or true sugar in whole blood. Opinions differ as to what is a dangerously low level, but most physicians agree that a glucose level of less than 45 mg.% is harmful to infants. Many times newborn infants may show transient hypoglycemia related to events of their delivery. Infants immediately after a normal delivery usually run slightly higher glucose levels than do their mothers, but important factors include whether or not the mother received glucose during labor and whether or not the infant suffered hypoxic episodes. If the infant did experience a difficult delivery, his glucose level is usually very low, since he used his energy stores for survival. Clinical signs of hypoglycemia are unspecific symptoms such as jitteriness, twitching, apnea, or a high-pitched cry. Initial treatment includes the immediate administration of 50% glucose, intravenously, and then continous infusions of 10% glucose so-

lutions.[2] Early feedings are also of benefit.

Umbilical catheters

A large number of infants in the intensive care nursery have umbilical catheters. The use of umbilical vein catheters began in 1956.[2] Since then the practice of catheterization of umbilical veins and arteries has become widespread despite some problems. The primary problems concerning the nurse are (1) to keep the catheter patent, (2) to decrease the chance of infection, (3) to detect signs of possible infarctions or clots in the vessel, and (4) to prevent accidental hemorrhage.

Catheterization of umbilical vessels is accomplished with a 3½ or 5 French soft plastic radiopaque catheter with a round-edged end hole. The catheter is inserted by a physician, using as close to sterile procedure as possible. The instrument he uses should be sterilized, the infant's abdomen and umbilical cord should be thoroughly cleansed, and the physician should wear sterile gloves. Once the catheter is sutured in place, a sterile dressing is applied to the umbilical stump where the catheter enters it. Some physicians like to apply a bacteriocidal ointment, such as Neospiran, as well as the dressing. An abdominal x-ray film should be taken to determine the position of the catheter. If the catheter is incorrectly placed, the physician should adjust it.

Once the catheter is properly placed, it may be used for obtaining blood samples and infusing fluids. The nurse should keep the catheter patent by irrigations with 0.5 ml. of either normal saline solution or a dilute heparin solution.* Irrigations should be done approximately every one to two hours.

To prevent hemorrhage great care must

---

*Heparinized saline solution may be made as follows: 24 ml. sterile water, 6 ml. normal saline solution, and 0.1 ml. sodium heparin (1000 unit/ml. strength).

be taken to prevent the catheter from coming apart at junctures or from accidentally becoming dislodged from the vessel. It must be remembered that, especially if this is an arterial catheter, the infant can bleed profusely and exsanguinate in a matter of seconds. The infant should have soft restraints placed on all extremities. The catheter should be removed by a physician as soon as possible when it is no longer essential to the infant's care.

Nutrition control

The infant who is ill cannot usually be fed by nipple. This leaves three alternate methods of feeding: (1) by indwelling nasogastric tube, (2) by intermittent nasogastric tube (placed only at feeding times and then removed), or (3) by gastrostomy. Whenever indwelling nasogastric tubes are left in place for longer than eight hours, there may be irritation of the nasopharynx and subsequent large production of mucus. Intermittent passing of nasogastric tubes may also cause irritation, but this is generally less irritating than are indwelling tubes. In both methods the nurse must check carefully to ensure the proper placement of the tube. She checks placement by either (1) placing the outer end of the tube into water (if bubbles appear at the same time as the infant's expirations, the tube is improperly placed) or (2) injecting 1 cc. of air into the tube while listening with a stethoscope over the infant's stomach (the nurse will hear the air entering the stomach if the tube is in place).

If the infant is on a respirator or is expected to be critically ill for a long time, gavage feedings are difficult and may lead to problems with aspiration of formula into the infant's lungs. Frequently, gastrostomies become the feeding method of choice for these infants, but they should not be used routinely if the infant can tolerate other means.

A gastrostomy is usually performed by a surgeon, who makes an incision in the abdominal and the stomach walls. An 8 to 12 French Foley catheter is then inserted, the balloon is inflated with approximately 2 ml. of sterile water, and the catheter is sutured into place. This procedure may be done in the infant's Isolette and generally does not require that he be sent to the operating room. A local anesthetic is usually preferred. The gastrostomy is not used for twelve to twenty-four hours to give the stomach a chance to recover, and then the infant is given dextrose water feedings per gastrostomy, and gradually is progressed to full strength infant formula as he tolerates the feedings. If an infant has a gastrostomy, it can serve as a route for decreasing abdominal distention caused by air in his stomach. For this reason the gastrostomy tube should be left open to air (not clamped between feedings). The outer tip of the gastrostomy tube should be no higher than 10 cm. above the level of the infant's abdomen to allow for liquid overflow as necessary. In other words, if the infant needs to regurgitate, the fluid can take the path of least resistance by refluxing into the gastrostomy tube instead of up the infant's esophagus.

If the infant does not move the formula from his stomach, that is, if large amounts are aspirated from his stomach prior to feedings, he should be offered a pacifier to suck and turned to his right side with the head of his bed elevated to help his stomach empty. X-ray studies show that infants have difficulty emptying their stomachs when they are supine and their beds are flat.

Blood gases

A critical infant's blood gases must be monitored frequently, especially if his condition is unstable. Blood samples, which may be drawn from his umbilical catheter, are analyzed on a blood gas machine by a trained laboratory technician, nurse, or physician. Arterial blood gas levels that are considered to be adequate are (1) a P_{O_2} greater than 50 mm. Hg and less than 120 mm. Hg, (2) a P_{CO_2} level greater than 20 mm. Hg and less than 50 mm. Hg, and (3) a pH from 7.28 to 7.35.[3] These values are to be considered as guidelines, since opinions of actual values differ. If the infant has abnormal blood gas values, the physician will want to correct them quickly. The pH, P_{O_2}, and P_{CO_2} levels can all be altered by improving the infant's ventilation. The use of a buffer such as sodium bicarbonate is beneficial in correcting severe acidosis.

Hyperbilirubinemia

There are basically two types of hyperbilirubinemia. The first is found in almost all newborn infants and is called physiological neonatal jaundice, which results as the infant's liver adjusts to performing functions that the mother's liver performed while the infant was in utero. The second type is hyperbilirubinemia secondary to such causes as infant infection, prematurity, or Rh or A-B-O blood incompatibilities. Many factors are involved in selecting a treatment if the physician determines that the infant has hyperbilirubinemia. Formerly the primary method of treatment was exchange transfusions, but currently some centers have found that exposure of an infant to daylightlike light helps to decrease the bilirubin level in cases where hemolytic disease is not the cause of the elevated bilirubin.

Neonatal infections

There is high risk that the critical infant will develop a systemic infection. The symptoms of such infections are nonspecific and include such signs as lethargy, poor sucking, poor weight gain, and poor temperature control. The infant's temperature may decrease instead of becoming elevated when he has a systemic infection. Diagnostic tests for systemic infections include cultures of cerebrospinal fluid, gastric contents, blood, urine, and stool. Which antibiotic to use in treatment differs from physician to physician, but the treatment for infections in newborn infants *must* begin immediately, even before the specific organism is identified. For this reason, wide-spectrum antibiotics usually are selected.

Respiratory distress

Many infants demonstrate periods of respiratory distress not associated with respiratory distress syndrome. The primary signs of respiratory distress are grunting, flaring, and retracting. Grunting is an audible sound like a short cry, which is made whenever the infant exhales. Flaring is the enlargement of the infant's nostrils on inspiration. Retractions are indrawing of the infant's chest wall between his ribs, above and below his sternum, and below his rib cage. All infants are abdominal breathers, but when an infant is having difficulty breathing, his movements become exaggerated and he appears to be really working at breathing. Sometimes an infant will show these symptoms merely because he is cold, but often they are the first signs of aspiration pneumonia, pneumothorax, or early respiratory distress syndrome.

Another respiratory problem that some infants demonstrate is apnea. The causes of apnea include prematurity, an elevated environmental temperature, or central nervous system damage.[4] One machine used to help detect apnea is called an apnea monitor. This electronic device is applied to the infant by means of external chest probes (electrodes), and the alarm sounds whenever the infant stops breathing. The nurse can attempt to stimulate the infant to begin breathing again by tapping his feet or by rubbing him; but if these attempts fail after a few seconds, the nurse will need to resuscitate the in-

fant with a positive pressure bag and mask.

Communicating with parents

One important staff function in an intensive care nursery is that of maintaining good communication with the parents of the infants. These parents are likely to be anxious and confused. They will ask many questions and will need not only answers to specific questions, but reassurance as well. The mother is likely to feel isolated from her infant, and she will want to know about how he is now and how he will be when he is discharged from the hospital.

A team approach of physicians, nurses, and social workers is helpful in providing the type of communication needed by the parents. However, it is essential that all members of this team know what the other members are telling the parents; therefore communication between physicians, nurses, and social workers is also important. Telephone conversations and direct conferences with parents are the best methods of communicating with them. The nurse should encourage the parents to visit their infant as often as possible, and when the infant is almost ready for discharge, the nurse should make sure the parents have many opportunities to handle and care for their infant.

• • •

In summary, the preceding section discussed the problems encountered by most all of the infants (or staff caring for those infants) in an intensive care nursery center.

Problems specific to some intensive care infants

The next section will discuss four specific patient problems including (1) infants with respiratory distress syndrome, (2) infants having surgery, (3) premature infants, and (4) infants small for gestational age.

Infants with respiratory distress syndrome (hyaline membrane disease)

One of the best ways to discuss the care of an infant with respiratory distress syndrome (RDS) is to describe a typical patient and his care. An infant with respiratory distress syndrome would typically be a premature infant of about 3½ to 4 pounds, with signs of grunting, flaring, and retracting. He is brought to the nursery, umbilical catheterization (usually arterial catheter) is done, and his first x-ray film shows the early lung changes of RDS. For the purpose of this discussion the patient will be followed through the stages of (1) hood, (2) bagging, (3) intubation, (4) respirator care, and (5) weaning from the respirator to home. Other problems such as pneumothorax and gastrostomy will be mentioned at the appropriate place.

When the infant is first brought to the nursery, if his color is dusky to cyanotic and he is grunting, flaring and retracting, he is placed into an environment of increased percent of oxygen (above room air) while his umbilical catheter is inserted. His first set of blood gases is done, and the physician orders him to be put in an oxygen concentration greater than 50%, for example 55%. Any oxygen concentration higher than 50% is very difficult to maintain in an Isolette, so the infant would need to be placed into a hood.

A hood is a Plexiglas box that has an opening for the infant's neck and that fits comfortably over his head. It has an oxygen-air inlet hole and a hole for exhaled gases. The oxygen-air mixture, which is flushed into the hood, needs to be at a flow rate of at least 7 liters/minute (which will mean the dilution of 100% oxygen with compressed air to obtain the oxygen concentration desired). This oxygen should also be warmed to approximately 32° C. and humidified to about 70%. The nurse must monitor the oxygen concentration carefully to make sure the infant does not receive a higher or lower concentration than was ordered. She monitors the concentration with an oxygen analyzer every hour if the oxygen level is stable, and as often as every 10 minutes if it is unstable. The hood may be removed from the infant's head for brief intervals, such as if the infant requires suctioning. Also, if condensation of moisture occurs on the inside of the hood, it should be removed with a cloth frequently, so that the infant's face can be observed for such signs as flaring or cyanosis.

Occasionally, despite vigorous care in the hood with the percent of oxygen gradually increased to 100%, the infant's condition does not stabilize. The physician might decide to begin "bagging" the baby. This procedure is done with an infant resuscitator bag and mask. The nurse holds the mask to seal the infant's mouth and nose, and hyperextends the infant's head. She then ventilates his lungs with whichever concentration of oxygen the physician has prescribed, using positive pressure applied by squeezing the resuscitator bag.

There are basically two techniques in bagging, depending on what result the physician desires accomplished. If the infant has a high level of carbon dioxide, as determined by a blood gas sample, the nurse will "bag" with quick, shallow breaths (sixty or more times per minute). If the infant's P_{O_2} level is low, the nurse will use deep, slow breaths (forty to fifty times per minute). Bagging might be done for 2 minutes every 30 minutes, 2 minutes every 15 minutes, or whatever amount of time the physician thinks is necessary to correct the infant's problem.

During the time the infant is bagged, the physician does several sets of blood gases. If the infant's condition continues to deteriorate, the physician will decide that the infant requires a respirator. Most intensive care nurseries utilize pressure controlled ventilators such as the Bennett or Bird intermittent positive pressure ventilators. Some centers use volume regulated respirators such as the Engstrom or Harvard respirators. There is also an infant negative pressure incubator, which is like the old-fashioned "iron lung," that is designed for infants; but in my opinion, based on personal experience, these respirators are difficult to work with, and the infant has many physical discomforts.

Nasotracheal intubation is performed by either a pediatrician or an anesthesiologist. The physician decides the proper sized tube and how long it should be. When the tube is prepared, the physician places an infant laryngoscope so that he can visualize the infant's vocal cords, and then the physician inserts the tube through the cords into the infant's trachea. The nurse should have suctioning equipment, a clock, materials for making the endotracheal tube secure once it is in place, and an infant resuscitator bag on hand. During the time the physician is intubating the infant, the nurse should time his attempts to make sure the infant goes for no longer than 1 minute without being ventilated. The nurse can also observe the infant and notify the physician if the infant is becoming cyanotic. (Many times the physician concentrates so intensely on the procedure of intubation that he loses track of the time and the infant's condition.) The infant's mouth and airway may need to be suctioned of secretions while the physician is trying to place the endotracheal tube. When the tube is in place, the physician will listen to the infant's breath sounds with a stethoscope to determine that the tube is in the trachea and not in the infant's esophagus.

Once the physician decides the tube is in the trachea, the tube should be tied in position (Fig. 11), so that it will not become dislodged, and the infant's head should be immobilized with wrapped sandbags on either side. The weight of the respirator tubing should be supported

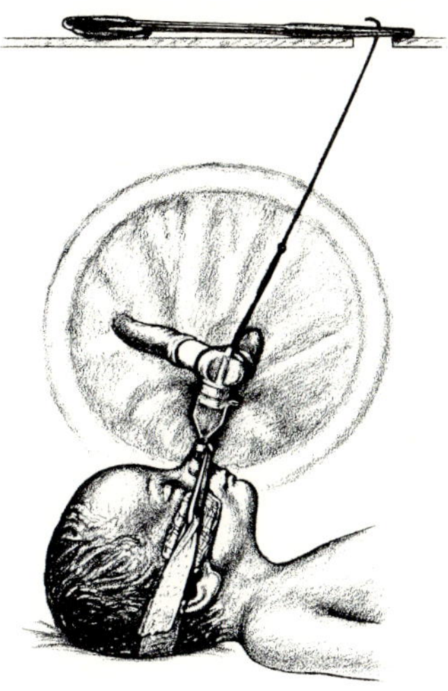

Fig. 11
Infant with endotracheal tube secured in place.

with either a string of rubber bands or tape, so that the weight does not rest on the infant's endotracheal tube. At this point the infant is connected to the respirator, and a thoracic x-ray film is taken to determine the endotracheal tube's placement.

Any infant who is placed on a respirator will often have secretions in his lungs that will need to be removed by suctioning through his endotracheal tube. He will also probably require percussion, vibration, and suction to remove the secretions from his bronchioli and alveoli. The nurse performs percussion by tapping her cupped fingers on the infant's chest. She accomplishes vibration by placing her cupped fingers on his chest and tensing her arm muscles to produce a fine vibrating movement. The infant is placed in a head-elevated position while percussion or vibration is being done to the upper lobes of his lungs; and he is placed in a foot-elevated position while the lower lobes of his lungs are receiving this treatment. His bed is then placed in a flat position while the nurse suctions the secretions from his endotracheal tube and mouth.

Suctioning is done while the infant is in a supine position. His head is held straight, then turned to the right, and then to the left. He is suctioned in each of these head positions. This removes the secretions from his right and left main stem bronchi.

The infant should not be suctioned for more than 10 seconds at a time without being placed back on the respirator for a brief rest. Suction catheters should be cut 2 cm. longer than the infant's endotracheal tube to prevent a plug from forming at the tip of the tube.

While the infant is on the respirator, the nurse will need to observe his condition carefully. If he has a sudden deterioration in his condition, she should listen to determine that his breath sounds are equal in all quadrants and are of good quality. If his breath sounds are diminished or unequal, he may have a dislodged or plugged endotracheal tube, or he may have developed a pneumothorax. The physician is notified, and if he thinks the breath sounds are not good, he will order a chest x-ray film. If the infant's tube is dislodged or plugged, it will need to be changed. If the infant does have a pneumothorax, chest tubes will be inserted through the chest wall by the physician to remove the air that has leaked into his pleural cavity.

An infant who is on the respirator is an excellent candidate for a gastrostomy, which was described earlier. Not only can his gastrostomy be used for his feedings, but it will also serve as a route for decompressing any air in the infant's stomach; and if he should regurgitate, his formula is more likely to go into his gastrostomy tube than into his esophagus. Infants on respirators can easily aspirate vomitus because they are in a supine position most of the time and they have an endotracheal tube through their vocal cords.

The infant may be on the respirator for several days or perhaps even a week or more; but at some point the physician decides to begin to wean the infant from the respirator. The nurse prepares a hood with the oxygen concentration prescribed by the physician (usually the concentration in the hood is higher than the infant has had on the respirator). The nurse suctions the infant while he is still on the respirator, gives him a few minutes back on the respirator, and then places him into the hood. During the time he is in the hood, she will check his apical pulse, respiratory rate, color, and condition continuously to decide how well he tolerates being off the respirator. Weaning will probably be accomplished gradually; 5 minutes each hour, then 10 minutes each hour, and so on until the infant is off the respirator all of the time. This period of weaning will probably have many setbacks; it is the rare infant who comes off the respirator without any difficulty. The physician will continue to monitor the infant's blood gases while he is being weaned to make sure he is tolerating the procedure.

Once the infant is off the respirator, his endotracheal tube is removed and the oxygen concentration in the hood is gradually decreased to room air oxygen concentration. He will continue to require nursing care including percussion, vibration, and suction (PVS), feedings, and rest while he recuperates. If all is well, he will gradually gain his strength, gain weight, and be ready to go home. If the infant's lung condition warrants PVS at home, his mother can be taught to do this, and she may use a bulb suction to remove the secretions from his mouth.

The preceding discussion involved nursing care of a typical infant with RDS. This complex patient is challenging, and it is rewarding when he does well. It should be remembered, that the mortality and morbidity rates in these infants are high, but their chances for normality are increased in high-risk centers.

Infants having surgery

Most infants who require surgery are those with congenital anomalies. The anomaly might be of the gastrointestinal tract such as bowel obstruction, tracheoesophogeal fistula, or omphalocele; it might be of the central nervous system such as a myelomeningocele; or it might be of the cardiovascular system such as tetralogy of Fallot. All of these infants will experience the hazards of anesthesia and the problems with hypothermia in operating rooms; all will require immediate postoperative care. The nurse should be aware of their specific situations and the signs of a deterioration in their condition so that she may intervene as necessary.

Premature infants

Premature infants are quite different from full-term infants. Premature infants range in size from 1½ to 4½ pounds, are immature, and require specialized care and equipment. They have less cartilage in their ears, less fatty deposits throughout their bodies, delicate skin, and poor muscle tone and coordination. They frequently have difficulty with temperature regulation, infection, and jaundice. They present difficulties in feeding. Their breathing patterns are usually irregular (periodic breathing), they frequently have periods of apnea, and they are more prone to developing RDS. Premature infants could easily be the subject of an entire book, but they can be mentioned only briefly here.

Infants small for gestational age

Infants who are small for gestational age are usually described as "small for dates" babies and are often mistakenly called premature infants. Quite often the mother had an infarction in her placenta that caused improper development of the fetus. The infant is usually more mature than his physical size would indicate. Some of these infants may have hypoglycemic episodes postpartum and should be watched for this; but most "small for dates" babies have only a problem of weight gain to overcome.

Mothers with predictable problems

Infants who are small for gestational age are one type of infant whose problem has a maternal cause. Other infants are affected by problems in their mothers; these infants will be the subject of the following discussion. There are many types of maternal problems, but only the most common will be described.

Low-income mothers

In all pregnancies, one important factor is the early detection of pregnancy to allow proper prenatal care for the mother and fetus. The mother who is from a low-economic background may not receive the proper care prenatally, and her infant may have difficulty when he is born. Her infant is likely to be a premature infant or to have signs of poor nutrition, such as anemia, poor development, or hypoglycemia. Greater efforts must be made to improve the socioeconomic status of some of our poorer population, to improve their nutrition and living conditions, and to increase the availability of medical attention, especially during pregnancy.

Maternal infections

Many infections that the mother contracts while she is pregnant can cause abnormalities in her infant. The three major ones are (1) rubella, (2) toxoplasmosis, and (3) cytomegalic inclusion disease (CID).[5] A mother who develops clinical rubella within the first 14 weeks of pregnancy has a higher risk of producing an infant with cataracts, deafness, congenital heart defects, mental retardation, or any combination of these abnormalities. Mothers who develop either toxoplasmosis or CID have higher incidences of infants with damaged retinas, damaged livers, and mental deficiencies. In the case of these three diseases that produce problems in infants, the mothers may have no clinical signs of disease, which makes it difficult to determine the cause of the infant's problem.

The mother with an infection at the time of delivery may be the source of the organism causing infection in the infant. Such conditions as herpes, syphilis, or a staphylococcal infection can cause a neonatal infection in the infant if during delivery he is exposed to the organism causing the infection.

Maternal diabetes

Mothers with signs of clinical diabetes during pregnancy have higher infant mortality rates than do nondiabetic mothers.[5] Infants of diabetic mothers tend to be large (9 pounds or more), and are frequently hypoglycemic postpartum. Although these infants are large, they are often notably immature. One theory about the cause of neonatal hypoglycemia in these infants is that regardless of how well the mother's diabetes was controlled, she probably had several episodes of *hyper-glycemia* during her pregnancy. At these times the infant produced large quantities of insulin and continues to do so after birth, leading to his periods of hypoglycemia. The nurse should watch the infant carefully for signs of hypoglycemia and respiratory distress, and notify the physician of difficulties.

Hemolytic disease of the newborn caused by Rh incompatibilities

A mother who has an Rh-negative blood type is at high risk of producing an infant with hemolytic disease of the newborn if the father is Rh positive. If the mother who is Rh negative produces a fetus who is Rh positive, she manufactures antibodies to his blood cells. These antibodies cross the placenta and destroy the infant's blood cells.

The infant's umbilical cord blood should be sent to the laboratory for a Coombs test and bilirubin determination, and he should be watched for signs of anemia, shock, and hyperbilirubinemia. With each successive pregnancy, the mother has in-creased chances of producing more severely affected infants.

History of repeated abortions

The mother with a history of repeated abortions during previous pregnancies has an increased risk of delivering an infant with anomalies. Early abortions (before 12 weeks' gestation) are often the result of poor implantation, infection in the mother, or defective chromosomes.[5] The latter group of mothers should receive counseling by their physician with the help of a geneticist. Genetic counseling requires a careful family history, and in some cases the preparation of chromosomal cultures obtained from blood samples of the parents. This latter procedure is usually only considered for parents with a history of previous problems, since the results are used to predict the likelihood of the parents producing a defective child.

• • •

In summary, the preceding five categories of infants are those whose mothers have a history of previous problems.

Mothers with unpredictable problems

Some mothers have a normal pregnancy, and then have some crisis at the time of labor and delivery that was unpredicted. The next few paragraphs will describe these mothers, and measures that can be taken to reduce problems in their infants.

Even if the mother has not demonstrated adverse symptoms during her pregnancy, there are crises that arise at the time of delivery that may produce hypoxia, anoxia, or other problems in the infants. Such crises include placenta previa, prolapsed cord, precipitous delivery, cephalopelvic disproportion, or analgesia and anesthesia received during labor and delivery. These crises must be recognized quickly and dealt with by competent obstetrical staff as they arise. Many of these problems require a cesarean section to be performed immediately.

Some problems can be anticipated by monitoring the fetus. Perhaps, ideally, every fetus should be monitored, but it is of the utmost importance that all high-risk mothers have their labors monitored. Formerly, the most common method of fetal monitoring was to listen to the infant's heart sounds with a fetal stethoscope. One disadvantage to this method is that it offers only spot checks and not continuous monitoring. Now there are methods for continuous monitoring of fetal heart activity during labor and delivery. There are also other methods of periodically evaluating the status of the infant such as amnioscopy and direct fetal blood sampling.[6]

Fetal cardiac monitoring of the infant's ECG is accomplished by either of two ways: (1) electrocardiography with abdominal leads on the mother and (2) electrocardiography with direct fetal leads. The second method is usually more accurate than is the first; however, the direct fetal leads are more difficult to place and cannot always be used. A scalp electrode is attached to the fetus with a surgical skin clip by a physician after the mother's membranes have been ruptured. This electrode is then connected to the monitor that records the infant's ECG, and the electrical impulses of the mother's uterine contractions.

Fetal blood sampling is accomplished by a physician who makes a small scratch on the infant's scalp and obtains a small quantity of blood that is analyzed for blood gases, hematocrit, or other blood tests which give an indication of the fetus' status. Direct amnioscopy is done with a small lighted instrument that is brought into direct contact with the mother's amniotic membranes. By noting the color of the membranes, the physician can determine the color of the amniotic fluid, and thereby detect such conditions as hyperbilirubinemia or meconium staining of the fluid.

Problems at the time of delivery

In the event of a crisis at the time of birth, it is important to have personnel, equipment, and areas provided for the physical care of the high-risk mother and her infant. If there is an emergency with the infant, the mother probably will have feelings of apprehension and fear about the procedures being done. If a nurse stands at the mother's head and gives simple explanations about what is being done, she can help to allay some of the mother's fears.

In many high-risk delivery centers it is not feasible to maintain a warm temperature in the entire room. These centers usually provide a warmed "microenvironment"[7] for the infant consisting of a radiant heating bed with the necessary resuscitative and emergency equipment and medications close at hand. The importance of decreasing heat loss in the infant cannot be stressed enough. If a radiant heating bed is not available, the infant should be wrapped in warm blankets and placed into a prewarmed bed.

During the delivery process, all infants undergo many physiological changes. Their bodies are compressed into a small space, and later reexpand as the infant emerges from the birth canal. The infant goes from a dependent state in utero to an independent state where he must support his own life. Many changes in the respiratory and cardiovascular systems occur. If the infant shows signs of respiratory distress or of cardiovascular difficulties, the nurse should consider such causes as obstruction of upper airways, pneumothorax, aspiration pneumonia, or cardiac anomalies; and she should act accordingly. If a pediatrician is not in the delivery area, she should summon him whenever a serious problem arises. Sometimes infants experience a traumatic delivery that may cause skull or other fractures, or periods of hypoxia. The nurse should also be alert to these possible problems.

The dying infant

The material covered in the first pages of this chapter has been concerned with the critical situations in the infant's life from birth through the following critical days. Besides critical infants, there are also dying infants and convalescing infants in the intensive care nursery. These two groups of patients will be discussed next.

The death of an infant is a time of upheaval for his parents and for the staff involved in his care. If he has been in the nursery for a long time, the staff will probably be emotionally attached to him and they will feel a great loss when he dies. If he was a very "important" baby to his parents, that is, if they had a difficult time producing him, the parents will be particularly distressed. These and other problems surround the death of an infant, making this a period of stress for all concerned.

The staff's reactions

The nurse frequently becomes quite emotionally involved with the infant, since she is often the one most closely associated with the patient for long periods of time. If the nurse believes the patient will die, she gives comfort until he dies without prolonging his life. However, if the nurse thinks the patient may live, even though the physician says he will die, the nurse will check vital signs frequently and will continue to give life-prolonging care.[8]

Deaths seem to occur in series, and therefore staff morale may be low for certain periods of time. If an infant who dies was a "favorite" of many of the nurses, they will be upset at his death. If the death was unexpected, they will show signs of disbelief and grief, and many times the staff feels guilty over the loss of an infant. They feel if only they had done

something differently, the infant might have lived. These feelings may hamper the staff's communications with the parents of the infant. Often group sessions with a psychiatrist help the staff air their feelings and help them determine how they can best help the parents. In these meetings the psychiatrist usually serves as a moderator, and the staff is free to discuss any feelings of frustration, anger, or depression.

There are instances where ethical, legal, or moral issues arise: for example, when an infant has been maintained for a long period of time on life-support therapy (such as respirator care); when he has probably sustained brain damage secondary to hypoxic or anoxic episodes; or when he has multiple serious congenital anomalies and a poor prognosis. In these situations the staff may wonder whether they should utilize heroic measures to save this infant's life. The question is, "If the infant had a cardiac arrest, what should be done?" This is a difficult question to answer, and ultimately the decision is the physician's. In all of the situations described, group sessions with a psychiatrist are beneficial to the whole team of physicians, nurses, and social workers in helping them accept the decision.

The parents' reactions

Different parents react differently to the news that their infant has died. Most parents are very sad; some may be confused and shocked. They need kindness and support when they learn of their infant's death and when they must make stressful decisions. It is important that parents be informed as soon as possible that their infant might die. Regardless of the amount of preparation they have had, however, they will still experience shock and grief at the time of the infant's death.

Most births are times of great joy and anticipation. Almost no one anticipates that an infant may be critically ill, and certainly no one really expects a newborn baby to die. When an infant dies, his parents must inform many people of his death. If the infant dies while the mother is still on the maternity floor, every effort must be made to move her away from the normal infants and mothers who are receiving their babies.

The parents of a deceased infant need comfort and support. Referring physicians and clergymen, who have known the parents under other circumstances, are of great help in satisfying these needs. Many painful decisions that the parents must make immediately following the death of their infant include whether or not to permit a postmortem examination, and the arrangements that need to be made for the infant's funeral. One of the best ways to handle these situations is for the physician and social worker or nurse to take the parents into a quiet room and calmly discuss these problems with them.

· · ·

In summary, caring for the dying infant is a stressful and depressing situation for all concerned. A team approach is necessary in helping the parents during their experience of grief. The staff may find it of benefit to discuss their feelings in a group meeting with a psychiatrist.

The convalescing infant

Infants who are in a convalescing stage need rest and the opportunity to gain weight and stamina. During this period the infant's mother should be taught how to care for her baby. She will need to learn feeding, bathing, and handling techniques. She will need opportunities to overcome her fears of inadequacy. If this is her first infant, the nurse should plan to spend more time instructing the mother. Some infants need special treatments, such as PVS, to be done at home. The mother should feel comfortable in doing all procedures before the infant is dis-

charged. The nurse should explain proper clothing and equipment to have on hand, and formula preparation should also be taught. Public health nurse referrals give the mother an additional teacher in her own home.

The nursery social worker is an invaluable aid in assessing the parents' financial resources and pressures. If there are financial difficulties, she can frequently provide information and channels for funds.

The infant should be in the best possible condition before he is discharged. He should be able to meet these criteria: (1) be able to maintain his temperature in an open crib in a room of 70° F., (2) be able to gain weight consistently, and (3) have good head movement (in the event he regurgitates at home, he should be able to move his head out of the way to prevent aspiration).

Regressions common during convalescence

Sometimes during an infant's convalescence, a medical problem is detected that had not been noted earlier, such as retrolental fibroplasia (RLF) or chronic lung changes.

At the time of this writing, the facts surrounding RLF are still unclear.[2] No one seems willing to state specific concentrations of oxygen or levels of P_{O_2} that should be considered dangerous levels leading to RLF. There have been rare reported cases of infants with RLF who were never in oxygen concentrations higher than 21%. However, the infants who are most prone to this disease are immature infants (with immature retinal vasculature) who are placed in oxygen levels greater than 21% for any length of time.

Follow-up thoracic x-ray films, done routinely on convalescing infants, frequently identify an infant who has signs of chronic lung disease that will make him more susceptible to bronchitis, pneumonia, and other lung problems throughout his infancy and childhood. These infants' mothers should be warned of symptoms to watch for, and they should be told that the physician will want to follow their infant's progress carefully.

Mother surrogate syndrome

A different but equally important problem is found in situations where there are convalescing infants. This is an emotional phenomenon of the nursing staff, which can be described as the "mother surrogate syndrome." Frequently, the nursing staff of intensive care nurseries consists of young nurses who do not have any children of their own. If an infant is critically ill and has required much nursing support, his nurses may find difficulty in relinquishing him to his mother when he recovers.

The nurses may attempt to delay the infant's discharge by deciding that the infant is "not ready" to go home. They may feel that the mother is incapable of caring for her infant, and they may lose their objectivity in determining the mother's abilities. These reactions of the nurses are more pronounced if the mother has not come to visit her infant, or if she shows signs of disinterest. It is especially trying when the mother really does not want the challenge of a potentially chronically ill child. Nursing personnel should be aware that the situation of "mother surrogate syndrome" does exist, and the staff may need to examine their attitudes carefully at times.

• • •

In summary, the convalescing infant does present challenges to the nursing staff, as does the critical infant and the dying infant. The nurse's primary responsibilities are to teach the mother how to care for her infant and to make arrangements preceding the infant's discharge so that he will continue to progress at home.

Problems in intensive care nurseries not associated with patient illnesses

Some problems in intensive care nurseries are not directly associated with patient illness problems, although they do involve the infants, their parents, and the staff of the nursery. The high cost of patient care, methods of transporting infants from surrounding hospitals, and research and teaching responsibilities will be discussed.

The high cost of patient care

Unless there are grant funds available, the cost of hospitalization for this group of infants is unbelievable. The exorbitant costs are difficult for well-established families who have saved money for medical treatment, and devastating for young families who have no reserve funds. Most insurance policies do not cover the infant's hospitalization costs until he is from 14 to 30 days of age. Present costs in most centers are well above $100 a day for critically ill infants (this does not include the cost of certain equipment and supplies). Infants may be hospitalized for 3 weeks or more, and their bills are likely to be beyond belief.

Transporting of infants to high-risk centers

The process of transporting infants can be a physically stressful situation for the infant. Even with the use of specially equipped ambulances or helicopters, many times conditions are not optimal during the actual transportation. Some high-risk centers are concentrating their efforts on solving the in-transit problems of temperature control, oxygen stability, and an environment in which emergency treatments may be performed.

Teaching and research responsibilities

Most intensive care nursery centers take the responsibility for training outside personnel in the techniques of intensive infant care. This means the development of a teaching program and designation of personnel to perform this function. In addition, in many centers there are active ongoing research programs that require accurate recording of data and sometimes additional procedures to be done by nursing personnel. These factors, coupled with the level of illness of the infants, necessitate high staffing ratios of nurses to infants. Finding qualified personnel to provide the necessary care may be difficult.

Conclusion

This chapter has included a presentation of various diseases and problems surrounding the nursing care of high-risk infants. The care of these infants is a highly specialized area of nursing, which requires knowledge of infant problems and methods of helping infants and their parents during the infant's hospitalization.

References

1. Mizrahi, A., London, R. D., and Gribetz, D.: Neonatal hypocalcemia—its causes and treatment, New Eng. J. Med. **278:**1163-1165, 1968.
2. Problems of neonatal intensive care units: Report of the Fifty-Ninth Ross Conference on Pediatric Research, Ross Laboratories, 1969.
3. Pringle, J. A.: Respiratory distress unit, Amer. J. Nurs. **68:**2370-2373, 1968.
4. Daily, W. J. R., Klaus, M., and Meyer, H. B.: Apnea in premature infants: monitoring, incidence, heart rate changes, and an effect of environmental temperature, Pediatrics **43:**510-518, 1969.
5. Bookmiller, M. M., and Bowen, G. L.: Textbook of obstetrics and obstetric nursing, Philadelphia, 1963, W. B. Saunders Co.
6. Saling, E.: Foetal and neonatal hypoxia in relation to clinical obstetric practice, Baltimore, 1968, The Williams & Wilkins Co.
7. Du, J. N. H., and Oliver, T. K.: The baby in the delivery room, a suitable microenvironment, J.A.M.A. **207:**1502-1504, 1969.
8. Glaser, B. G., and Strauss, A. L.: Time for dying, Chicago, 1968, Aldine Publishing Co.

Bibliography

Babson, S. G., and Benson, R. C.: Primer on prematurity and high-risk pregnancy, St. Louis, 1966, The C. V. Mosby Co.
Butler, N. R., and Alberman, E. D., editors: Perinatal problems, Edinburgh, 1969, E. & S. Livingston, Ltd.
Haller, J. A., editor: The hospitalized child and his family, Baltimore, 1967, The Johns Hopkins Press.
James, S. L., editor: The pediatric clinics of North America, Philadelphia, 1966, W. B. Saunders Co.
Schaffer, A. J.: Diseases of the newborn, Philadelphia, 1965, W. B. Saunders Co.

Chapter 9

Retarded babies and the nursing challenge*

Martha Adams

Picture a busy pediatric ward with several toddlers free to interact with one another and to help themselves to the many playthings available. One child, however, is alone in his crib in a cubicle away from the other children. This boy with Down's syndrome sits rocking and playing with his toes. Two nurses pass and one says to the other, "See, that's typically Mongoloid behavior." The child had been given no toys to play with, yet his attempts to pass the time with the only materials available to him were labeled "typically Mongoloid behavior."

This is a dramatic example of a nurse's failure to meet her challenge of providing appropriate play activities to stimulate a child to further development. A contingent part of this challenge is her opportunity to help mothers recognize the growth potential of their infants and the great maternal joy that can replace the initial despair at the diagnosis of mental retardation.

Learning to be a mother

Rubin[1] states that the ability to mother successfully does not develop automatically with the birth of the baby but rather must be learned in interaction with the infant. Every new mother must gain a feeling of competency in the maternal role. To do this, she must work hard in getting to know her baby. She needs continued observation, practice, and trial and error in "reading" the behavioral cues of her infant. She often sees the best proof of her mothering abilities in the behavior of her infant, that is, eating well, gaining weight, developing regular sleeping patterns, and crying little. Also, she must discover the temperament or behavioral style of her infant.

*The author wishes to express her appreciation to Miss Lee Patterson for editorial help under U. S. Public Health Service Grant No. NU-00-177. She is also most appreciative of contributions of many students including Miss Nancy Parry who worked with Dena and her mother and to Mrs. Marcia Westmoreland for sharing her experiences with the F family. The author appreciates the assistance of Mrs. Mary Ann Newcomb, presently Educational Coordinator, Contra Costa School, for planning and orientation to the project.

Recent research indicates a wide variability within the normal limits of infant behavior. The New York Longitudinal Study,[2] initiated in 1956, stresses the innate differences of infants and the effect of this individuality on the mother and her care-giving behavior. The focus of the study is on the temperament or behavioral styles of infants; temperament is defined as the "characteristic tempo, energy expenditure, focus, mood and rhythmicity that typify the behaviors of an individual child, independently of their contents."[2] Parents of 136 children were interviewed every three months during the infant's first year and every six months to the age of 5 years to gain information about the child's daily behavior. Standard test-play interviews and observations of the children in various settings were also used to obtain data on the children.

Individual behavior styles of the infants were assessed based on the following categories: reactivity, rhythmicity, approach-withdrawal, adaptability, intensity of reaction, threshhold of responsiveness, quality of mood, distractibility and attention span, and persistence. A number of behavioral styles were identified from analysis of the data. The "easy child" is described as one whose feeding and sleeping patterns are regular, who takes new foods easily, smiles in response to strangers, adjusts to new situations easily, and is not easily frustrated. A child with somewhat opposite characteristics is described as the "difficult child." Temperamental styles of infants tend to persist and to exert a large degree of influence on maternal care.

On being the mother of a retarded child

The new mother of a retarded child especially needs to gain a feeling of maternal competence. Rubin,[3] in observing families having children with congenital handicaps, concludes that these mothers are themselves handicapped in the development of normal mothering by their babies' inabilities to respond normally.

This mother experiences a feeling of failure at not having produced a perfect child. She, along with the father, must grieve the loss of the dreamed-of perfect child.[4] This takes time during which the mother needs physical rest, opportunity to talk of the wished-for child, and, through thinking and feeling, time to be able to work toward a more realistic view of the newborn infant.

Kubler-Ross[5] describes the grieving process as having certain predictable stages—denial, anger, bargaining, depression, and hope versus stark reality. These seem pertinent to the parent's loss of the dreamed-of child and the birth of the retarded child.

The following quote from this writer's interview with the mother of a boy with Down's syndrome illustrates the denial stage.

Unless you have had such an experience you can't imagine my feelings as my pediatrician talked to me about Bobby. I couldn't have heard him correctly. We have only well-developed, intelligent children. I even harbored the thought that the babies may have been switched. This child was short and fat, and not at all like our other babies. For three days I didn't eat or sleep. I was in a world of misery all my own. I paced the floor at night. Sedatives did not faze the torture. I wept when anyone spoke to me. How could they understand? I have always felt that if I were handicapped physically I'd make out but without my mind I'd be dead, and, now, I have given birth to a son who would be both physically and mentally handicapped.

This, too, was a most difficult time for John. We decided our children had to know some cause for their father's agony but what should he tell them? Was this more than we should expect them to bear? Would this make their feelings toward the new baby strained and unnatural? No one seemed to have the answers, so John blurted out the entire situation to them as soon as he returned to the car. To say that he was disturbed by their matter-of-fact acceptance of the sad news is an understatement. They quickly returned to their play as if this was no matter. By their infrequent questions about the baby we knew they heard and understood, but were able to accept this with ease.

Denial on part of the parents seems to operate not only in the initial stage upon the birth of the retarded child but from time to time throughout his life. A mother spoke of her 6-year-old daughter, describing in detail the diagnostic procedure and the signs the doctor had pointed out to her. It was clear she had understood the diagnosis well. Then, in the next breath she said, "You know Joan, the retarded child, fell down the other day and we thought this might shock her back to normal."

The second stage as described by Kubler-Ross is anger. Parents often ask, "Why did this have to happen to us?" They need to be able to express their anger and to be helped in recognizing that they are angry.

The third stage is that of bargaining. "If God would only let this pass from us we would. . . ." Parents of retarded children seem to be bargaining for the most favorable diagnosis for their child in their shopping around from doctor to doctor. They also seem to be saying, "Let this be anything but mental retardation, for we can handle anything else our child may have."

Finally when parents are faced with the irreversible fact that the child is retarded, the next stage, depression, will be likely to follow. It is often with the diagnosis of mental retardation that the parent feels that he is on a dead-end road, and that the child can learn nothing. Acceptance follows with further realization of the irreversibility of the condition.

The last step is hope versus stark reality. From the realization that their child is retarded and, often, with an assumption that this means their child can learn nothing, parents must be brought to see there is growth potential of some sort in every human being. They must be shown that their child will develop, but more slowly than other children and to a less advanced ceiling.

Hopelessness or despair is characterized by lack of energy, an orientation to the present, hostility, inability to act, and a feeling one cannot act on his environment effectively. Hope, on the other hand, is characterized by activity and willingness to expend energy because there is some possibility of accomplishment. Stotland[6] cites the importance of hope as a prerequisite for action.

The nursing challenge

An important part of nursing is to assist mothers in gaining confidence and skill in early mothering. Intervention is crucial to future health and growth of both mother and child and for the unfolding interrelationship between them. For example, in the first feeding experience it is important that the mother finds the most comfortable position for herself and the baby and that the nurse encourages the mother by being available and nearby. The goal is to build in success for this and all early experiences.

The first twenty-four hours at home is a special time of need for new parents because so much energy goes into "reading" the baby's cues in behavior. When he cries, is he wet, hungry, or what? What are the unusual sounds he makes at night? Is he even breathing?

Mothers need to know the sequences of child development whether through previous experience or through education. Miss Mary E. Boyle, head of Merrill Palmer Institute's Infant Services, is an outstanding example of a nurse who, for more than fifteen years, has been dedicated to helping young mothers enjoy their developing infants. Through casual laboratory sessions mothers and infants share in teaching students from colleges and universities. Together Miss Boyle, mothers, and students record the baby's growth from birth to two years. An extremely helpful aid is a record of locomotor development that the mother keeps and shares with the group when she comes to the institute. This record diagrams and describes normal locomotor development in a progressive manner and includes two columns in which the mother records the date on which new behavior first appears and the age of her infant when this happens. An important advantage of this tool is that while the mother records she learns about progression in motor development and is looking at her own infant's development in relation to himself, rather than comparing him to other infants.

Observing infants and young children for the presence of deviations in development is another nursing function. The value of discovering deviations early cannot be overstressed. The accurate assessment of both potential and limitations helps parents achieve a more realistic idea of what can and cannot be expected in their child. So often handicapped children are not helped to develop the growth potential they possess because parents do not realize that these children can develop and need appropriate stimulation to do so.

A number of excellent assessment tools are available. *A Developmental Approach to Casefinding*[7] by Mrs. Una Haynes focuses on the basic neurological reflex patterns and the maturation of the central nervous system. It is a thorough aid in detecting early deviations in infants and young children. A chart in the form of a wheel, included in the book, offers a ready guide to observing children up to 36 months of age for presence or absence of various reflexes.

Another tool useful in alerting professionals to developmental lag is the *Denver Developmental Screening Test.*[8] This screening test looks at behavior in four major areas of development, that is, gross motor, fine motor, personal-social, and language. It is not an I.Q. test, but it is useful in spotting delays in development that may indicate if the child needs to be referred for further psychological testing. This test was standardized on 1,036 normal children in Denver and includes items that illustrate behaviors which occur at various ages from 2 weeks to slightly over 6 years. An easily carried play kit contains a skein of red wool, a box of raisins, a rattle with a narrow handle, 1-inch colored cubes, a small glass bottle with ⅝-inch opening, a small bell, and a tennis ball, which are used in administering the test. The manual that accompanies the play kit and test forms gives information about the development of the test and specific directions for administering the test.

Approaches in early intervention

The retarded infant cannot easily reach out for stimulation from his environment; therefore stimuli must be brought to him.

As with any infant, he needs to develop a smile, since many more people respond to a smiling infant. This is one way he can elicit attention and assurance that his needs will be met. John Watson[9] called a baby's smile "social currency." Through studying smiling in infants he concluded that probably face-to-face smiling and vocalization are the best ways to elicit the infant's smile. How simple it is to encourage mothers—especially of retarded infants—to use face-to-face smiling and vocalization in as many care-taking activities as possible.

The infant also needs to feel some control over his environment. This trust is partially developed when the infant finds his needs being met by his mother. Further control is felt when mobiles are placed close enough so that he can kick them or balloons are tied with short strings to his arms or legs so he can bat at them. The baby initiates the action and something happens that reinforces the action, and the infant's sense of control is increased. Changing the position of his crib and placing him in positions that will increase his visual field increase sensory stimulation. The use of soft music near the crib increases auditory input.

Consideration of temperamental styles is important because of the direct bearing that temperament has on adaptive reactions and responses to environment. An exuberant, impulsive child may not stop to consider alternative approaches to a solution in a learning situation. He needs to have alternatives explicitly pointed out or to have verbal instructions to "slow down." A sensitive or fearful child requires special encouragement, slower introduction into the learning situation, and "muted" reactions by those working with him because of the child's tendency to overreact to minimal stimuli.

Preparation of nurses to meet their challenge

One example of how nurses can be prepared to meet the challenges of working with retarded children and their families is given below. Members of the faculty of the University of California School of Nursing, San Francisco, identified three educational goals that they deemed would help to prepare nurses to care for children with handicapping conditions (including mental retardation). Specifically, these goals are (1) early recognition and identification of deviations in development, (2) skill and confidence in working with atypical infants and their families, and (3) ability to assist mothers of these babies to recognize developmental levels of their children and to provide appropriate activities to stimulate growth potentials.

Classroom and clinical experiences were developed to aid the students toward these goals.

Early recognition of deviations is based on knowledge of normal child development. Although tools are useful, none can measure the complexities of child behavior nor give an appreciation of the innate need for growth. Facility in assessment comes by continually observing children. Ultimately, each nurse must develop her own systematic observation of on-the-spot cues in maternal-infant interaction. Much of her success will depend on her trust of her own clinical judgment. Thus, opportunity for students to attain knowledge of normal child development and to use that knowledge in clinical situations was provided.

Many current studies stress the importance of early environmental enrichment as a stimulus in teaching infants how to learn and in promoting later cognitive development.[10, 11] Thus, much attention goes to prekindergarten youth and their acquisition of emotional, cognitive, and social abilities. The University of California program has a basic assumption that such early enrichment is more important to the infant with a developmental deviation than to a child who normally explores as widely as he is allowed. When infants lack positive response, mothers need encouragement to continue stimulation despite this rather unrewarding behavior.

Student experiences with atypical infants

In exploring areas for clinical experiences, the planners found an atypical infant project across San Francisco Bay in Contra Costa County. The interdisciplinary project staff worked with infants from birth to 3 years of age with a wide variety of handicapping conditions. The prime goal was early developmental assessment and intervention by working with these babies and their families in providing growth promoting activities. The project included a seven-hour daily nursery program conducted by a registered nurse and a program of home visiting for those infants who were not ready to participate in the daily program at the center. A permeating message of the center seemed to be, "These are children who can learn, and we who care about them can help them to learn."

Since the goals of the Contra Costa project and for student experiences were so similar, this seemed like an ideal setting for clinical experience for students. Furthermore, the director was receptive to the idea of student nurses taking part in both school and home care. Mutual planning for learning experiences for students and for orientation to the project was carried out jointly by the project staff and the author.

Orientation started in early afternoon with discussions or demonstrations, or both, by the director, occupational therapist, physical therapist, and nurse. In the evening students attended a parents' meeting and met the families with whom they were to work. Students had experience in the center and also functioned as home visitors.

Levels of infant functioning were determined with tools previously mentioned after initial rapport had been built with the families. Approaches in intervention varied according to cues in behaviors of the infants. Experiences were shared in weekly seminars. Students were often helpful to one another in comparing and sharing new approaches. An instance of this was when one nurse discussed her futile attempts that week to teach the child with whom she was working to chew. Another student reported she had found pectin gum drops helpful in developing chewing with her child.

The following is an account of the experience of a second year basic student. During this time she worked with Dena W, an 18-month-old child with Down's syndrome, and her family.

The W family lived in a comfortable home near San Francisco. The student recorded her early observations and reactions:

Dena is a cute blonde little girl, a little small for her age, happy, but not particularly responsive to people. She bears only a few of the physical characteristics of Down's syndrome. I found her cute and fun to play with, much more than I expected. Dena and I played on the floor with some of her toys while Mrs. W and I talked.

From my observations during this period, and from comments from Mrs. W I learned the following: Dena is kept in her playpen most of the day; therefore, her environment is quite limited. She lacks a variety of experiences. I discussed with Mrs. W the value of placing Dena in a prone position on the floor. She creeps on her tummy quite well, but doesn't get up on her hands and knees. She moves around quite a bit on her bottom, propelling herself with her hands and feet.

Dena does not finger feed or drink from a cup. She holds her own bottle and is fed junior foods. Apparently she is given little opportunity to try, since her first few attempts were quite unsuccessful. I wonder if she might have trouble in swallowing. This is an area in which I need to make further assessment, and it seems to be a good area to work on.

I feel that because Dena is so easy to care for and is such a pleasant child that she actually lacks much stimulation and is rarely put into situations where she can learn new things. So much is being done for her that she could be learning to do for herself. I plan to do some motor therapy with Dena to assist in crawling and to observe her eating to determine what can be done to assist her in this area.

On her next visit, ten days later, Mrs. W greeted the student nurse by telling her, first of all, that Dena's playpen had broken so the little girl had to spend all her time on the floor. By doing so, she at times got up on her hands and knees to crawl and spent less time pushing herself on her bottom. Both Mrs. W and the student were delighted with this new step in motor development. The student nurse showed Mrs. W how a towel under Dena's abdomen, held from above, could help support her while crawling and how toys placed in front of Dena could motivate her to move forward. The student nurse also demonstrated for the mother the technique of using various textured materials while rubbing and naming body parts to teach Dena the location and names of parts of her body.

Mrs. W also gave Dena a deep bowl with some cereal in it, and Dena ate several spoonfuls of the cereal. Together Mrs. W and the student nurse made a list of finger foods of increasingly different textures and tastes.

The student's main goals in working with the W family were to increase the family awareness of what could be done to help Dena and, primarily, to work with her crawling and feeding. After the student's final visit 3 months later, she reported:

When I first started with Dena, she was creeping on her tummy and propelling herself on her bottom. Thanks to getting rid of her playpen, Dena now spends most of her time on the floor, crawling in a normal pattern quite extensively, and exhibits little of her old pattern of locomotion. Dena is still being fed junior foods and drinks from a bottle. We have begun to give her some finger foods, and started her drinking from a cup. She really doesn't like the new textures because she makes faces but she will eat cereal and crackers and has increased the number of hand to mouth gestures. She grasps a cup quite well and with assistance drinks a small amount of liquid.

The W's provide excellent care for Dena and give her a great deal of love. I really feel that I have started them to stimulate her more and I think more encouragement is needed in this area. However, Mrs. W is so pleased with Dena's progress, as a result of her own efforts, that she seems enthusiastic to continue to use new approaches. I can't get over how quickly Dena learned—the timing was so perfect.

One can conclude from this student's report that Dena was ready to learn many new things when in an environment that not only allowed, but encouraged, her development. An important outcome for her mother was that, although she knew Dena was retarded, she found her daughter capable of learning on her own developmental level with maternal help supplying suitable activities. Mrs. W was rewarded and further motivated by seeing change and growth as a result of her own efforts.

A graduate nurse student's recording of interactions with a 20-month-old retarded child and his family illustrates the nurse's functions in providing a role model for the mother and, at times, actually mothering the mother.

The F family consisted of the father, 23, the mother, 21, and Paul, 20 months. Both parents were of Cantonese origin, but the son was born in San Francisco. At birth his Apgar ratings were one and three for 1 and 5 minutes, respectively, and a diagnosis was made of aspiration pneumonia.

The graduate student first met the family in the developmental clinic where Paul was being seen for "slow development." At 14 months he could sit with support for a short time, had good head control, and could roll from front to back.

Due to the Cantonese custom of child rearing by servants and the fact that Mrs. F was the last sibling to be born, she was unfamiliar with the attitudes of mothering and the emotional energy of motherliness that are required in our culture. Added to this was her lack of close family members who could assist in the care of her infant. Although she carried on routine activities, the quality of her relationship with her infant indicated a lack of self-trust in her own abilities. She was apprehensive in handling the baby and displayed an unfamiliarity with children and their development.

In observation, the nurse noted:

Mrs. F holds the baby stiffly on her lap away from her body. There is little face-to-face interaction and I have never seen her kiss him or call him by name. She does not use her arms to enfold Paul and care is given in a rather mechanical, impersonal manner. The mother has not yet progressed to the point where contact with her infant is sought for the sheer enjoyment of contact. In fact, Paul spends most of his time in a walker in front of a colored TV.

From these observations the nurse's initial assessment was "slow development, especially gross motor, under stimulation, and a poor quality of mothering."

The importance of a healthy male heir cannot be overlooked in the Chinese civilization and of the additional status a baby boy affords the wife and mother. Mrs. F was handicapped by feelings provoked by having produced an imperfect child, by lack of positive feedback in Paul's behavior, and by lack of knowing how children grow and develop. For instance, when the nurse suggested Mrs. F play more with Paul, Mrs. F replied, "Play, I don't know how to play with baby."

The nurse's goals for intervention were to give Mrs. F positive ideas and meet her dependency needs so that she would be better able to meet her child's needs. Second, the nurse functioned as a resource of knowledge of Paul's condition and his potential and developmental needs. Most importantly the nurse was a role model to the mother in holding Paul close, talking to him, utilizing face-to-face interaction, and, generally, in providing additional stimulation.

Mrs. F is slowly showing evidence of increasing trust and skill in her mothering abilities with much patience, encouragement, and understanding on the part of the nurse.

Summary

Every child needs activities appropriate to his developmental level for growth. This is especially true for infants and children with developmental deviations. Nurses need theory, experience in assessment of development, and approaches in intervention to prepare them to assist the mother in determining the child's level and in initiating appropriate activities to attain developmental potential. The University of California School of Nursing Training Project to prepare nurses for these tasks is a successful example of how this may be done.

References

1. Rubin, R.: Basic maternal behavior, Nurs. Outlook 9:683-686, Nov., 1961.
2. Chess, S.: Temperament in the normal infant. In Hellmuth, J., editor: Exceptional infant, vol. 1, The normal infant, New York, 1967, Brunner/Mazel, Inc.
3. Rubin, R.: Maternal touch, Nurs. Outlook 11:828-831, Nov., 1963.
4. Solnit, A., and Stark, M.: Mourning and the birth of a defective child, Psychoanal. Stud. Child 16:523-527, 1961.
5. Kubler-Ross, E.: On death and dying, New York, 1969, The Macmillan Co.
6. Stotland, E.: The psychology of hope, San Francisco, 1969, Jossey Bass Inc.
7. Haynes, U.: A developmental approach to casefinding, Washington, D. C., 1967, U. S. Government Printing Office.
8. Frankenburg, W., and Dodds, J.: Denver developmental screening test, Denver, 1967, University of Colorado Medical Center.
9. Watson, J.: Why is a smile? Trans-action 4:36-39, May, 1967.
10. Gordon, I.: Home stimulation for disadvantaged infants, unpublished manuscript, 1967.
11. Schaefer, E., and Furfey, P.: Intellectual stimulation of culturally deprived infants, unpublished progress report, 1968.

Bibliography

ANA Committee on Education: American Nurses' Association's first position on nursing education, Amer. J. Nurs. 65:106-111, Dec., 1965.

Blake, Florence, Wright, F. H., and Waechter, E. H.: Nursing care of children, Philadelphia, 1970, J. B. Lippincot Co.

Fromm, Erich: The art of loving, New York, 1956, Harper & Brothers.

Lorenzen, Elizabeth: The clinical specialist role model change agent, University of Colorado School of Nursing, 1969 (unpublished independent study).

Nightingale, Florence: Notes on nursing, London, 1859, Harrison & Sons.

Tournier, Paul: The meaning of persons, New York, 1959, Harper & Brothers.

Vaillot, Sister Madeleine Clemence: Commitment to nursing, Philadelphia, 1962, J. B. Lippincott Co.

Wiedenbach, Ernestine: Clinical nursing: a helping art, New York, 1964, Springer Publishing Co., Inc.

Yura, Helen, and Walsh, Mary B.: The nursing process, Washington, D. C., 1967, The Catholic University of America Press.

Chapter 10

Caring—a priority in pediatric nursing

Boonie Ford and Maxine Berlinger

The major focus in nursing has been to provide nursing care to individuals and their families. Many authors, including Florence Nightingale, have written about it. In 1966 The American Nurses' Association adopted a position paper in which care, cure, and coordination were stated to be the components of nursing care. In this chapter we want to discuss the caring part of nursing care. The reason for this focus is that we believe caring to be the foundation in nursing of children.

Nursing process of caring

For the reader to understand the nursing process of caring as used in this chapter, it is necessary for us to define caring and the nursing process. Caring is the personal expression of concern for and about another in a meaningful way. Caring in this context is the giving of oneself in such a way that the person receiving the care knows that the one giving the care is concerned about him and what happens to him. Commitment and involvement are the essential components of caring. Commitment implies a concern for and a belief that children are individuals with certain rights and needs. It also implies that the nurse cannot be concerned with the child without expressing concern for those who are important in the life of the child. Involvement means the nurse empathizes with the child and his family because she recognizes and seeks to understand the motivation underlying their behavior and feelings as reflections of needs. Our belief is that caring for children should be demonstrated wherever children are encountered. The nurse knows that caring is the key to her effectiveness in working with children and their families.

The nursing process is the systematic, orderly manner of carrying out the steps of sensory encounter, validation, intervention, and evaluation.

Sensory encounter, the first step in the nursing process, is an overall observation including what is seen, what is heard, what is touched, and what can be smelled. This initial step is a basis for all further steps and provides the basis for the setting of priorities. It is the foundation for any further nursing care with the child.

Validation is the second step in the process. Validation includes confirmation or disconfirmation of the interpretation of the encounter; therefore, it requires the nurse to seek out more information. Her validation may include further encounter with the child, encounter with the family, significant others, colleagues, peers, and numerous other people. Her validation could also include going out beyond the proximity of the child at the current time. For instance, she may have to go into the home or the school to know more about the child's culture. This process may take some time if the nurse is to intervene appropriately. Based on the validation, priorities are determined for the next step of intervention.

Intervention, the third step in the nursing process, involves purposeful behaviors and skillful application of techniques by the nurse for maintenance or change, or both, relative to the child's health or illness. Intervention is based on the sensory encounter and validation. The formulation of objectives is an explicit part of intervention. Objectives may be directed toward biological, behavioral, or social maintenance or change. Interventions are also based on priority of need. This step is the key to the nursing process, since her skill and behavior are the art of caring. Effective verbal and nonverbal communication based on accumulated data is essential to this step.

Evaluation becomes the last step in the process; however, it is by no means the end. Having stated objectives, it then becomes necessary to evaluate the outcomes of the interventions. Behavioral and physical changes are excellent evaluative dimensions and perhaps the major dimensions necessary to the nursing process.

The nursing process of caring is based on the assumption that the nurse has a comprehensive knowledge of the physiological, psychological, cultural, and environmental aspects of child growth and development. The knowledge includes the recognition that children are not miniature adults; they are developing, they are vulnerable, and they are in a period of crisis just from the standpoint of their physiological and psychological growth.

Examples of the nursing process

Some examples demonstrating the nursing process may be seen in the following illustrations.

If when the nurse enters a child's room, she observes that the child is sleeping quietly, is calm, has good respiration, but she smells an odor, sees a cluttered, unkept room, then her initial response may be that of looking at the environment. Validation is immediate; her intervention and also objectives are directed toward seeing that the room is cleaned to make the environment conducive to the child's recuperation. Her evaluation would come later as she further observes the child in his environment.

If, however, the nurse enters the room and finds the child crying, thrashing around the bed, and perhaps even banging his head on the side rail, she, after her sensory encounter, makes certain inferences concerning pain, separation anxiety, and physical discomforts such as wetness or hunger, which involve priority setting. She then must validate her inferences. Validation may be done by seeking the answers to certain questions by closer examination of the child, by reading the nursing notes or physicians orders, or by talking with the child's parents. She may then set objectives and carry out actions that are conducive to achievement of the objectives, that is, intervene.

If the nurse determines that the child has not eaten, she may feed him, and when indeed he stops crying, she may evaluate this as an accomplishment of an objective. However, if she determines that the crying, etc., is due to separation anxiety, several objectives could be stated and evaluation postponed until all interventions are completed. Each objective could be pursued individually. This latter approach could call for a complete recycling of the nursing process.

In some cases, upon the initial sensory encounter, the nurse may find that quick validation is required and immediate intervention is needed. In this situation all steps in the process may be accomplished immediately. For instance, if upon entering a room she would find a child in acute respiratory distress, immediate on-the-spot validation is needed, and immediate intervention is necessary on the nurse's part. The effectiveness of the intervention will be evaluated when the crisis is over. This crisis having been handled would then require her to recycle to the initial step of sensory encounter for further intervention.

Caring for Mary

The following is a description of how one pediatric nurse demonstrated her commitment to caring and applied this commitment in her nursing process.

When I first met Mary, a 13-year-old Mexican-American girl with a diagnosis of acute uremia, she had been transferred from the adolescent ward to the intensive care unit for peritoneal dialysis. Mary was brought to my attention by the nursing staff because she was "depressed and noncommunicative." Mary was heavily sedated and was quite toxic from her uremia, causing almost complete lack of consciousness. I did not feel this was the time to introduce myself, but I did discuss with her mother my desire to work with Mary and her family while she was hospitalized. During this conversation Mary's mother brought out that Mary was a quiet girl even at home, and that she was getting quite disturbed by the nurses constantly probing her about her "feelings and depression."

After this conversation I decided my approach with Mary would have to be slow and would involve constant evaluation concerning what she was ready to talk about. So our relationship moved gradually from my giving physical care in the intensive care setting, to social conversation, to very deep discussion of her fears of bleeding to death, dying, her dislike of being hospitalized, and frustrations with the unknown in her diagnosis and future treatment. Eventually I could confront her with verbal cues I was picking up, and she would be able to talk about these problems and fears. This took much time and effort at first, but she did not avoid my confrontation. Soon she was able to see that I could understand she had a right to these feelings and that I would not criticize her for them. During this time she was also able to transfer this relationship, to a certain degree, to other nurses who became more interested in her as she began to respond.

My goal at this time was also to help Mary put her fears into perspective. I could not and would not make them vanish, but by preparing her for procedures and treatments, she grew less fearful. We discussed dying, transplantation, and bleeding. All were very real possibilities and the unknown qualities of each increased the anxieties she felt. For much of the time the diagnosis of acute glomerulonephritis was unknown. Several delays of a biopsy perpetuated the frustration. It was after her biopsy that one of her greatest fears almost came true—that of bleeding to death.

It was at a time when Mary and I were trying to make her low-protein diet more appetizing and, to her way of thinking, more fun to eat. We made a sandwich out of her tiny piece of meat and stole the lettuce from under her salad. At this time Mary was slumped down in her chair and complaining that her stiches were pulling, so I said I'd fix the pillow behind her if she would sit up straighter. I looked down and noticed a large amount of serosanguinous drainage on her robe. I told her that there was some drainage coming through her dressing and that I thought the doctor should know, so I had one of the other nurses call him. I went back to Mary, helped her into bed, and when she saw the drainage she became panicky. I reinforced the wound as I was helping to calm her by saying that I would stay with her through this and that we would get the bleeding stopped. I talked softly to her and constantly encouraged her to be as still as possible. I said I knew it must hurt, but that we were helping her even though at times it probably did not seem so to her. This last comment applied when the doctor told her to stop complaining and crying and to act her age while he was drawing blood from her arm and was starting an intravenous infusion. It was essential for me to stay close to her and to hold her hand. Mary had lost about 300 ml. of blood, and blood and equipment were everywhere. In general it was very gory and frightening to her. I remained with Mary until the bleeding was stopped and she was almost asleep. Then I emphasized that the nurses who were working there would take good care of her when I left. I also informed her that I would return after she had rested.

After this experience several people expressed their gratitude for my being with Mary during this time. Mary, herself, said she was terribly afraid and was glad that I had been with her. Her mother expressed her relief, and the staff nurse on the ward felt similarly because she was very busy with her other patients and was not used to emergency situations.

In general, there were several crisis situations during Mary's hospitalization that provoked more concentrated effort on my part. These included helping Mary work through feelings of receiving a kidney transplant and of accepting one from a member of her family. Because of Mary's constant fears, the many pros and cons about this were discussed. At this point the staff members also became interested in helping Mary. This interest was met with positive responses by Mary which created excitement in the staff.

An unexpected circumstance (the premature birth of my baby) prevented my visiting Mary for a period of two weeks. I feel this added as well as detracted from our relationship to a certain extent. Throughout this time Mary and I maintained contact by telephone. I assured her that I was still interested in her and would again continue to work with her. It seemed to give our relationship a new perspective because she was thinking about my welfare in addition to her own. Perhaps she could see I was experiencing some similar feelings and worries to those that she was having. This may have enriched our understanding.

Mary is at home now after having had a right nephrectomy, which was precipitated by the bleeding. She is to have her left kidney removed at an unknown future date and will receive a kidney from some undetermined member of her family. Until then, twice a week she comes to the hospital for approximately six hours of dialysis. It is in the dialysis room that I maintain contact.

While visiting with Mary in this room, she appears much more tired—only wanting to sleep. This she attributes to getting up early in the morning in order for her parents to drive a great distance and to being in such an awesome and unaesthetic room. It has been hard for us to discuss anything in this particular room because of the lack of privacy, and immediately after her dialysis we are hampered because her family has a long drive home and they want to leave right away. But I do plan to find a conducive time and place to discuss more of her feelings about being kept alive on this machine, about receiving a kidney from a member of her family, and about the uncertainty of timing for the transplant to come.

I am a firm believer in family involvement and have maintained close contact with Mary's mother and sister and some contact with her father. My role with these family members has included clarification and interpretation of what her mother has discussed with the doctor, discussion of

Mary's concerns so the family can help her with these, and by being a resource person and coordinator for certain problems such as finances and diet. I contacted the dietitian who helped the mother with preparing a low-protein diet at home. The social worker helped Mary's mother find housing while in the city and discussed with her the financing of Mary's hospitalization and transplant. My role has also been supportive to the family, since they are allowed to vent their feelings of concern about Mary and the impact of her illness on the family.

Analysis of caring for Mary

Because of the nurse's concern about Mary's behavior, the nurse felt the need to approach Mary's mother to obtain a picture of her life at home and also what behavior Mary usually exhibits. The nurse in this approach displays to the parents an interest in Mary as a person, not just a patient. She also is telling the parents, "I need your help to know Mary," involving the parents in the process and denoting I *care*.

She also realized that to establish a relationship with Mary, the first objective would be to establish nonverbal communication by showing Mary that she is skillful in application of techniques. She also realized the objective of assisting Mary in expressing her concerns and fears by the establishment of a trust relationship that would be enhanced by the nurse's demonstration of skillful application of techniques and physical care. By this demonstration, she expressed, nonverbally, *I care* enough to provide nursing care that is effective and efficient. One cannot negate the effect of "laying on of hands" as one valuable communication tool. This also provides the nurse with contact and makes her available to Mary in a continuity experience. *She is there when needed.*

Having shown care through giving, the nurse allows Mary to move at her own pace. Mary's feelings of trust for the nurse provide both the nurse and Mary with a basis for them to verbally communicate. The result of these interactions assisted

Mary in expressing her desires, concerns, and fears. The nurse, in allowing Mary to express herself, did not deny that these feelings were present. She encouraged her through listening, not commenting inappropriately, and indicating she understood. The nurse also helped her to see that others have similar feelings. Being able to verbalize these fears and concerns assisted Mary in becoming aware of the reality of the situation. The interventions of the nurse helped Mary make this awareness a growth experience.

Throughout this continuous professional involvement with Mary, the nurse communicated with the staff to keep them appraised of her progress, thereby assisting them to increase their understanding of Mary. This, in turn, helped the staff to approach Mary in a more consistent manner and gave them a basis from which to demonstrate care. The nurse continually involved Mary's parents by encouraging them to assist in her care and by providing information to them to increase their understanding about Mary's condition and needs.

It is interesting to note that Mary's interest in the nurse changed to one of also caring about the nurse as a person. If caring does indeed take place, the patient is able to move from concern of self to concern for others.

It is essential that the nurse is free to provide continuity by moving from one area to another when the needs of the patient warrant this. This freedom of movement assists the nurse to consistently express concern for and about the patient. This constant contact also provides the nurse with data on which to base further intervention as new needs arise.

Summary

In this chapter we have focused on the caring part of the nursing process in pediatric nursing. Caring is the manner in which the nurse demonstrates her personal concern and warmth for children and their families in carrying out the steps of sensory encounter, validation, intervention, and evaluation. The nursing process of caring is continuous, each step occurs or reoccurs separately or simultaneously with one of the others. The nurse also must experience that someone cares about and for her so she in turn can express care for others. Caring is a continuous learning and sharing of the nurse's commitment and involvement. It is a life-long professional commitment. It does not start and stop. It cannot be turned off. It becomes her philosophy of nursing. Caring puts the personal and meaningful touch back into what has become the scientific, technical emphasis in nursing. We believe it is the heart of nursing. In pediatric nursing, to consistently care for and about the child is the true art of nursing.

Chapter 11

The therapeutic use of separation during hospitalization: an alternative to pediatric rooming-in

Maxine Rubin*

Children and parents belong to each other. The "belonging" is always legal, usually biological, and continuously emotional. To remove a child from his legal parents requires court action and to surrender a child for adoption requires the mother's and sometimes the father's consent and another court action. But whatever its quality, there is always some kind of ongoing emotional relationship between the child and his parents, whether the latter are natural, adoptive, or foster parents. Most children are born into, or soon acquire, families; it is with these children that this chapter is concerned.

The mother is the first significant "thing" the infant comes to know. The quality of his relationship with his mother affects the child's perception of himself, his mother, and ultimately his family and the world. The quality of the mother-child relationship determines the child's growth and development through the "eight ages of man" as described by Erikson.[1] Of course, the functioning of the mother and the other family members among themselves and with the child will be affected by their own developmental progress. The family is the primary socialization agent for the child. As a family member he learns what he is, how to behave, how to grow and develop, how to function within its structure, and how to perceive and behave in the world outside the family. As the infant interacts with his mother, he develops a sense of trust[1] about himself and the world around him as she meets his needs and makes him comfortable. On the basis of this sense of trust will be built the subsequent stages of development. As he develops within the family, he will imitate the behavior of its members, for they are his frame of reference as he tries on new roles, skills, and ways of coping with "life." Necessary to his growth and

____

*Written while a student in the Master of Arts program in the School of Nursing, Boston University; supported under Professional Nurse Training Grant No. 3 A11 NU0053-1383.

his imitative behavior is that he receive the stimulus in the first place, and, second, that his attempts at imitation be encouraged.

This positive growth and development of the child is postulated on a healthy mother-child relationship. Caplan[2] states:

A healthy mother-child relationship can be defined as one in which the mother reacts to the child *primarily* on the basis of her perception of the child's needs as a person in his own right, respect for those needs, and her attempts to satisfy them to the best of her ability, in line with the accepted practices of her culture and society. There are four elements, (a) perception, (b) respect, (c) satisfaction of the child's needs, and (d) the child being seen as person in his own right.*

Symonds[3] discusses the essentials of good parent-child relations. He says that the foundation is a sound, stable marriage and two good parents who had their own good and secure parents. He describes the following characteristics to be found in the parents: they have a concept of the child as "good" and show sincere love to the child for himself and not as a doer of "what is expected"; they make fair demands on the child in line with his maturity and achieve satisfaction as he grows toward independence; they are honest and straightforward, tolerant and accepting while they plan for mature growth; they are sincere, outgoing, and immediate in their emotional responses to the child, both positive and negative, while their control is firm, quiet, and consistent; they honestly share the child's pleasures and activities. A child of such parents is described as basically secure; as a socialized child who is cooperative and loyal and fits into his milieu; as honest and straightforward without guilt or deceit; and as friendly, outgoing, interested, and with good morale.

---

*By permission from Caplan, Gerald: An approach to community mental health, New York, 1961, Grune & Stratton, Inc.

Sometimes, however, children do not live and grow up within the concentric circles of a good mother-child, parent-child, family-child relationship. Bowlby, in his pioneering study, describes at great length the adverse effects on the physical and mental growth and health of " . . . children who are orphaned or separated from their families for other reasons and need care in foster homes, institutions, or other types of group care" and so experience "maternal deprivation,"[4] especially in their early years. Robertson related the maternal deprivation due to separation of the child from his mother to the behavior of children hospitalized for illness, both during the hospitalization and after discharge.[5]

Robertson[5] states that the young child has a primary need for a continuous warm relationship with his mother, which both find satisfying, and that it is a serious matter to separate a young child from his mother. He maintains that a hospitalization for illness without adequate contact with the mother creates two dangers for the child: (1) Traumatic, in which the shock of separation is associated with the pain of illness, examination, and treatment and is more than the child's immature mental structures can control. This produces feelings of insecurity and hostility toward the environment that may be lifelong. (2) Deprivational, in which the lengthy separation in a traditionally organized hospital unit causes prolonged deprivation of maternal type care and produces consequent and serious impoverishment of personality.[5] He states that as the separated child "settles in" on the hospital unit, he passes through stages of protest, in which he cries for mother, shows confusion, and rejects comfort; of despair, in which his hopeless need for mother causes him to withdraw and become apathetic; and of denial, in which he represses his feelings for mother, appears happy, and hardly seems to know his mother. The admission to the hospital of the mother with her child is stated as the optimum provision for the mental health of young children in hospitals.

On this thesis many studies have been done on the deleterious effects of hospitalization of children. Vernon[6] reviews a large number of studies and comes to several interesting conclusions.

> . . . there has been a tendency to use long separation and institutionalization as a basis for generalizations about the dire effects of such experiences. There has been little recognition of the possibility that these generalizations may not be entirely applicable to separation occasioned by short term hospitalization. Perhaps illness and pain contribute to upset and their effects should not be confused with effects of separation.*

He also questions the Bowlby-Robertson formulation that suggests that the diminution of upset in the child as he remains in the hospital is pathological in nature and reflects undesirable defensive processes; he argues that this diminution of upset may reflect positive factors such as the child's adaptive coping with experience or an improvement in health that results in fewer painful treatments. This he calls a "true adjustment hypothesis."[6]

Vernon[6] questions the reliability and validity of much of the research on separation and also the extent to which the conclusions of the research are applicable at present. In the last fifteen years many persons have become aware of the possibility that children may be upset by hospitalization. Consequently, many changes have occurred such as liberal visiting hours, programs for preparation for surgery, play rooms, and more liberal rules concerning bed rest. Much of the data he reviewed was gathered prior to the introduction of these changes. He anticipates that new data, collected in these ameliorating circumstances, might indicate hospitalization is not as traumatic as previous literature indicated.

Two other interesting points were made by Richmond and Lipton.[7] They state that it is probably not the separation per se, but rather the degree of sensory deprivation that is of significance in understanding the varied results in the literature reported as a consequence of separation. It seems reasonable to think of the continuity and quality of the experience as significant factors rather than just the separation. They also mention that mastery of separating experiences is a normal developmental task for the child as he grows. Much of his later adaptive potential depends on his capacity to deal with separating experiences. Therefore, one can have a more positive view of separation as a developmental task, and a hospitalization experience need not be seen in an entirely negative context.

In any context the hospitalization of a child is a crisis to that child and his family. The presence of an illness so severe that it cannot be treated at home by the mother is indeed threatening to her and to the family. Caplan says that the essential factor in defining a crisis is that there is an imbalance between the difficulty of the problem and the resources available to deal with it; the usual does not work and the problem cannot be avoided.[8] The mother is ineffectual and upset, since she is no longer adequate to cope with her child but must relinquish his care and safety to others. The mother feels inadequate in the face of the omnipotent and infallible hospital and feels she has somehow failed as a mother.[5] The child is frightened or at least impressed by the fact that he is ill and no longer in his home. He is faced with a variety of strangers who manipulate his body and often hurt him. He, too, has no reliable coping

---

*From Vernon, David, Foley, J. M., Sipowicz, R. R., and Schulman, J. L.: The psychological responses of children to hospitalization and illness, Springfield, Ill., 1965, Charles C Thomas, Publisher, p. 50.

mechanism to deal with the crisis as he perceives it.

Since mother and child are used to being together, since the mother has always helped her child cope by using her maternal skills of comforting and physical presence, and since being with her child to minister to his usual needs will help the mother actively participate in his care and so feel "motherly," rooming-in of mothers with their sick children or at least unlimited visiting hours seem essential to mitigate the impact of the crisis. Success of some familiar coping responses will help reduce tension. The advantages of rooming-in have been well stated by Robertson,[5] Bowlby,[4] and many others.

However, this is still a crisis situation, since the child remains ill and hospitalized. Therefore, there will be a continuation of tension and a stimulation of internal and external reserves until new behaviors are developed[8] to deal with the place and the personnel of the hospital and with the reality of the illness. Clinical experience abounds with examples of families who rise to the occasion and master the current stress.[9]

Caplan[8] lists three aspects of crisis that have particular significance to a positive outcome. (1) The resolution of the crisis depends not on antecedent factors but rather on the interplay of intrinsic and extrinsic forces in the course of the crisis. Extrinsic intervention may counteract antecedent factors and yield unexpected results, good or bad. (2) During a crisis an individual feels an increased desire for help and stimulates a helping response in others. (3) During the tension and disequilibrium of the crisis, the individual is more susceptible to influence by others so that even minor intervention can alter the resolution of the crisis.

These aspects of crisis have an enormous implication for the nurse who cares for the child in the hospital. As she cares for the child or assists the mother in providing care, she can observe and interpret their crisis-coping behavior in the mother-child interactions. The positive ways the nurse aids the mother and child to learn helping, coping behavior will surely result in healthy crisis resolution. Through her presence, her awareness, and her active participation with the mother-child unit, the nurse can influence their reduction of anxiety. Caplan states that the interpersonal action helpful in crisis coping deals with individually focused methods to ensure that the persons in crisis choose effective, reality based ways of handling their crisis tasks so that they emerge with a decreased vulnerability to mental disorder. The nurse can then help the mother and child plan actively for participation in treatment and for ongoing care after discharge. With relatively simple, but not always easy, intervention the nurse can usually help most children and parents cope with hospitalization; this is true for those who room-in and also for those who do not. With assistance from nurses most mothers can successfully room-in with their sick child if they so desire and thus prevent the stress of separation from adding to the stress of illness. A crisis situation involves both danger and opportunity.[10] While caring for hospitalized children, the nurse must seize the opportunity to eliminate the danger.

The value of pediatric rooming-in is postulated upon a healthy mother-child relationship as defined earlier. This healthy relationship is in direct contrast to

. . . an unhealthy, or potentially pathogenic relationship in which the mother perceives and reacts to her child *primarily* on the basis of her own needs, and attempts to satisfy these by means of her behavior through the child. The child is not perceived by her as a person in his own right; and even if he is occasionally so perceived, his needs are not respected; and certainly, of course, his needs are not satisfied.*

---

*By permission from Caplan, Gerald: An approach to community mental health, New York, 1961, Grune & Stratton, Inc., p. 103.

For these mothers and children pediatric rooming-in or unlimited visiting will not bring about a better adjusted child. The mother who relates to her child primarily on the basis of satisfying her own non-maternal needs, rather than on that of satisfying the needs she perceives in the child, is likely to deprive him of his essential psychological supplies and to promote unhealthy personality development in him.[8] In this crisis of illness and hospitalization she will use old, unsatisfactory coping mechanisms that will not only be ineffective for her and the child but may also be life threatening. For example, in her need to see her child as "perfect" she may deny that his symptoms exist.[11] Is the tight physical and perceptual union of this child and his rooming-in mother an authentic defense against the anxiety of illness and hospitalization or is it representative of an enduring pattern of chronic infantilism depriving the child of ego nurture? Is it constructive support to the child or pathological regressed symbiosis?[12]

Some mothers, because of their anxiety, guilt, and other attitudes associated with their child, his hospitalization, and his illness, may adversely affect his reactions to these experiences because they are incapable at present of providing him support and a sense of security.[6] They may undergo undesirable changes in behavior toward the child, becoming oversolicitous, rejecting, or inconsistent.[6] Mothers handicapped by such anxieties, guilts, and behaviors may be unable to prepare their children for admission, exercise mothering skills, or perceive the advice of the pediatrician.[11]

The child is in an emotional environment which affects him, for good or ill, every moment of the day. . . . It is often possible to change this emotional environment so that at least relief is given to the child and, under favorable conditions, even recuperation follows. An adverse emotional climate for children is often the product of emotionally handicapped parents. To bring about a change in the climate will, sometimes, involve making a break in the physical link between the child and the parents.[*]

For this reason I believe, with Rose and Sonis, that structured, nonpunitive, and participating separation of child and parent (mother) and separate assistance to each would permit the emergence of a constructive experience for both parent (mother) and child.[12]

The major point here is that the circumstances surrounding the separation are the most important factors in determining whether or not the child is deprived of the right care, rather than the separation itself.[13] The right care for a child can sometimes be most advantageously supplied apart from either of the parents. A significant fact to overcome in arriving at this conclusion is that the literature tends to treat separation and deprivation as synonymous. Howells sees this as fallacious and differentiates between the terms.[13] Separation implies being physically apart from the love object. Deprivation implies loss of parenting, the necessary care for emotional growth; this can occur with or apart from the parents. In fact, the child from an unstable home and family may find in the hospital gratification of his need to be loved and accepted that may lead to additional problems when he is returned to his family setting.[14]

When the crisis of the child's illness and hospitalization is compounded by parental inability to cope with the situation or by parentally caused deprivation, ways must be formulated in which to use separation therapeutically to reduce trauma to the child. Careful safeguards must be applied so that separation does not create additional deprivation; the separation must

---

[*]From Howells, J. G.: Child-parent separation as a therapeutic procedure, Amer. J. Psychiat. **119:** 922, April, 1963.

supply what is lacking in the mother's care. Either partial or complete separation can be used. In any case the nurse is a key member of the team who will use separation as a therapeutic measure.

The nurse is the one who has the most frequent and sustained contact with the child and his mother. Alert to their interactions and to their behavior in the various situations that occur, she may be the one to suspect the need for therapeutic separation. When the efforts of the nursing team to help the mother and child to cope with the hospitalization crisis do not bear fruit, then the skill of the entire medical and paramedical team will be enlisted to intervene. The separation must be structured, that is, partial or complete, and set within some time limits. The separation must be presented to and perceived by the mother and the child as nonpunitive; they must have some participation in the arrangements or else their anxiety and hostility will preclude positive results. And, most importantly, both the mother and the child must have separate assistance so that the separation will have constructive results.

Perhaps the nurse, who is already known to him, is the best one to provide support to the child. She can provide him with media for guided play, with explanation and support during treatments and procedures, with company during meals, with guidance in appropriate behavior in the ward situation, and with the reassurance of her concerned presence at "difficult" hours such as bedtime.

I do not believe that the same nurse who works intensively with the child should also be primarily involved in assisting the mother. Perhaps it would be best if no nurse from the unit was *actively* involved with the mother *at this time*. The anxious and struggling ego of the mother might respond more easily to the help of someone not engaged in the current daily care of her child. The social worker might be the best choice to help the mother in

the crisis. At this time the mother might interpret extra time spent with her by the child's nurse or doctor as depriving the child of their time and care. Because of her own needs she may respond best with someone who is "all her own."

As the mother's reality view of her child and of the crisis situation develops, she will gradually spend more time with him. Guided contact with the child will help her to see his new functioning and to test her new modes of behavior. At all times the attitude of the team must actively communicate that the child and the mother belong to each other and that the team is simply trying to help them to be more successful and happy when together.

There are several other times when limitation of visiting is appropriate, even desirable. It is in the nature of the mother-child relationship that both are more relaxed when they are not together constantly. Mother and child need to be helped to "take a break." There are times when a mother needs to feel that limited visiting hours are a regular and accepted thing; otherwise she will be torn between her desire to stay and the knowledge that the rest of her family needs her at home.[15] Adolescents, whose developmental task it is to establish independence, need help in interpreting this to overprotective mothers.

Finally, the exhausted mother needs help to go home for a rest away from the constant demands of her ill child. I take umbrage as a mother, a nurse, and a human being each time I read Spence's[40] oft-quoted statements regarding the advantages of a mother rooming-in with her hospitalized child:

She needs little or no off-duty time, because the sleep requirements of a mother fall to near zero when her child is acutely ill.*

---

*From Spence, James C.: The care of children in hospitals, Brit. Med. J. 1:125, 1947.

Obviously Sir James has never spent several days without sleep in an attempt to comfort his own sick child. It is physically and emotionally exhausting. Mothers need the support and encouragement of nurses so that they can leave their children to get proper rest. Only then will the mothers be able to continue to adequately and positively care for their children.

Most children have relatively healthy relationships with their mothers. Rooming-in during hospitalization or at least unlimited visiting, with support and help from the nurse, will help these children and their mothers grow during the crisis of illness and hospitalization. Exceptions to the rule indicate that separation of a special type may be necessary in order for the experience to provide growth. Planned separation does allow for exceptions—that all children are not better off with their own parent(s). A structured and realistic separation is not inevitably traumatic; separation is available as a relieving and therapeutic tool.

References

1. Erikson, Erik: Childhood and society, New York, 1963, W. W. Norton & Co.
2. Caplan, Gerald: An approach to community mental health, New York, 1961, Grune & Stratton, Inc.
3. Symonds, Percival M.: The dynamics of parent-child relationships, New York, 1949, Bureau of Publications, Teachers College, Columbia University.
4. Bowlby, John: Maternal care and mental health, Geneva, 1952, World Health Organization.
5. Robertson, James: Young children in hospitals, New York, 1958, Basic Books, Inc., Publishers.
6. Vernon, David, Foley, J. M., Sipowicz, R. R., and Schulman, J. L.: The psychological responses of children to hospitalization and illness, Springfield, Ill., 1965, Charles C Thomas, Publisher.
7. Richmond, Julius B., and Lipton, Earle L.: Studies on mental health of children with specific implication for pediatricians. In Caplan, Gerald, editor: Prevention of mental disorders in children, New York, 1961, Basic Books, Inc., Publishers.
8. Caplan, Gerald: Principles of preventive psychiatry, New York, 1964, Basic Books, Inc., Publishers.
9. Parad, Howard J., and Caplan, Gerald: A framework for studying families in crisis. In Parad, Howard J., editor: Crisis intervention, New York, 1965, Family Service Association of America.
10. Caplan, Gerald: Emotional problems of early childhood, New York, 1955, Basic Books, Inc., Publishers.
11. Lewis, Melvin: The management of parents of acutely ill children in the hospital, Amer. J. Orthopsychiat. 32:60, 1962.
12. Rose, John, and Sonis, Meyer: The use of separation as a diagnostic measure in the parent-child emotional crisis, Amer. J. Psychiat. 116:409, 1959.
13. Howells, J. G.: Child-parent separation as a therapeutic procedure, Amer. J. Psychiat. 119:922, 1963.
14. Blom, Gaston E.: The reactions of hospitalized children to illness, Pediatrics 22:590, 1958.
15. Baty, James, and Tisza, Veronica: The impact of illness on the child and his family, Child Study 34:14, 1956.
16. Spence, James C.: The care of children in hospitals, Brit. Med. J. 1:125, 1947.

Bibliography

Aubuchon, Marie: To stay or not to stay—parents are the question, Hosp. Prog. 39:170-177, May, 1958.

Fagin, Claire M.: Pediatric rooming-in: its meaning for the nurse, Nurs. Clin. N. Amer. 1:83, March, 1966.

Faust, O. A.: Stop scaring the children, Mod. Hosp. 80:94-96, May, 1953.

Heavenrich, Richard: Viewpoint on children in hospitals, Hospitals 37:40, May 16, 1963.

Henning, Emilie: Crisis intervention theory applied to nursing. In Clark, Ann, et al., editors: Parent-child relations: role of the nurse, New Brunswick, N. J., 1968, Rutgers, the State University of New Jersey.

Irvine, Elizabeth E.: Children at risk. In Parad, Howard J. editor: Crisis intervention, New York, 1965, Family Service Association of America.

Roy, Sister M. C.: Role cues and mothers of hospitalized children, Nurs. Res. 16:178-182, Spring, 1967.

Smith, Margo: Ego support for the child patient, Amer. J. Nurs. 63:90-95, Oct., 1963.

Chapter 12

Black child—white nurse: a nursing challenge and privilege

Ruth E. Redmann

A black child's experience in a hospital can be one in which he gains increased self-esteem and pride in himself as a black child. Nursing ministrations can be instrumental in helping him achieve this goal. To help a black child acquire increased self-respect during a hospital experience is no easy task for the nurse, but with inner motivation it can be accomplished. It requires readiness on the part of the nurse to increase her knowledge of the commonalities and differences in the physical and psychosocial characteristics of each black child she encounters. It also requires willingness on the part of the nurse to explore deeply and forthrightly her own feelings, misconceptions, prejudices, and stereotyped thinking not only about black people but also about each black child and his family. Then she needs to probe deeply and honestly into all the emotional and intellectual responses she has as she ministers to each of the family members. Lastly, she needs motivation to change those behaviors that prevent her from delivering the best possible nursing services to black children and their families.

A dark skin may not be the only characteristic of the black American that evokes prejudiced and derogatory responses from white Americans. Yet it is the characteristic that can by its sole presence so effect the life of a child that he thinks less of himself because he is dark skinned.

Admittedly, recent socioeconomic and legislative trends directed toward lessening the subsidiary roles of black people in our society will aid in changing the self-concept of black children from that of dislike of black skin to that of acceptance and pride in their skin color. But it will take time and emotional reeducation for the goal to be reached. Meanwhile pediatric nurses have the opportunity, privilege, and responsibility to modify the hospital environment in the particular ways necessary to enable each black child to master feelings aroused by threatening situations. Then he can emerge from the experience with strengthened inner resources. Implied in this concept is respect for and admiration of the uniqueness of each person. When attitudes of this kind exist in white nurses, appropriate environmental modifications will be made and the black child will feel loved for what he is. Communication of such attitudes in all that is said and done for and with a black child strengthens his capacity to cope with threats from within or from a strange world.

Health statistics demonstrate that children of low-income black families have many unmet health needs. When resources for the care of all children are expanded as they need to be, it can be expected that pediatric wards will become even more populated with black children who are suffering from chronic and long-term illnesses. Within the hospital milieu changes in self-concepts can be wrought by the ways in which nurses work with the black child and his family. To bring about this change nurses need to be cognizant of the strengths and limitations all members of the family bring to the experience and the way in which they view the white environment of the hospital and its white inhabitants. Nurses also need to be aware of their own perceptions of the black child and his family. They need to recognize the reciprocal effects that these subtle factors may have on the child's, his parents, and the nurse's behavior.

Black children's feelings about being black

As each young black child develops, he discovers through a variety of experiences that to have dark skin is to be different from the majority of people living in the United States. At what age awareness of racial characteristics most frequently occurs and what other feelings the child develops concerning his minority membership have been studied by many investigators.

It is generally agreed that the ability to identify black and white racial characteristics occurs as early as the age of 3 years.[1-4] What is of more crucial value is the realization that children are developing racial preference and racial rejection during this same preschool period of development. Clark and Clark[1] found direct evidence of this when they asked these questions of 253 2- to 7-year-old black children: "Which doll looks nice?" "Which doll looks bad?" "Which doll is a nice color?" The majority of the children picked the white doll as the one who "looked nice" and had a "nice color" and chose the black doll as the one who "looked bad." Further evidence of racial preference and rejection is provided by Clark and Clark who gave 160 black subjects ages 5, 6, and 7 a coloring-task procedure. In the second part of the experiment, the children were given the usual assortment of crayons and asked to color the little boy or girl the color they like boys or girls to be. While 48% of the 160 black children colored the child brown or black, 36% colored him white or yellow. The remaining children made bizarre responses to the task.

The above data suggest that many black children, although able to identify their racial characteristics correctly at this early age, show a clear preference for white skin color. The child thus identifies with that which he rejects. He is what he would rather not be; he would rather be what he is not. The child who feels repulsion for his own race actually feels repulsion for himself. Although the child, as he grows older, identifies less with the white race and rejects his own race less, these conflicting feelings have become implanted in his basic personality structure.[2] They can breed subsequent feelings of inadequacy, ambivalence, and self-doubt.

The child's self-concept arises not only from the way he perceives himself but also from his perception of the way others see him. The black child who is ill, and must also simultaneously face a white hospital world, is extremely vulnerable to the responses of others to him. Such a position provides the white nurse with the opportunity to provide experiences in which his feelings of worth about himself as a black child can increase in positiveness through his perceptions of her perceptions of him.

Black children's perceptions of hospital experiences

For many black children admission to the hospital can be their first encounter with a predominantly white environment. The doctors and nurses wear white uniforms. The linen is white, the walls in many institutions are white, but, and not of least importance, the majority of the personnel are white skinned. The aseptic-looking hospital environment partially evolved from scientific advances in bacteriology and microbiology. It can be surmised that in an effort to accentuate to the public that the hospital environment and personnel were clean and safe, white became the color of choice. There are institutions that have changed their policy and permit personnel in pediatric units to wear multicolored uniforms. Although this may be of benefit to all children, it may be of greatest benefit to black children. To the black child who has already been enculturated to the "rightness of whiteness," the traditional white hospital environment can accentuate what he has already learned, that is, to be white is to be pure, angelic, clean, and free of germs; to be black is to be dirty, germ laden, infected, and sinful.[5]

Another factor that may contribute to the black child's fear of the hospital is the preponderance of white nurses and doctors. In homes and neighborhoods black children learn that "white people can hurt you." Such indoctrination causes black children to acquire a fear of white people. Those children who are reared in the ghetto may have had few or no direct associations with white people wherein their pain inflicting or helpful qualities could be determined realistically by the child. If this is the case, entrance into the hospital burdens the black child with an additional stress. He not only has to deal with the stresses that are common to all children—illness, intrusive procedures, pain, separation from his home, peers, or family, and the gratification which they provide—but he must also concern himself with the fear of white people and what they might do to him. In many instances it will be white nurses or doctors who will give him unpalatable medications, painful injections, and frightening tests and treatments. He may believe that each treatment given by the white nurse or doctor is leading to his ultimate destruction Under such circumstances feelings of fear and aggression may overtax his coping capacities and overwhelm him with anxiety.

The black employees in the pediatric ward may present an added dilemma to the black child. He may notice that the black workers are most frequently the persons who do the menial tasks; they are janitors, nurse's aides, maids, etc. They hold positions of low status in the hospital hierarchy; they receive their orders from white employees who rank above them in position and in the respect afforded them. Observations of this kind cannot help but influence the child's perception of the status of black people in the hospital. Such perceptions will not only influence his feelings about the status of black people in our society, but they may also reduce his self-confidence and increase his apprehension about his own position as a patient in the ward.

Every child in the hospital suffers from a loss of familiar and satisfying experiences. He is also confronted with the task of trying to understand and to cope with a new world that includes a host of strange activities, people, and equipment. The economically deprived black child's problems may be greater in magnitude because what he has known at home has less similarity to what he meets in the hospital. The eating, sleeping, and play routines that he enjoyed at home may be vastly different from those in the hospital. The preparation of food and the way it is served, a bath in a tub alone, as well as sleeping alone in a single room may break all the customs that have become familiar and comfortable. The vocabulary and pronunciation of hospital personnel may strike his ears as peculiar or foreign. The amount and type of stimulation the poverty stricken black child receives in his home is in vivid contrast to that which he receives in the hospital. Periods of silence may be painful for him; crying children may upset him, and the play materials and activities provided in the ward may be completely strange to him. If this child loses most of what is familiar to him and is confronted with a host of situations that are new and strange, he cannot help but be grief-stricken and fearful; his losses are great and a multitude of fear-provoking unknowns have replaced that which was familiar. Supporting him in the expression of sorrow and reduction of fear is imperative to conserve his energy for recuperation and for coping with threatening new experiences. To accomplish this goal the black child, like any other child, needs to learn that his caretakers will accept his unique way of expressing sorrow and fear and will provide the supportive nursing measures he requires to cope with his feelings and new experiences.

The black child who is unable to trust his white nurse to respond to his needs may be burdened with grief and fears throughout his hospitalization. He may believe that his expression of grief and fear could cause her to harm him. Such a misperception can frustrate a child's need to grieve and to overcome his fear by talking with an understanding person and by having opportunities to learn, through exploration, that his environment is less destructive than he imagined it to be.

The ill child who learns to trust in his caretakers quickly and who is able to al-low himself to be dependent on them will have more energy to invest in the healing process and in coping with all the other problems that he faces when hospitalized. Only a hypothesis can be made about the amount of energy a black child might utilize to his disadvantage before learning to trust a white nurse. To conserve his energy the black child needs to learn that a white nurse will not hurt him unnecessarily, that she sincerely desires to be helpful and comforting to him, and that he can depend on her to meet his needs for gratification as well as to help him tolerate all the frustrations he must bear to reach a higher level of health. When painful treatments are necessary, he needs to know the real purpose of the treatment and be encouraged to vent his feelings about it. Unless he vents his feelings forthrightly, he may never learn that treatments are healing measures and not retaliatory attacks, and that open expression of feeling is justifiable, acceptable, and helpful to him.

Black children's responses to white nurses

If a black child believes that white nurses wish him harm, he may exhibit behaviors that are a deterrent not only to developing relationships with nurses but also to his ability to learn to cope with new experiences in a realistic and growth-producing manner. To lessen the stimuli with which he has to deal, the black child may try to control his environment by withdrawing from it. He remains silent when approached and his motility may be limited to careful, slow movements while his gaze is ever watchful. He behaves as if he were trying hard to camouflage his very presence in the ward. At a time when his energy supply is depleted from illness, he may expend what surplus energy he has available to him in maintaining rigid control of his feelings.

A child who is unable to maintain such

strict control of his turbulent emotions may deal with his feelings with angry, acting-out behavior. With a feeling of being "cornered" and unable to take flight, he resorts to fighting the white nurses. He may fight with shouted angry directives, temper-tantrum-like behavior, and retaliative retorts. These behaviors are indicative of his attempts to control his environment—to ward off the destructiveness he feels is embodied in the white nurse. They communicate the level of his fear and anxiety and are a cry for help.

Prior to the renewed efforts to give the black man the same rights as white Americans, it was not unusual to note compliant, polite behavior in black youngsters. Instances of this response are still in evidence today. Nurses' questions are answered with "Yes, M'am" or "No, M'am." The child who utilizes this mode of dealing with the questions posed to him has denied his angry feelings toward whites or is too frightened to express them or even to try to communicate his thoughts to others. He behaves in ways that he believes are most acceptable to those people whom he thinks discredit him. In this way he attempts to ward off real or imagined hostility toward him, but in the process, he dissipates, in nonconstructive defensive behavior, some of his energy that would otherwise be available for the healing process. This behavior also prevents the reception of pleasure that is derived from verbal communications with others. Unless white nurses can prove the sincerity of their wish to be helpful by staying close by to identify signals of need from nonverbal behavior and to provide physical care and emotional support when he needs it, they will be deprived of the pleasure that comes from helping children overcome their fear of them. Increased verbal communication of feelings and needs manifests a decreasing fear of people; if this communication can be sustained, the development of satisfying and growth-producing relationships may result for both children and nurses.

White nurses' responses to black children

White nurses can communicate to children and to hospital personnel with both words and deeds their false generalizations, stereotyped thinking, attitudes, feelings, and selective perceptions about black Americans. Each nurse develops a characteristic style of dealing with situations that are unfamiliar or threatening to her in some particular way. Care of the black child and working with his parents is an example of a situation that, if threatening, will call into play the nurse's individualized style of dealing with stressful events.

There are nurses who use avoidance to deal with new or threatening situations. The lack of actual touch of the child may evidence avoidance, or the nurse's response to him may be as overt as to avoid entering his room except when duty demands. Her avoidance response may emanate from feelings that make her perceive the child with black skin as unclean, dirty, and infected. She may even feel that "it will rub off on her." Evidence to support this assumption is the frequency with which the author has heard inexperienced students or young graduates in their first experience in caring for black persons make such statements as: "I washed him twice and the washcloth still looks dirty the second time."

Other instances of avoidance are exemplified by the nurse who can accept the child but not his family. Black adults may arouse fear in her due to feelings of repulsion, feelings that make her perceive black adults as inferior to white people, unintelligent, and consequently unworthy of the time she usually spends conferring with parents. "They wouldn't understand what I was talking about!" was one remark which was overheard when the author observed the undergraduate students talking together. The second nurse's response was equally derogatory as she said, "I sure don't understand their lingo either."

Failure to invest energy in learning to understand the speech patterns of the black person is one more covert, rationalized way of avoiding the child and his family. This question arises: Would the same avoidance be practiced as frequently if the child were Italian, German, or French? The individual needs of the child and family are not adequately met when verbal communication is ignored. Clear pronunciation and range of vocabulary are often less well developed in the black ghetto–reared youngster. Avoiding verbal communication with the child and his family reduces their self-esteem and prevents nurses from collecting the data they need to be of real help to them.

In so many ways false generalizations about black people are made that decrease the nurse's ability to fulfill the health needs of the growing individual. This comment said in a debasing tone, was heard by the author, "I can't even tell those two kids apart. They're just black kids to me. And all black kids look alike!" They illustrate one nurse's unreadiness to differentiate between the physical characteristics of two children. Since she was the nurse who was assigned to them, it is doubtful that services to them consisted of more than the most routinized kind of nursing care.

There are other nurses whose characteristic style of dealing with new or threatening situations is to respond to them and the persons involved with hostility. Hostility may be overtly expressed by isolating a black child in a room by himself when other rooms housing children of his own age have vacant beds. Judgmental comments are often made more frequently about black families. Clearly recalled are the comments of two nurses as they watched the arrival of a black mother and child. "Just look at the way she's dressed —and the way she dresses that kid! I wish I could afford to dress like that!" Closer scrutiny would have shown those nurses that although the style was mod, the clothing was of an inexpensive quality. Since the author had made several home visits to this family prior to the child's second admission, she was aware that the boy was dressed in his best outfit and the dress on the mother was one of the few she owned. (They were dressed in their finest because they wanted to look their best when coming to the hospital.) Equally judgmental comments are made when black or poor people are dressed slovenly. "Soap and water is cheap" is a commonly heard remark in pediatric clinics and wards. It would seem that these people are chastised if they do and if they do not dress well.

Nurses may also overprotect as a means of alleviating their discomfort when nursing of the black child presents a new or threatening situation to them. Deeply buried in their unconscious may lie feelings of the uncleanliness and unworthiness of blacks or of feelings of fear that the blacks are evil and will hurt them in some way. The nurse's intellect may tell her that there is no rational basis for these feelings and that white people share the responsibility for thwarting black citizens in their struggle to develop optimally in our society. In an effort to eradicate her guilt and deny her irrational feelings the white nurse may overprotect the hospitalized black child. This response may be evidenced by overfondling of the child, or the inability of the nurse to set limits that the child needs to feel secure and to learn to meet the expectations of his new world. Or it may be reflected by inconsistent responses to the child's demands. An example of overprotectiveness in the care of the black child was observed recently when a 2-year-old girl was admitted to the ward. During the child's four-day stay in the hospital, she was continually held and fondled by various white nurses. When her mother was there she walked and played in the halls and playroom.

The child and his parents quickly recognize ambivalence when it exists in the nurse's feelings about them and their child. One black mother's preparation of her young boy for his pending hospitalization demonstrated awareness of the overprotectiveness she had seen in some nurses. She prepared him for it this way: "The white people in the hospital will pat you on the head a lot and want to cuddle you in their laps. They just don't stop to think how it makes you feel." The mother expressed to the author the feelings that these were degrading gestures; she said that they reminded her of the way people respond to puppies.

True acceptance of the black child and family is evidenced in the behavioral responses of many nurses. Although the situation presenting itself may be new or even threatening to them, they respond with respect for and sensitivity to black youngsters' common human needs and the particular ways in which they seek gratification of them. They are aware that this family brings to the situation their unique genetic endowment, cultural background, and life experiences as does any other family. The following vignette is a composite of nursing behaviors perceived by the author to be some of those that are an expression of sincere acceptance of black people. It includes examples of nursing behaviors that could enhance the black child's acceptance of himself and his black heritage.

Darryl, age 4, was admitted to the hospital for surgical removal of scars and keloid formations acquired from burns on his face and neck when he was 3 years of age. It was his second experience in a hospital where the population of the pediatric ward averaged a high percentage of black children. The nurses in this hospital had sought assistance many times to learn about the beliefs, value systems, and social practices of members of the black race living in the area. Ward conferences and in-service programs initiated by staff nurses had increased their understanding of the children and families in their care. Scheduled conferences with a resident in psychiatry pertaining to children who presented nursing problems to the staff were utilized to explore nurses' feelings and responses to black patients.

On his second admission, Darryl, clasping his mother's hand, pulled her out of the elevator toward the nurse's station. Upon reaching it, he held his slender, tall body erect, searched expectantly for a familiar face and called out above the din of the busy ward, "Hi, Nurses!" Three white-capped heads turned and returned his greeting with smiles of welcome. Darryl's behavior suggested that his previous hospital experience had helped him to master many of the trials and tribulations that had confronted him then. Certainly his familiarity with the people, the environment, and the procedures lessened the unknowns and, hence, his fears. Additionally, his hand was held tightly to a great source of security for Darryl—his mother.

With the admission procedure completed, Darryl's nurse brought forth the surprise she had promised him on her last home visit. It was a case of toys that had been especially prepared for him. The case contained the usual paints, crayons, paper, scissors, playdough, clay, and family figures. The nurse had added to it those items that she felt would be most appropriate for Darryl to use at 4 years of age, as a member of the black race, and as a child about to have plastic surgery performed on his chin and neck. These items of play material included black family figures of the number and size of his own family, cars and trucks, figures of a nurse and doctor, an intravenous bottle, tubing, and needle, bandages and tape, several sizes of sandbags, various sizes of syringes and needles, stethoscope, anesthesia mask, and rubber dolls both black and white.

With excitement, Darryl opened the case and quickly examined each item of play material while removing it from the case to the floor beside him. During the play period Darryl gave the white nurse and doctor figures injections; he taped the intravenous needle to the black doll's arm, gave it an injection, and listened to its heart as well as to his nurse's and mother's heart with the stethoscope. Initially his eyes frequently sought his mother's face when he handled the syringe. He acted as if he were seeking her permission to play with such dangerous instruments. However, after he had gently stuck the doll three or four times with the needle, his movements became swifter and more aggressive. He stabbed both rubber dolls. His nurse also wondered if he were seeking permission to exhibit angry, aggressive behavior.

The play session was interrupted by the arrival of the intern and resident who explained that they wanted to do a physical examination of Darryl. They turned to Darryl and listened as his nurse explained exactly what the doctors would do. Swiftly Darryl disposed of his shirt and extended his bare chest toward them. When the doctors had finished examining him, Darryl said matter-of-factly, "I listen yo' heart now!" He proceeded to do so much to the delight of the intern and resident. Darryl completed his examination of their hearts. Then he used the flashlight and tongue blades in appropriate doctorlike fashion to examine each of their throats.

Later that same evening, before Darryl's mother made preparations to leave, he sought the help he needed, "Yo' get my toy box, nurse? Yo' stay 'n play with me?" While Darryl fingered the various play materials, his nurse prepared a neck and chin bandage for the black doll. She handled the doll gently as she explained in a quiet, steady voice what she was doing and her reasons for it. Her tone of voice and her touch communicated sym-

pathy and understanding. Darryl watched all of her movements closely; he listened intently. "Dat doll's gonna cry!" he blurted out his warning. His nurse took his cue, reassured the doll, and gave it permission to cry. Simultaneously her arm encircled the doll's head as her empathic mutterings continued: "It hurts to have those bandages on and to have an operation. It's frightening to many boys and girls. The hurt will go away. Each day it will feel better!" The nurse's glance toward Darryl assured her that he sensed her understanding; his furrowed brow and intense gaze softened as his muscles relaxed. Then slowly and carefully Darryl placed sandbags around the head of the doll. He had learned from past experience that head immobilization was required for healing.

When his mother informed him that she was leaving and would be back before he went to the operating room in the morning, Darryl's tightened lips emitted muted sobs. It was as if he were fighting with all his strength to keep his feelings under control. His mother reassured Darryl of her return and added, "Your nurse will stay with you until bedtime." Darryl's mother was asked to wave from the front walk of the hospital as she left. The purpose was twofold. Not only would waving to her from a distance aid Darryl in mastering his feelings about separation, but it would also give his nurse a chance to touch and hold this child so he could view his mother. By so doing his nurse hoped that she could provide him with the comfort of her touch and help him to know that it was available to him if he felt a need for it. His body remained rigid in her arms as he waved and yelled "goodbye" to his mother. He shouted imperatively: "Yo' come back 'fore surgery, Mama!" She assured him that she would. Then he pushed away from the nurse as he said, "Yo' stay 'n play wi' me?" The need to control his feelings, not to cry, appeared important to Darryl. Perhaps the body contact with the nurse tempted him to cry or perhaps the body contact with a white nurse was frightening to him.

A preoperative pHisoHex bath was necessary that evening. In simple, short phrases, the procedure and its purpose were described to Darryl. He walked with his nurse as he helped her collect the soap and pajamas. He controlled the faucets to fill the tub and added the pHiso-Hex. The toys the nurse brought from the toy box consisted of one syringe, the doctor and nurse figures, and the black doll. Darryl bathed himself proudly and smiled as his nurse complimented him about his ability to do so. She took advantage of the opportunity to demonstrate her concern for the care of his body by washing his back. While doing so she was aware that the soft brown of his skin was caused by the amount of melanin manufactured by the epidermal cells; she was also aware that epidermal cells desquamate constantly and that desquamated cells can color washcloths. The bath ended after Darryl had held the floatable figures of the nurse and doctor under water several times and after he had washed the rubber doll vigorously. Darryl dried and dressed himself. When handed the hairbrush, he pulled a chair in front of the mirror, climbed to a standing position, and tried in vain to brush his hair into Afro style. "Yo' fix it, nurse. Fix it like Jeff's!" he said. (Jeff, his teen-age brother, wore his hair in Afro style and Darryl sincerely admired Jeff's hairdo.) Darryl's short curled hair could barely be brushed up. His nurse explained that his hair would have to grow longer and that it would do so as he grew.

Two children's books, both of which had illustrations of children of many races, were read to Darryl before he relaxed and slept. Four times before falling asleep he repeated, "Yo' goin' be here when I go to surgery. Yo' goin' with me to surgery."

The nurse's knowledge of Darryl's needs which were the outgrowth of his developmental level, of his pending operation, and of his racial characteristics, was utilized in her nursing interventions. The availability of toys and books that were of interest to black children provided more opportunities for the expression of feelings. The nurse's familiarity with Afro hair style and her capacity to understand the speech of black children and the physiologic cause of skin coloring were evident in her interactions with him. As a consequence of her understanding, Darryl's behavior demonstrated that a helping relationship had begun to be established. Such a relationship between a black child and a white nurse provides the medium through which a child gains increased feelings of pride and self-worth.

References

1. Clark, K. B., and Clark, M. P.: Racial identification and preference in Negro children. In Newcomb, T. M., and Hartley, E. L., editors: Readings in social psychology, New York, 1947, Holt, Rinehart & Winston, Inc.
2. Stevenson, H. W., and Stewart, E. C.: A developmental study of racial awareness in young children, Child Develop. 29:399-410, 1958.
3. Moreland, J. K.: Racial recognition by nursery school children in Lynchburg, Virginia, Social Forces 37:132-137, 1958.
4. Goodman, M. E.: Race awareness in young children, New York, 1965, The Macmillan Co.
5. Citron, A. F.: Rightness of whiteness, Detroit, 1969, Michigan-Ohio Regional Educational Laboratory (pamphlet).

Bibliography

Blake, F. G., Wright, F. H., and Waechter, E. H.: Nursing care of children, Philadelphia, 1970, J. B. Lippincott Co.
Brink, W., and Harris, L.: The Negro revolution in America, New York, 1964, Simon and Schuster, Inc., Publishers.
Deutsch, M., Katz, I., and Jensen, A. R.: Social class, race, and psychological development, New York, 1968, Holt, Rinehart & Winston, Inc.
Miel, A., with Kiester, E.: The shortchanged children of suburbia, New York, 1967, Institute of Human Relations Press (pamphlet).

Eugenia H. Waechter

Chapter *13*

The responses of children to fatal illness

Anger, fear, anxiety, and depression are expected emotions in adults who are faced with life-threatening illnesses. Such emotions are far less commonly anticipated in children who are so threatened. Since children seldom have opportunities to discuss their diagnoses and prognoses, due to parental and professional efforts to protect them from such knowledge, it is often assumed that they cannot know what is occurring within their bodies and are unperceptive to the changes in their environments that herald the onset or progression of their illnesses. It is also frequently assumed that the defense of denial effectively insulates against suspicions that may be aroused from clues the child receives from within his body or from alterations in parental behavior.

During the preschool years most children have encountered death, and by the age of 8 or 9 years they have learned that ultimately everyone must die. Although a mature concept of death is rare before the age of 9, anxiety related to death may begin as early as 3 years of age in the well child, and during the late preschool and early school years most children are deeply concerned with attempts to comprehend cessation of life. They are also frequently fearful and anxious regarding the possibility of loss of those whom they love and on whom they must depend, or of their own eventual demise. Many magical practices may arise to reduce such anxiety.

The need and efforts of children to work through their concerns related to death by play or ritual burials, singly or in peer groups, has been influenced by the decided change in cultural attitudes toward death that have evolved in America during this century. Prudery has shifted from disgust with the natural processes of reproduction to disgust with the corruption and decay of death.

Our culture has been historically future oriented. In the framework of the Protestant ethic and of frontier experience, the subordination of the present for future goals was underlined as an American ideal. This was upheld by the religious orientation that stressed preparation for the future and of a life after death as the transcendent goal. In the future-oriented tradition also, America learned to admire young and youthful energy and vigor, thus providing the basis for the child-centered family unit of the present middle class.

The child also has been enculturated

with the death taboo in the socialization process and has learned through many small encounters that this topic elicits evasion from adults and is surrounded by a special aura of anxiety. Thus, he is unlikely to initiate conversations related to this topic. In addition, from infancy onward he is imbued with the value of mature behavior and receives pressure to avoid whining, complaining, or weeping when physically hurt or frightened regarding the environment or future.

Hospitalization produces a discontinuity, often accompanied with fear and pain, which makes experiences unforgettable, and underlines cultural values and attitudes communicated to the child by professional personnel. In this atmosphere the child may feel vulnerable and sensitive to unconscious motivations transmitted to him by those with whom he comes in contact.

When a child is hospitalized for a fatal illness, the nurse has grave responsibilities because she is a constant figure in the environment of the child. Unless she is perceptive, knowledgeable, and empathetic, she may imply expectations regarding the avoidance of painful topics of conversation and orientation to the future. Under such conditions, children with long-term illnesses and poor prognoses may not directly express fears for the future, anxiety, or anger at what is occurring within their bodies and may hesitate to question the changes they perceive in their environments.

The problem, purpose, and methodology of the study

Observation has indicated that circumstances of death and dying are often circumvented by professional personnel, themselves products of the culture and imbued with the death taboo in the socialization process. This results in progressive lessening of involvement and contacts with a child as his condition becomes terminal. The nature of the profession is dedicated to the preservation of life so that death can be seen as a professional challenge and a failure. When children between the ages of 6 and 10 years who are hospitalized with conditions for which death is predicted are studied, many of them demonstrate symptoms of depression, withdrawal, or anxiety that are proportionately greater than those indicated by children with good prognoses, but with similar physical functioning.

As an educational problem this issue has also become pressing. The education of the nurse is primarily concerned with illness and health, life and death. Teachers of pediatric nurses are becoming aware of the difficulties involved in helping students to work with dying children and in assisting them to understand and to cope with their own anxieties. The importance of the problem concerns not only the current responsibilities of the nurse, but also her future sense of competency and confidence when faced with similar situations.

The problem involves several questions. What factors lie behind the behaviors and anxieties of adults in the face of death? Although children are rarely specifically told of their imminent deaths, do adults, in fact, communicate this anxiety to children in nonverbal ways, thus arousing fear in the child that is demonstrated by the observed behavior? Lastly, if the answer to the second question is positive, is this death anxiety present in the school-aged child and can it be measured or demonstrated through use of available psychological techniques?

In order to study this problem 64 children, between the ages of 6 and 10 years inclusive, were studied. The sample included four categories of children: (1) children with chronic diseases for which death was predicted, (2) children with chronic diseases where early death was not anticipated, (3) children hospitalized

Table 1. Projective test pictures

Code	Description	Source
Form A	Two boys in adjoining beds	Designed for the study
Form B	Small child in hallway outside closed door to ICU	Designed for the study
Form C	Boy in front of mural depicting operation	TAT* 8 BM
Form D	Small child in bed, nurse nearby with back turned	Designed for the study
Form E	Figure outlined in open window	TAT 14
Form F	Child in bed, parents and doctor outside door	Designed for the study
Form G	Woman entering room, hand on face .	TAT 3 GF
Form H	Small child sitting in doorway of cabin	TAT 13 B

*Thematic apperception test.

with minor illnesses or conditions, and (4) normal, well children. The children in all groups were matched on the basis of age, sex, social class, and family background.

The major instrument of the study was a projective test administered to each child in the study. This test consisted of eight pictures that were shown to the children individually. The experimenter asked each child to tell a story based on the clues he perceived in the picture, including what he saw as occurring, the thoughts and feelings of the characters, and the events preceding and following the scene depicted in the presented picture. Four of these pictures were designed for this study and included more clues relating to hospitalization and four were selected from the thematic apperception test in which clues were more vague. Table 1 describes the pictures utilized and their source.

The stories told by the children were later scored independently by two judges. No interpretation was attempted, and only actual statements made by the children were examined for content relating to fantasy expression of anxiety regarding present or future body integrity and functioning, the manner in which the characters in the story coped with threat, and the feelings expressed throughout the stories.

In addition, each hospitalized child in the study answered a questionnaire which measured anxiety in aspects of everyday living.[1] This test, termed "the general anxiety scale for children," was not specifically aimed toward measuring fear relating to body functioning and was administered to determine whether a child who is fearful of the future also has a higher level of anxiety in many aspects of current life experiences.

Since it was felt that such variables as previous experiences with death, amount and manner of religious education, the warmth of the mother-child relationship, and the relative opportunities the child had been given to discuss his concerns may well affect the child's responses, a tape-recorded interview was held with one or both parents of each hospitalized child to elicit this information. These interviews were also scored independently by two judges, based on rating scales that were developed to assess and code the information received.

Results

Since no inter-judge decisions were required in determining the score on the general anxiety scale for children, a simple check of computations was done. Previous standardization of the test with normal, well children resulted in a mean score of 12.00. In this study the mean score for the children within the fatal group was 36.50, whereas children in the chronic group had a mean score of 18.56 and children with brief illness had a mean score of 19.44. These findings suggest that the anxiety of children with a fatal illness may also be expressed in areas of living not associated with hospitalization. This is understandable in terms of generalization of uncertainty and fear; a spreading of insecurity into areas where the child may have had little discomfort previously.

The insignificant differences between the two hospitalized groups with nonfatal illnesses led to the speculation that although the children with chronic illnesses had been under stress for a longer period of time, knowledge and experience with hospital routine and with professional personnel may have provided a sense of competency and mastery that lessens anxiety to some extent.

Concern regarding death as related to previous experience

Interviews with parents were conducted on the ward during their child's hospitalization and provided parents with an opportunity to discuss their feelings and concerns, both about hospital practices and about the prognosis of their child. Many parents indicated their intense need for understanding and support while undergoing this poignant, frightening, and chronically stressful experience.

Effects of religious education

In assessing the effects of religious education that the child had received, it became evident that such experience, while not lessening appreciably the amount of anxiety expressed, did affect the *meaning* of death to the children in this study. A concept of immortality implies departure to another world rather than complete cessation of existence. It had previously been speculated that children who had been taught that hell is the final destination of sinners may suffer a greater fear of death as a result of a sense of guilt for past real

or imagined misdeeds. None of the children in the present study indicated direct concern. It certainly may be that such a concept is too frightening to face directly.

The quality of expression in the stories of children coming from religiously devout families did reflect a sense of continuance. On the other hand, it was frequently evident that heaven could also be a frightening unknown that they might need to face without the support of the meaningful adults in their lives. Some children voiced the thought that it would be better to remain on earth. Such feelings can be seen in excerpts from some of the stories:

Just bad people go to heaven—good people stay here on earth.

He does get killed. He dies. He goes to heaven. He doesn't do anything in heaven. He has a special God, like Holy. There are angels in heaven. The man paints the angels, so they'll be pretty. He didn't like it in heaven. He would rather be back here—he has a little boy he'd rather be with.

An overriding sense of loneliness was also seen to permeate stories containing religious themes. One girl of 8 concluded a story with the comment, "This little girl in the picture died, and they buried her. And then she went up to heaven. She didn't like it there—because God wasn't there."

Other children voiced a wish to see the God about whom they had learned, and reflected a sense of continuation of activity following the cessation of mortal existence. Following are illustrations of such expressions:

She's very sick. She's got a very sick heart. She's thinking about God. She would like to see him. She gets dead. She's going to get dead. A nurse is in the picture too. She's checking her. The little girl doesn't get well—she gets dead. She's going to heaven—and then she sees God there.

They're thinking about God. They're thinking about God and where he lives—up in heaven. They're thinking about when they die and go up to heaven. They want to go there, to help other people. They can help other people by watching over them. That's what people do in heaven—they're souls. God turns their soul into an angel and they watch the people below.

Although the number of mentions of death and the fear of loneliness and mutilation were as frequent in the stories of the religious children as in the nonreligious, the parents with faith in an afterlife unanimously commented on the comfort that religious beliefs gave to them and the support they received from the prayers and understanding of the friends within their churches.

Previous experience with severe illness and death

Although it had been predicted that children who have experienced the death of a significant person would indicate a greater anxiety regarding their own future, conclusions could not be reached in this study due to the subjects' almost complete lack of such experience.

One 9-year-old girl with cystic fibrosis who had had a number of traumatic encounters with death did indicate considerable preoccupation with the concomitants of death—the immobility, coldness, and lack of responsiveness and awareness. Further research with larger numbers of children involving a greater variability in experience may shed some light on this question. It is possible that the significant variable may not be the mere fact of the experiencing the death of someone to the child, but the quality of support and understanding received during and after such a stressful situation.

Maternal warmth

It is difficult to make valid judgments regarding the warmth of family relationships after a diagnosis of fatal illness is made. Under the tremendous threat of losing a child, most parents understandably view their child in the past and pres-

ent much differently than they did previous to the diagnosis. Acknowledgment of negative qualities or behavior can be threatening in terms of present and future comfort. Also, the very threat of loss highlights all that is admirable and lovable, and the frightening prospects of forcible separation make the loved one infinitely more valuable. This was illustrated in this study by the fact that as the condition of the child deteriorated, parents were less able to express anger or ambivalent feelings in their relationship with their child.

Despite difficulties of appraisal of warmth in the mother-child relationship, enough variability existed between parents in this dimension to make an analysis. No relationship was found between the warmth of the mother's feeling toward her child and the amount of anxiety the child expressed specific to insecurity regarding body integrity and functioning. However, a significant relationship did exist with the score the child received on the general anxiety scale for children. Since this test measured generalized anxiety, this finding suggests that although the security and love the child receives from family relationships may not mitigate specific anxiety about death, it can minimize fears and insecurities relative to the general environment.

The child's awareness of the nature of his illness

Few children are either specifically given their diagnoses or prognoses or have opportunities to discuss their fears and concerns relative to the future. Until the fairly recent past, few studies have been designed to assess the concerns of the fatally ill child. Strong resistance to such studies may illustrate the avoidance by professional personnel, along with the feeling that death as a topic of conversation with the dying can lead only to increased anxiety. In addition, it has long been felt by physicians and nurses that the defense of denial was adequate in protecting the fatally ill from awareness and anxiety relative to their prognoses.

Knudson and Natterson[2] concluded from their study that children were not fearful of their own impending deaths until after the age of 10. They felt their data indicated that under the age of 6 years, fears of separation are paramount, whereas from 6 to 10 years, fears related to physical injury are foremost. These findings were later corroborated by Morrissey[3] who based his conclusions on medical charts and conferences with hospital personnel.

It is possible, however, that the complete alteration in the environment of the child may convey to him that a situation exists which is too terrible to discuss. Anxiety of parents that is not directly verbalized may yet be effectively transmitted because of the perceptiveness of children to nonverbal clues. General apprehensiveness gained from clues within and without may not be manifested overtly, in that such specific verbalization may threaten a loss of contact with the meaningful people in the child's environment. Fear of separation or loneliness and fear of mutilation, intrusive procedures, and pain may be substituted in overt expression of a basic anxiety regarding survival.

Awareness of diagnosis and prognosis is not an absolute in that a child either realizes fully that he is facing death or he does not. The children in this study indicated differing degrees of awareness, although only two had had overt discussions with their parents or professional personnel regarding the future. These two children had diagnoses of cystic fibrosis. It appeared that it was less difficult for parents to discuss the child's illness with him when death was less imminent and less immediately threatening.

The question of whether and how to have such a discussion with their child is very real and disturbing to parents of all fatally ill children. Many felt strongly that their child should never know his diagnosis. Others felt that such a discussion could be helpful to their child, but that enduring such a situation would be more than they could bear. Some went to great lengths to assure that their child did not learn of his diagnosis inadvertently, and others felt the stigma that society still places on diagnoses such as leukemia or cancer. Parents of children with these diagnoses often felt that the child's playmates might avoid him should they learn of the prognosis.

One mother of an 8-year-old girl who had recently been diagnosed as having Ewing's tumor of the hip, commented:

> Oh, we don't talk about it with Mary. We would never use the word 'cancer' to her. She knows what it is. When she was in the hospital last time, Mary had a friend who had the same thing—cancer of the hip. Mary knew what she had, but of course, the girl didn't. This girl had had x-ray therapy which hadn't done any good, and Mary knows this. The girl was obviously dying, and it affected Mary quite a bit. So we don't ever want her to know what she has, or hear the word 'cancer.' Why should we make her suffer by telling her? It's much better that she doesn't know . . . we will think of some way of protecting her from knowing.

A mother of a 9-year-old girl who had terminal leukemia stated:

> Well, I feel that it's cruel to take away all hope. We have not told Beth that she has leukemia. Not that I'm adverse to the word, but to the connotation it holds. . . . Yet, I think she is catching on . . . she is suspecting.

Reflecting the concern many parents expressed relative to the reaction of others to their child, the mother of a 6-year-old boy with medulloblastoma commented:

> Well, in Donie's case—it's a cancer, and it's incurable. If I say . . . to anyone in his presence 'he has cancer' their immediate reaction would be one that would be completely disheartening to him. If he saw their faces! Because it is to me when I see their faces. And I've gotten used to it. But now I've decided it's the time to [tell him] —I'm sure many parents think I'm an idealist very

strongly. I just couldn't quite bear having another child saying to him 'you have *cancer?*' You know —that way.

Many parents wished to discuss at some length the relative merits both to themselves and to their children of frank answers to the child's questions. Some felt that such answers would be of benefit but that such a discussion could be better done by a professional person or clergyman who was not as anxious as they or as deeply emotionally concerned.

Another factor entering into their decision appeared to be the extent to which the child's cooperation was necessary in treatment aspects. Parents of children with cystic fibrosis were more openly frank with their children in order to persuade them to cooperate in the many therapeutic efforts.

Certainly all parents could not totally avoid some discussion of treatment aspects with their children, since these children were of school age and all were of normal intelligence. Such procedures as blood transfusions and surgery merited explanation. However, these explanations about the purpose of the treatments were often seriously incomplete or misleading.

One of the most striking findings of this study related to the dichotomy between the parents' belief of their child's awareness, and the stories told by the child that gave evidence of his understanding, fears, and concerns. As mentioned previously, only two of these children had previously discussed their diagnoses and prognoses with their parents. Most of the other parents felt quite certain that their child could not know that his life was threatened. Yet, in analyzing the stories told by these children, 63% of those stories dealing with threat to body integrity included statements regarding death or the fear of death.

In all of the stories the degree to which the characters in the story had been given the child's own diagnosis and symptoms was clearly apparent. Often the character thus identified with the child died of the child's own illness.

The mother of one 6-year-old boy with leukemia felt assured that her son had never heard the word "leukemia" and had always spoken to her of his "tired blood." Yet, he told the following story when shown the picture of a woman with her face on her hands:

> This is about a woman. She's somebody's mother. She's crying because her son was in the hospital, and he died. He had leukemia. He just had a heart attack. It just happened. He died. Then they took him away to a cemetery to bury him, and his soul went up to heaven.
> The woman is crying. But she forgets about it when she goes to bed. Because she relaxes and her brain relaxes. She's very sad. But she sees her little boy again when she goes up to heaven. She's looking forward to that. She won't find anybody else in heaven—just her boy that she knows.

The mother of an 8-year-old boy, also with leukemia, reported that he did not know that he had a serious illness, that he asked few questions, and that they had told him only that "something in his blood didn't keep up where it should and that the doctor had to keep checking." To the same picture as in the previous illustration, this boy also told a story to the effect that the woman depicted had a little boy in the hospital and that she thought he was going to die. The little boy had a disease "that was very, very bad" and he also was afraid that he would die. In another story, this child described the child in the picture as in the process of dying, " . . . he just keeps laying there and mumbling that he wants to get well, but he never does."

A 6-year-old boy with astrocytoma commented in one of his stories, "He gets an operation on his head. He wanted the operation so he could get better . . . the little boy doesn't get well. He dies and they have to bury him."

One 7-year-old girl who had surgery for astrocytoma, and whose parents had not told her of the surgery, told the following tale:

It's at a doctor's place, 'cause that's the nurse. It's a hospital. And that's a little girl—she's sick. Her head hurts her bad. She has a lot of pain. She's thinking that she hopes she gets well. She's afraid she might die. The nurse is looking at a little table—she helps the little girl. They have to put stitches in the little girl's head. She had an operation and she didn't want the stitches because it hurts. They take care of the little girl. Her mother comes to see her. This little girl doesn't get well—she keeps on having pain in her head like me. She finally dies. She goes home from the hospital, but she has to keep coming back for treatment and x-rays to her head.

In another of her stories, this same girl commented, "The girl in the picture is in the hospital. Something's wrong with her head. They had to operate and take her to surgery. They took something out of her head. . . . She's dreaming that she gets better and doesn't die. . . ."

An 8-year-old girl who had very recently been diagnosed as having a malignant tumor of the femur and whose mother made the comments previously cited to the effect that her daughter should never hear the word "cancer," nevertheless also indicated preoccupation with death in all eight of her imaginative stories. In the following illustration, she also indicates a loneliness which extends to heaven itself:

She's in the hospital, and the doctor is talking to her mother and father. She's sick—she's got cancer. She's very, very sick. She's thinking that she wishes she could go home. She had an operation at the hospital—but she didn't want it, because she wanted to get out of the hospital. This little girl dies—so she doesn't get better. Poor little girl. This girl at the hospital—she has cancer. Her hip's swollen and her bone's broken. This little girl in the picture died, and then they buried her. And then she went up to heaven. She didn't like it there—because God wasn't there.

The loneliness of perceiving prohibitions against discussing her fears and concerns could be seen in the concluding comments to many of the stories told by this

child wherein the main character died, and "nobody cared—not even her mother."

Some of the children also gave other indications of awareness of what was occurring. One 10-year-old boy spent much time in drawing and painting while hospitalized. On one occasion, he drew a picture of a graveyard with his name on the gravestone. The loneliness he felt was also indicated somewhat later when he drew a picture of a tree on a knoll. When the picture was praised, the boy responded, "But it's very lonely. It's all by itself." The child who had not been told that she had had brain surgery nevertheless commented to the investigator that she "wasn't afraid to die."

It seems possible from the stories these children told that fear of death from inside the body may be partially denied, but externalized and displaced to fear from without. Thus, the inner sphere may be altered to an outer sphere of threat so that the environment itself appears to be menacing. Fears of separation, loneliness, mutilation, intrusive procedures, and pain may substitute for an underlying general apprehensiveness about survival. Certainly, death is the ultimate in separation, and loneliness may be increased when children sense that their parents and the adults around them, on whom they must depend, are keeping something from them —evading honest and frank answers to their questions or discussions about their fears and concerns. Loneliness may also stem from the sense of not being understood. Many children with terminal illness experience a real sense of loneliness in that they are more often isolated from other children and have fewer actual contacts with professional personnel and less emotional involvement with them.

In many of the stories told by the children, loneliness was a major theme. Also, in analyzing the differences in mentions of separation and loneliness between the four groups of children, the children within the fatal group mentioned the emotion in 27.73% of their stories dealing with threat to body integrity as compared with 6.76% in the stories of children with chronic illness and of children with brief illness, whereas well children mentioned loneliness only 1.64% of the time.

Some comments from the actual stories may illustrate these findings. The following statements in a story told by a 6-year-old boy with leukemia make the point very poignantly: "He looks very lonesome, all by himself. Maybe he's sick. Maybe he wishes somebody would take care of him and he wishes he would be better. But there's nobody to take care of him and that's why he's sad. He gets very sick all alone and dies and goes to heaven."

The fact that time seems to stretch interminably for young children separated from their parents also adds to the child's depression. A 6-year-old girl with cystic fibrosis commented, "She has to be in the hospital for long days and never gets to see her Mommy and Daddy. She's very lonesome."

The child's separation from his siblings, from playmates, and from the security of a known and predictable environment is also a real aspect in the hospitalized child's loneliness. A 6-year-old boy with astrocytoma told the following story about the picture of a small boy sitting alone:

> This is a little boy. It's my little brother, Mark. He's thinking about me. He's lonesome for me. He wishes I'd come home. He's thinking that I am going to come home pretty soon and then we'll have a party. Mark is thinking that we'll have ice cream and that he's glad I'm coming home.

This story illustrates also the manner in which young children can use projection in expressing their own emotions and the use of wish fulfillment in relieving anxiety for the future. Fear of the future and of coming surgery in this instance is translated into joyful reunion.

Although many of the stories expressed the children's dependence on hospital personnel to alleviate the threat to body integrity, indications of the children's perception of the hospital environment as menacing were also apparent. Certainly many procedures are viewed as punishing by children and retributive for real or imagined misdeeds. A sense of personal guilt over the illness itself was frequently noted.

Externalization of inner threat could certainly be another aspect of indications in the stories that the children perceived therapeutic efforts on the part of professional personnel as hostile. Several excerpts from the stories may illustrate the viewpoint of the children. One 7-year-old boy indicated both inner and outer spheres of threat, a sense of body inadequacy, and fear of death in these words: "The little boy got a shot in the back; a big needle! He was scared of shots, and didn't want it. And the doctor did it hard! His lungs are gone and he can't breathe. His lungs got worse and he didn't get well. He died. He was buried with a big shovel." His concern about a hostile environment was also apparent in later stories with such comments as: "They put a tent on him and freeze him too," and "The nurse turned off all the lights and closed the door and he was lonesome and scared."

An 8-year-old girl with cystic fibrosis who was afraid that she would be subjected to surgery commented: "So they called the doctor and they had to take her to the hospital, and they jerked her into the operation room and made her go to sleep. She didn't like that at all. She didn't want the operation. And so they started cutting . . . . Then she waked up. She thought, 'They'll do it again!' "

Certainly, such expressions from children give strong indications that along with a deep concern regarding body integrity and the future, many also see the current environment as threatening and punishing; they feel isolated, alone, and lonely. They may fear that their illness is retributive for their misdeeds and may be concerned that few care deeply or that they may be facing death alone and unsupported.

Another striking finding of this study is related to the amount of opportunity the child had had to discuss his fears and concerns and the amount of anxiety expressed in his fantasy stories. The correlation found between the total score the child received on the protocols of eight stories, and the rating of degree to which his parents had discussed his questions and concerns frankly was found to be .633, which is significant at the .01 level. This finding indicates that contrary to much parental and professional conviction, allowing the child to discuss his fears of the present and for the future does not heighten anxiety, but decreases insecurity related to loneliness, isolation, and alienation, concern regarding the intent and purpose of therapeutic efforts, guilt related to the origin of the illness, and fear that cessation of life may be retributive.

Other findings regarding death anxiety

Each protocol of eight stories was scored by two judges independently on a scoring system designed to determine both the total amount of preoccupation with threat and the "fear-related motivation score" and to provide comparative data on specific aspects, such as causality and perceived patterns of adaptation. The measurement of fear was based on the same general rationale utilized in the scoring of other motives under the view that fear of bodily harm is a motive. Many of the categories utilized were an adaptation from the scoring manual for the achievement motive as outlined by McClelland and associates.[4] The general behavior sequence that followed differed somewhat in that the focus related to analysis of threat and of avoidance of threat.

In comparing the total score (fear-related motivation score) received by the four groups of children, it was found that there was minimal overlap between the scores of subjects with fatal illness and the scores of subjects in the comparison groups. Table 2 presents the range, mean, and standard deviations of the four groups.

The results are as predicted, that is, children with fatal illness indicated significantly greater preoccupation with death, loneliness, and mutilation than did other hospitalized children, and all hospitalized groups indicated significantly more concern with threats to body integrity than did the normal group of children.

Children with fatal illnesses told substantially more stories relating to threat to body integrity than did the three comparison groups (p = .01). Such a finding would support the prediction that children with fatal illnesses are more preoccupied with threat to body integrity, since they did more readily perceive and utilize the clues in the pictures presented to them. This would suggest that the defense of denial was not completely effective in blocking perception of clues to threat. It was, however, noted that children with

Table 2. Means, standard deviations, and difference—projective test

Group	Range	Mean	Standard deviation	p*
Fatal	33-65	53.31	10.29	.01
Chronic	5-36	17.75	7.87	N.S.
Brief	8-29	18.19	5.94	.05
Normal	−1-29	11.06	8.92	

*Kolmogorov-Smirnov test of significance of difference.

diagnoses of fatal illness displayed more symptoms of stress while telling stories than did the subjects in the comparison groups, as indicated by long hesitations before beginning a threat-related story, delays and blockings, and other manifestations of tension.

In further analysis of the stories told, it was found that children with fatal illnesses discussed death and loneliness as a threat more frequently than did all comparison groups at a significance level of .001. All of the children perceived the threat to proceed more often from the environment than it did from the person involved in the threat. This suggests that externalization of threat may be fairly general in children, although the children within the fatal group seemed to externalize somewhat more than did the comparison groups of children. Children with poor prognoses also more often spontaneously expressed statements to the effect that the heroes in their stories met with obstacles emanating from the environment in achieving recovery or in reduction of threat. Such a finding could indicate that these children expressed depressive feelings in fantasy regarding the subjects of their imaginative stories.

The term "adaptive maneuvers" was given to those various methods that the child described as used by the subject in his story to relieve the threat or to reduce the anxiety caused by threats to his body integrity.

"Wish fulfillment" was noted whenever a child indicated that the character in his story "wished to get well" or desired reduction of anxiety but did not relate any personal effort on the part of the threatened individual—a reflection of a direct statement of desire for reduction of anxiety. Subjects within the fatal group made such statements significantly more often (p = .001), which would correspond to an intensification of need.

Children with poor prognoses also more often saw the personal efforts of the threatened individual as unsuccessful (p = .02). This suggests that these children more often expressed feelings in fantasy of being overwhelmed by the environment and events over which they could exert no control.

The chief difference between groups when the stories were analyzed for statements of affective feelings was that children with fatal illnesses more often noted negative affective feelings in their characters (p = .01); they did so more consistently and to more situations described.

Positive anticipations for the future predominated in the stories of all groups except for the group of subjects with fatal illnesses. These children more often ascribed negative or doubtful anticipations of the future, including a fear or certainty of death as the final outcome or a certainty that the threat or anxiety would not be alleviated by any of the adaptive maneuvers mentioned in the story (p = .001).

Children with poor prognoses also ended their stories with a less favorable outcome, that is, death of the main character or nonreduction of threat or anxiety, significantly more often than did the three comparison groups of children. Although "happy endings" were more frequent than were anxiety outcomes for all of the children, over one fourth of the stories told by children with fatal illnesses concluded on a note of pessimism or aura of hopelessness (p = .001). There appeared to be a difference in the manner in which these children coped with their personal threat; there appeared to be a consistency in the way individual children ended their stories. Some repeatedly pronounced death to their main character, whereas others consistently lifted the sentence, almost at the conclusion of the tale, with minimal indications of manner of resolution. Many of the children expressed a quality of hostility or defiance in their fatal pronouncements. Feelings of anger with respect to their diagnoses have previously been documented in children with fatal illnesses[3] as have the effects of submission and hopelessness.[5] In addition, anger can be aroused through the realization that meaningful adults evade discussions of importance to the child, and hostility may arise from an increasing sense of loneliness and isolation.

Implications for nursing

Contrary to much popular conception, the findings of this study indicate that children with fatal illness who are between the ages of 6 and 10 years do indicate considerable preoccupation with death and loneliness as expressed through fantasy. This suggests that physicians, nurses, and other adults may be blinded to the child's anxiety because of personal affect, unresolved feelings surrounding death, and a sense of professional helplessness related to the child's diagnosis. Previous failure experiences in providing the optimum support for the dying child and his parents adds to the response of avoidance of such situations in the future. Lack of guided experience and support during basic education when confronted with such a stressful situation may also contribute to conscious or unconscious withdrawal from emotional involvements with terminally ill children.

This study also supports the findings of previous research in relation to the therapeutic effectiveness of permissiveness and honesty in discussions with individuals facing the end of their lives. It also corroborates the findings of others to the effect that hospitalized children often feel a lack of control over the forces impinging on them and an incapacity to alter events in their environments, along with great dependency on the adults surrounding them to assist in the alleviation of anxiety.

Large differences exist, however, in the experiences of individual children; in the procedures, therapy, and pain they must face; in the coping capacities they have acquired in their early years; in the meaning death may hold for them personally because of prior experiences and religious education; and in the amount of parental support and warmth they have received in the past and during their current experiences. Nursing intervention, therefore, must be planned on an individualized and continuous basis.

Such planning can only be effective through communication with the child that results from a trusting relationship in which the child feels free to discuss his concerns, fears, and anxieties. It seems clear that the question, "Should a child be told of his diagnosis?" seems to have little meaning. Rather, the conscious fears and concerns of a fatally ill child should be dealt with in such a way that he does not feel further isolated, lonely, or alienated from others. Fears and concerns about facing the future with minimal support, or fear that serious illness is the result of personal wrongdoing can be frightening and painful.

Keeping the child on pediatric wards close to others both spatially and emotionally can help to relieve the utter loneliness of the child when he most needs closeness.

Assisting parents who are anticipating the loss of a child can be both difficult and challenging for the nurse who is in contact with them. Parents also need closeness, support, and frankness regarding their child's physical symptoms, treatment, and his day-to-day behavior and concerns. Taking the time to listen to their concerns, worries, and fears can be an important aspect of nursing care and provides them with more energy that they can devote to their child.

In addition, this research has indicated that many parents feel incapable of dealing directly with their child's questions or of coping with their own anxiety raised by these questions, and they may feel a need for knowledge of the methods and words to utilize that could be most supportive to their child. Parents who do not feel that they have the energy or capacity for this type of conversation with their child should not be subjected to further pressure to do so. An empathetic physician, nurse, or social worker, who has himself faced his anxiety regarding death, could be of help to both parents and child when such a need is communicated.

To be of maximum help to terminally ill children and their parents, however, nurses also need the support of their instructors, colleagues, and other professionals while engaged in such an experience. Team conferences and collaborative discussions with physicians, social workers, or psychiatrists can often be of great help to nurses in providing the optimal environment for the child and in recognizing and mastering their own feelings.

Dealing with such a tragic circumstance in childhood can never be easy for the child, his parents, or the professional staff. Yet if all professional personnel surrounding the child have given of their best efforts, the final loss may be felt keenly and deeply, but will not result in a sense of depression.

References

1. Sarason, S. B., Lighthall, F. F., Davidson, K. S., Waite, R. R., and Ruebush, B. K.: Anxiety in elementary school children, New York, 1960, John Wiley & Sons, Inc.
2. Knudson, A. G., and Natterson, J. M.: Participation of parents in the hospital care of their fatally ill children, Pediatrics 26:482-490, 1960.
3. Morrissey, J. R.: Death anxiety in children with a fatal illness. In Parod, H., editor: Crisis intervention, New York, 1965, Family Service Association of America.
4. McClelland, D., Atkinson, J. W., Clark, R., and Lowell, E. L.: A scoring manual for the achievement motive. In Atkinson, J. W., editor: Motives in fantasy, action and society, Princeton, 1958, D. Van Nostrand Co., Inc.
5. Bozeman, M., Arbach, C., and Sutherland, A.: The adaptation of mothers to the threatened loss of their children through leukemia, part I, Cancer 8:1-19, 1955.

Chapter 14

The changing role of the nurse in well-child care

Loretta C. Ford

We must start with this Nation's children. We must expand and accelerate our present efforts. We must find new solutions to the age-old problems. Philip Lee[1]

Finding new solutions to age-old problems in child care ought to have high priority in nursing. Meeting the needs of children and minimizing threats to their very existence are well within the purview of professional nursing practice, but nursing alone cannot solve the problems. The goal of optimal health for each child is articulated and documented in current literature.[2-4] What is not well defined are the specific responsibilities that each concerned group of health professionals will assume. Nor have the potential contributions of each group been explored.

This nation is a long way from reaching a stated goal of continuous, comprehensive family-centered child care. Reaching this goal—if indeed it is a possibility—will take a commitment as well as creative and courageous action on the part of nurses and other health professionals.

Many people express concern about the health of the nation's children. This strength of interest ought to form the flying wedge for bringing about constructive changes in patterns of delivery of service and in the preparation of those in the helping professions. To marshall this strength requires taking a hard look at current issues in the health-care crisis, exploding some myths in manpower utilization, and courageously planning future directions. What *are* the current forces in today's health crisis? Dr. Ward Darley[5] labels them as inevitabilities of the phenomenon of change in the health and medical care systems and says:

The components of this change, all of which are inevitables in themselves, constitute a chain reaction, the links of which arrange themselves in the following sequence: (1) increasing knowledge, (2) increasing specialism, (3) increasing demands for service, (4) increasing costs of service, (5) increasing shortages of personnel, (6) increasing complexity and efficiency in data processing and communication, and (7) increasing institutionalization (organization).*

---

*From Darley, Ward: American medicine and the inevitables in the future, J.A.M.A. **196:**267, 1966.

These inevitabilities are the realities that must be dealt with in evolving a health-care system which will serve all segments of our population, demonstrate concern for wellness and illness, and be founded on a commitment that ensures every individual the right to high-level wellness and comprehensive health care. Within this framework, current and future concepts for well-child care must be evolved.

This nation's future depends on its children and the mature adults who guide and nurture the young. In their concern for their own futures the young are challenging society's systems in disruptive and sometimes violent ways. Their messages are not always clear, but they do know their future is at stake. The young today are concerned with quick alleviation of old problems. They are impatient and rightly so. Soon health-care systems will experience this impatience.

Nursing must be responsive if it is to survive. Nursing's history is one of dynamic change. However, previously tasks and functions were added without much thought to changing roles. Acceptance of some past role changes, such as demonstrated by midwifery, has been relatively slow in gaining the profession's recognition. The fact remains, however, that changes are demanded—and now.

From these understandings of the past the health-care crisis today and their implications for child health, an exploration of nursing's potential for meeting needs of children in ambulatory care settings is in order. The posture of this author is that professional nurses have competencies and can acquire additional ones to expand their roles in child care, particularly well-child care, and thereby increase appreciably the quality of health care delivered to children in this country. Freeman supports this view as she calls for the application of the criterion of relevance. From her statement that in maternal and child care "the major problems revolve around edu-

cation, emotional support, careful observation, anticipatory guidance with relation to growth and development and feeding habits,"[6] she concludes nurses can provide most of the care needed.

Several studies on the role of the nurse in ambulatory child care settings have been reported.[7-9] All of these studies show that the nurse is competent to make sophisticated clinical judgments, can function effectively in team delivery of care, and is highly acceptable to consumers. Further, nurses express great satisfaction in fulfilling this role in clinical practice.

A recently completed study at the University of Colorado adds some interesting insights to the contribution nurses are making in well-child care. The pediatric nurse practitioner project was designed to expand the role of the professional nurse in child care in community settings. On a grant from the Commonwealth Fund, co-directors of the project, Loretta C. Ford, R.N., Ed.D., Professor of Community Health Nursing, University of Colorado School of Nursing, and Henry K. Silver, M.D., Professor of Pediatrics, University of Colorado School of Medicine, conducted a five-year (1965-1969) demonstration project in a specially designed educational and practice sequence.

The uniqueness of the pediatric nurse practitioner (P.N.P.) project emanated from the joint sponsorship and cooperative efforts of the School of Nursing and School of Medicine faculty at the University of Colorado, the articulation of the educational institution with the health-care delivery systems in community settings, and the recognition of the nurse's potential contribution in an expanded role within the system. A description of the pediatric nurse practitioner project follows.

The purposes of the project were (1) to prepare professional nurses in an educational program to assume an expanded role in child care in community settings within the scope of the Colorado Nurse Practice Act; (2) to provide opportunities in health stations, neighborhood health centers, and pediatrician's offices for the nurses to practice their newly learned roles as autonomous practitioners of nursing and interdependent health team professionals; and (3) to evaluate the child health needs of specific target populations, the competencies of the nurses, and the acceptance of the nurse's expanded role by nurses, physicians, and consumers (patients and families).*

To accomplish these purposes, the project design included two phases. Phase I, the educational part, was a four-month period of learning for the nurses at the University of Colorado Medical Center. As graduate students enrolled in two courses in the School of Nursing, the nurses increased their competencies in a clinically oriented educational program. Content included management of the well child, identification and care of acute and chronic conditions of children, and care of childhood emergencies. Major emphasis was focused on the well child. From these three major components, student learning experiences (both theory and practice) were provided in assessing the psychosocial and physical development of well children in family settings; studying varying life-styles and patterns of child rearing; learning to perform developmental tests and evaluative procedures, such as the Denver development test, health histories, basic physical appraisal, and selected laboratory procedures; increasing the nurses' understanding of family dynamics; and counseling parents regarding care of their children and family and carrying out immunizations. Systematic physical appraisal of children involved in-

spection, percussion, auscultation, and palpation. Utilization of the otoscope and stethoscope was included also. With these tools and techniques nurses collect meaningful, relevant data, assess its importance, and make sophisticated clinical judgments.

Knowledge of the well child preceded the nurse's learning experiences about the sick child. Nurses learned to competently assess the severity of illness and its potential for progression so that parents could be counseled to deal with the current condition and prevent future illness. The goal of the nurse is to help parents make astute judgments about their children and seek appropriate types of care. This increased their competency and self-confidence as parents. Further, they learned to use wisely the health-care resources.

Care of children following poisonings, injuries, and accidents also became an integral part of the program. Nurses would be based at strategic points of entry into the community health-care system and therefore would be called upon to give first aid if an emergency occurred.

After the nurses completed their four-month educational experience in phase I, they entered phase II—a year's assignment as a practitioner in a community setting. This afforded the nurses an opportunity to establish their role. It permitted time to experiment with placement and utilization, and further, it allowed opportunities to evaluate certain aspects of the project.

All of the nurses who entered the project held baccalaureate (or higher) degrees from National League for Nursing accredited schools of nursing and qualified for entry into graduate school. Thirteen nurses had master's degrees in maternal and child nursing or public health nursing. Most of them had experience in public health nursing. Some had served in the Peace Corps in foreign lands. All of them were committed to fulfilling a clinical role in nursing. The mean

---

*Evaluation of this project was conducted by the Institute of Behavioral Sciences at the University of Colorado and funded by the United States Public Health Association.

age of the group of forty-eight nurses prepared between 1965 and 1969 was 29; their ages ranged from 23 to 62 years.

Early in the educational phase it was noted that P.N.P.s were experiencing role confusion and anxieties about their potential to practice. Their struggles with their own evolving role and that of the health-care system required constant adaptive and coping behaviors related to the phenomenon of change.

One interesting observation emerged as the nurses altered their perception of their new role. Many candidates, prior to entry into the health-care system, had been assessing the physical status of children, making clinical judgments about levels of wellness and severity of illness, and counseling families. Once in the project the nurses became quite anxious about the clinical decisions they had been making. The realization of the degree of responsibility they had been assuming without adequate preparation was frightening to them. They questioned their capabilities and potential to accomplish project goals and fulfill the P.N.P. role. This anxiety was alleviated as the nurses became competent in synthesizing advanced scientific knowledge into nursing practice. However, an important corollary to this insight was that the nurse's socialization in the role was facilitated by her student status and faculty support. As a learner the nurse had the freedom to try and the right to succeed or fail. She became involved with faculty and classmates in planning, implementing, and evaluating her own learning. She was held accountable as a self-directed learner for her own performance. Faculty expectations were high and encouragement was generous. Invariably the student gathered strength from the support and rose admirably to the expectations. Challenging the student with clinical problems, supporting her through role reorientation, using positive reinforcement in learning experiences, and releasing the

student to the world of work as a professional practitioner with specialized knowledge and skill in child care were faculty responsibilities.

Originally, the project was designated to provide health services to relatively isolated, deprived populations. The first project nurse was placed in Trinidad, Colorado. Later, through the development of an urban project in child care and the cooperative efforts of the Denver Visiting Nurse Service, project nurses were placed in health stations and neighborhood health centers in Denver.[10] Pediatricians' offices were also used as a testing arena for this new role, since it soon became obvious that utilization of both nurses' and pediatricians' competencies could be improved through colleagueships.

The process of change in the role relationships of the nurse and the physician in the pediatrician's office was facilitated by planning for alterations in the system and in the expectations of co-workers and recipients of care. Sensitization of the patient population was accomplished by informing the group by letter of the preparation and functions of the P.N.P. and the plans for her entry into the private or group medical practice. In some pediatricians' offices the P.N.P. was introduced personally to each new mother at the time of delivery during her hospitalization. Establishing a relationship with the mother (and father if he were present) and offering support in her new role began before an office visit was made became part of the P.N.P.'s responsibility. Other patients and parents were introduced to the nurse upon their visit to the office. Parents participated in deciding whether or not they wanted care from the nurse, the physician, or a combination of the two. Personal preference, types of health problems, and particular situations were considered in developing the plan of care with the family.

Orientation of the office staff—other

nurses and clerical people—usually was accomplished by the doctor prior to the arrival of the P.N.P. It continued as she evolved her role in that setting and other changes became necessary to facilitate the P.N.P.'s functioning. Physical rearrangements were required to accommodate the nurse's practice as she made assessments and counseled parents. Policies relating to telephone calls, ordering certain laboratory tests, and patient visits were altered to permit increasing autonomy in practice on the part of the P.N.P. Acceptance of the P.N.P.'s role by co-workers was assured as she was observed in action and as the physician and the nurse developed an adequate colleagueship. Interdependence in practice for the nurse and the physician directed by a patient-centered philosophy was the optimal goal sought.

Well-child visits to the experienced nurse practitioner usually require 30 minutes, although time ranges upward to an hour depending on the complexity of daily living patterns, the ensuing problems, and the family's coping potential. On a typical visit of a young child, the nurse takes a complete health history (a combination of medical and nursing histories), assesses the physical and psychosocial growth and development of a child, and counsels the parent regarding individual and family problems. Details of such a visit are described by Schiff, Fraser, and Walters[11]:

> . . . the nurse will discuss feeding (the ingredients of the formula; number, volume, and interval between feedings; acceptance; regurgitation), solid foods (when and how to introduce, variety), developmental milestones, bowel and urinary patterns, play habits, sleep patterns, mother's feelings about the infant, relationship with siblings, father's role in care, recent illnesses, accident prevention, immunizations (type, need, reactions, management), minor problems such as thumb sucking, and any other items that may be pertinent. Height, weight, and head circumference are measured for all children when indicated. Vision is tested with the Snellen 'E' chart or the Sloan letter chart for children over the age of 5 years and the Titmus Stereotests or the Guibor Nearpoint 'E' chart for those below the age of 5 years. As part of a thorough assessment, the nurse performs a developmental evaluation using the Denver Developmental Screening Test for children under 6 years. A complete physical examination is then carried out (including funduscopic and otoscopic examination and use of the stethoscope for appropriate regions of the body). Blood pressure determination and urinalysis are included as routine procedures. Gross testing of hearing and localization of sounds is accomplished in infants by use of high and low frequency noise makers.*

Mothers quickly learn to astutely use the skills of each professional wisely, having less confusion in understanding the respective roles of each than the professionals have themselves.

As soon as the P.N.P. entered the domain of the private physician, an interesting aspect of medical practice that the nurse immediately shared was the use of the telephone in dealing with clinical problems. One nurse reported that the amount of time she spent daily on the telephone ranged from 35 minutes to two hours. Further, she had observed differences in her nursing practice in that the characteristics of the population served altered the decision making in regard to handling of problems. Mothers in the middle and higher income brackets were articulate about their observations and concerns. Their telephone skills were well developed, easy, and natural. Intensive telephone history taking and assessment of the child's problem and the family's perception of it were possible. Nursing intervention was facilitated by this collection of meaningful data. In this manner the nurse not only helped mothers handle many of the daily care problems of children and families, but also paved the way for direct access to community resources

---

*From Schiff, D. W., Fraser, C. H., and Walters, H.: The pediatric nurse practitioner in the office of pediatricians in private practice, Pediatrics 44:62-68, 1969.

if referral was necessary. On the telephone the P.N.P. served primarily as a caring, comforting, and helping person. She functioned also as a health counselor and teacher, teaching the mother to make astute decisions about levels of wellness and severity of illness and injury as she fulfilled her mothering role. One example follows.

A mother called her pediatrician's office for help. Her physician was unavailable. She was told the P.N.P. was in her office if the mother would like to talk with her—the mother agreed to talk with the nurse. The P.N.P. had not met the mother prior to the phone call so the P.N.P. briefly explained her role and offered to help. The mother poured out her story. She was pregnant, 2 weeks away from delivery. Her husband was having the house remodeled. Carpenters, electricians, and plumbers were swarming all around demanding consultation regarding their work. John, her 2-year-old son, started crying soon after lunch and now, two hours later, she "couldn't take it any longer." Her final comment to the nurse was, "Look, can you help me?" The nurse suggested that the mother sit down comfortably by the phone and hold John on her lap. His crying was audible in the background. The conversation continued. Listening to the tenseness, desperation, and urgency in the mother's voice and cognitively recognizing the mother's and the child's physical and emotional growth and development stage, state, and needs, the nurse began listening and making notes for the eventual specific assessment of the mother's high level of anxiety, the child's condition, and the other problems in the family setting. John's whining, irritable cry continued in the background. After actively listening to the mother, the nurse asked, "What is upsetting you most right now?" The mother answered "John's crying—I think he may be coming down with something." Taking this clue as a point of departure, the nurse began a history-taking process that included specific questions about appetite, sleep and rest, play, elimination, etc. No abnormalities were found. Using the information to review the situation for the mother—both to validate the current data and to help her in the future to make these judgments—the nurse moved skillfully into discussing the mother's feelings and needs as they related to her pregnancy and finally back to some anticipatory guidance in understanding the growth and development of her 2-year-old son. During the course of the conversation, the mother's voice became calm and her speaking tones were low and even. The nurse noticed that John had stopped crying. The nurse commented on this to the mother, supported her handling of the problem, and directed the mother's attention to herself. In this particular situation the mother was extremely fatigued and was facing the final stages of pregnancy with ambivalence.

The nurse's recognition of this, other factors in the mother-child relationship, the growth and development of the child, and the family setting enabled the nurse to be immediately helpful on the telephone. The nurse did not suggest bringing the child to the physician's office. She could find no abnormalities that required medical referral. She predicted that an unnecessary visit to the office would increase the mother's anxiety and fatigue. The child's subsequent irritability would have been intolerable for the family. Also, it may have served to increase the family's dependency on professional help unnecessarily. Further, it could have deprived the mother and child of an important coping experience that could be transferred to other life situations. A follow-up phone call the next day revealed that the family had once more returned to an even keel.

Pediatric nurse practitioners and mothers have noted that tension in child care problems can be markedly reduced by contacting the nurse by telephone. Mothers are reluctant to call the physician about minor problems that are worrisome, distressing, and fatiguing for the mother and family and often uncomfortable for the youngster. The mother, however, is not reluctant to call the nurse. Immediate alleviation of stress is often accomplished through telephone discussion of the mother's problem. Quick entry into the health-care system is also possible if the pediatric nurse practitioner judges the problem to be medically or otherwise significant.

Positive responses of patients and families to the nurse practitioner are presented in the discussion on the project's evaluation which follows. Three major components of the evaluation design were (1) the identification of health needs and practices of specific target populations, (2) the competencies of the nurse in assessment, and (3) the acceptance of this expanded role of the nurse by nurses, physicians, and consumers of the service. Two surveys of health needs and practices were conducted, one in rural Trinidad, the other in urban Denver. In both studies it was evident that health needs and practices were based on definitions of health and illness common to low socioeconomic groups. In other words, recognition of deviations from health and ensuing action to seek care were prompted by severe, catastrophic situations while other conditions and preventive health practices were virtually nonexistent.[12]

Other research reports corroborate these findings. The competency of the project nurse to conduct a physical assessment of children was also tested. Pre- and post-educational testing was done on a small sample (N = 13) of project nurses using video tape recordings and written reports. Findings of this study confirmed the nurses' verbal reports. The nurses increased "the degree of comprehensiveness of their physical assessments of well children from pre-program to post-program testing, and systematicity of the assessments is extended concomitantly with comprehensiveness."[13] The most extensive part of the evaluation design was that of levels of approval of the nurse's expanding role. Jackson's return potential model[14] was used to develop a sixty-four-item questionnaire. Items were evolved from project faculty members' prescriptions and proscriptions within the role. The following findings[15] were reported:

The role of the Pediatric Nurse Practitioner is approved by nurses, doctors and consumers of service in Colorado. Differences within and among these groups of respondents are noted:

Public health nurses and teaching faculty members approved the role more than office, school and hospital nurses;

Pediatricians acquainted with the University of Colorado faculty approved the role more than did pediatricians in private practice, general practitioners or other physicians at the Medical Center. Nurses generally have higher agreement about the role than do doctors;

The variables of age influenced acceptance of the role. The younger nurse approved the role more than the older nurse. With physicians it was reversed. The older doctor expressed more approval for the role than the younger doctor;

Information about the program made a difference in acceptance too. The respondents who were most accepting of the role were well informed and knowledgeable about the project.*

Consumer acceptance of the expanded role of the nurse has been phenomenal, especially in view of the predictions of negative consumer response by some health professionals. In a study conducted in a community clinic in Colorado, Bellaire[16] reported:

. . . (1) patients seen regularly by the pediatric nurse practitioner had a much lower failure rate for return well child appointments—nine per cent in pediatric nurse practitioner clinics; 25-40% failure rate in other clinics; (2) field public health nurses reported mothers were following through on the advice given them by the pediatric nurse practitioner, and (3) patients seen by the pediatric nurse practitioner had a far lower failure rate in attending a consultant's clinic which was established for screening children for speech, hearing, dental and nutrition defects.†

In this same community, a survey conducted by indigenous workers on consumer acceptance of the pediatric nurse practitioner, findings indicated that:

(1) Mothers especially viewed counselling concerning child care problems such as feeding, toileting, growth and development as the responsibility of nurses and consequently felt more comfortable in bringing these problems to the nurse; (2) Parents tended to feel that the pediatric nurse practitioner provided them with more

---

*From Hunter, R. M.: Notes on findings: pediatric nurse practitioner study, Boulder, Colo., 1969, University of Colorado Institute of Behavioral Sciences (unpublished report).

†From Bellaire, J. M.: Paper presented at the Thirty-eighth Annual Meeting of The Academy of Pediatrics, Chicago, Ill., Oct. 23, 1969.

specific and individualized health counselling for their child than they had received from nurses not having this type of preparation; (3) A physical assessment with the "laying on of hands" so to speak was considered by parents as an important aspect of well child management and increased their confidence in the health professionals' decision as to the "wellness" of their child.*

Similar reactions are reported from patients and families of private pediatricians' offices.[11]

At the completion of the special pediatric nurse practitioner project, the findings of the research and the demands for these nurses gave overwhelming evidence that continuing the educational portion of the project (phase I) was paramount. The Continuing Education Services of the School of Nursing at the University of Colorado now assumes major responsibilities for the preparation of nurse practitioners. Other programs preparing or using nurses in an expanded role in pediatrics and in other areas of nursing practice are reported frequently.[9, 17, 18] The challenges and opportunities for nursing to assume creative leadership in well-child care remain. Nursing education and nursing service must look at the patterns of preparation and utilization of the nation's young talent in nursing. The new and now generation of nurses is looking for dynamic preparation and job enrichment beyond that which the past has offered.

The outcomes of our experience in the pediatric nurse practitioner project are congruent with the nursing profession's espoused goals for nursing. A clinical (person-side) nursing role, elimination of nonnursing tasks, colleagialities with physicians and other health professionals, team delivery of care, opportunities for clinical research, autonomy in nursing practice,

and differentiations for accountability commensurate with advanced preparation are all desirable directions.

Furthermore, nursing is seeking to influence and change the patterns of health-care delivery. These are also being realized. The special competencies of the pediatric nurse practitioner are used wisely in neighborhood health centers, health stations, and pediatricians' offices. Duplication and fragmentation of services can be prevented by careful articulation of the various workers and team planning. Service to people can be efficient and effective when the nurse is sophisticated and competent in her clinical judgment as shown in the following account of one family's experience.

Pediatric nurse practitioners in some agencies conduct child clinics in health stations. In these clinics, nurses provide comprehensive care for well children and children who have medically stabilized chronic conditions. Acutely ill children are also seen by the nurse. She determines whether or not she and the mother can manage the situation or if medical or other referrals are required. She also decides whether or not immediate or delayed referrals are in order. The Kelly family story demonstrates the P.N.P.'s decision to delay referral.

One morning, two young parents, the Kellys, brought their 6-month-old son in for a well child check. During the history-taking process the nurse had an opportunity to listen to the parents, to observe their interactions, and to collect meaningful data about them as a family. Both Mr. and Mrs. Kelly participated in the interview by responding to questions and offering information about their own daily living pattern and the care of the infant. They talked with each other and the nurse openly and rather eagerly. They revealed that the family's daily living patterns were extremely quiet and placid since the baby's arrival. The father

---

*From Bellaire, J. M.: Paper presented at the Thirty-eighth Annual Meeting of The Academy of Pediatrics, Chicago, Ill., Oct. 23, 1969.

worked long hours, mother and child were at home alone much of the time. Mrs. Kelly became an avid reader during baby's first months of life and maintained this habit as the baby grew. Noise was kept to a minimum so as not to "disturb the baby" and relatives and friends were not encouraged to visit frequently.

The child's nutritional intake, sleep and rest pattern, excretory functioning, and physical care were well understood and managed. The nurse noted that while both parents handled the baby lovingly and with close body contacts, neither parent talked directly to the child. The P.N.P. made a mental note of this and other observations about the parent-child relationships as she proceeded with the exploration of the family's daily living activities and the specific assessment (physical, social, emotional, and mental) of the child.

The assessment tools included the Denver Developmental Screening Test (D.D.S.T.). This standardized screening test was devised to help professionals determine whether or not a child's development is advancing within established ranges of normal. It serves as an indicator for (1) continuing specific observations of some aspects of growth and (2) the need for further, extensive diagnostic work. The nurses have found it is a useful mechanism for teaching parents about growth and development, for involving them in observation and responses to the child's growth, and in helping parents to understand and enjoy their parenting role. The D.D.S.T. extends opportunities for the nurse to support parents in their efforts to grow as a family. Specifically, the D.D.S.T. is a systematic approach to evaluating a child's fine and gross motor development, language, and personal-social growth. Testing of problem-solving ability is included for older children.

As the nurse conducted the test on the Kelly child, she involved the parents in observing the growth and development of the child, providing specific instruction to help them understand their child's current and future growth. The Kellys showed great interest in the process and its interpretation, which the nurse shared with them. From all the data that the nurse gathered by observation, interviewing, and assessment processes she determined that the Kellys' baby had a slight developmental lag in his personal-social development. His responses to self-feeding and resisting the pull of a toy away from him and his language development fell in the lower percentile for his age. He lacked spontaneity in reactions. Discussing the daily care of the infant revealed that the parents lacked an understanding of the need for stimuli of a personal-social nature for their child. They viewed their child as an ornament, to be cared for, admired, and cherished. Their interactions with him were limited somewhat by these perceptions.

Clinical judgment of the nurse regarding the developmental lag ended in the conclusion that the nature of the family's life pattern, mother's personal fulfillment through reading, and the misconception that normal sounds would be disturbing to the infant resulted in the developmental lag from lack of environmental and personal-social stimuli. The nurse predicted that (1) altering the situation would result in normal personal-social development of the child, (2) the parents had the potential and the interests in changing their life-style to a more lively one, and (3) growth and development of the child and family would be enhanced by these changes.

Some discussion with the Kellys regarding alterations of their patterns of living to provide opportunities for cultural stimulation of the child followed. In concert with the parents the P.N.P. prescribed (1) rearrangements of the physical environment to permit the child to see and hear his mother as she went about her household duties, (2) expanding family interactions during bathing, feeding, playing, handling, talking, and laughing with the child, (3) additions of action and sound in the environment, for example, hanging mobiles, playing the radio and television set at normal volume, and increasing social activities with friends and family, which included the child and other children. Scheduling a recheck in two weeks, the P.N.P. was able to validate her prediction that given external stimuli, the personal and social growth of the infant would fall within the expected range for his age. Further, the child's reactions would provide encouragement for the parents to continue to seek ways to help their child develop and increase their own competence and confidence as parents. Subsequent visits with parents and developmental testing revealed that the child's personal-social development was markedly increased. Parental interest and enjoyment were heightened by their understanding and participation in the growth and development process.

Despite some of the unknowns early in the project—such as levels of competency of the nurses, interdependent relationships in practice, and potential legal hazards—relatively few serious problems emerged. Nurses developed a competent and confident base in their educational phase and further enriched this in practice. Most of the operational difficulties occurred in the introduction of the project nurses into established systems of care. In the early part of the project, nurses were generally more threatened by the pediatric nurse practitioner than were other categories of health workers.

Stresses and strains in both phases of the project became a routine part of daily operations. Withdrawal, abuse, and harassment from nurse colleagues in both the educational and the service settings were a rather common occurrence. Man-

agement of these conflicts often took time, energy, and patience on the part of the project staff and service agencies. Essentially we were challenging territorialities, questioning the status quo, evolving channels and phraseology in communication, confronting traditionalism in functioning institutions, and establishing new and unorthodox relationships.

As the P.N.P.s entered the health-care system to practice their new role, it was recognized that they needed some preparation in understanding social change and dealing constructively with resistance. With the help of a social scientist, students began studying types of change, resistance to change factors, and the influence of bureaucratic and power structures. Strategies, logistics, and tactics of change were explored.

Introduction of the pediatric nurse practitioner into the health care system required constant interpretation of the role. A community nursing service committee was established to facilitate communication between the agencies interested in trying out new roles for nurses and the project staff. The purposes of this committee were to exchange ideas, review progress, plan for recruitment and placement of the pediatric nurse practitioner in the health-care system, and prevent problems or solve them if they occurred.

Operational guidelines developed to integrate the pediatric nurse practitioners into the current health-care delivery system prevented overlapping, duplication, and fragmentation of family service. In some agencies, pediatric nurse practitioners were assigned to health stations and functioned in a designated clinic setting. Agency public health nurses served in their usual district nursing roles. All the nurses talked together about specific family problems, used each other appropriately as consultants and as members of a multidiscipline health team, and offered continuous comprehensive health care to people.

Those agencies participating in the project pledged to provide opportunities for pediatric nurse practitioners to continually develop their specialized skills in child care and family counseling. Clinical conferences held weekly at the University Medical Center and the agency's inservice program enhanced the pediatric nurse practitioner's continuing growth. Efforts were made to avoid heavily scheduled clinics and assignment of nonnursing activities so that the pediatric nurse practitioners would not be divested of time and energy. These agencies helped in the transition of the pediatric nurse practitioner to the practice arena by communicating with them prior to their field assignment. An intensive and extensive orientation to the agency was conducted. Pediatric nurse practitioners functioned under the agency's program of nursing supervision and consultation. For some of the specialized competencies of the nurse, such as physical assessment and medical aspects of patient problems, pediatricians served as consultants.

Undoubtedly, this expanded role was not well explained or understood in the beginning. Sometimes this new role was referred to erroneously as a physician-assistant role. Clarification came about as the nurse's role became an autonomous clinical nursing one differing markedly from the physician-assistant in basic educational preparation, philosophy, scientific background, decision-making competencies, autonomy, and responsibility. The nurse's relationships with patients and families, with physicians and other health workers, and within the health care system changed. Its nature and scope became more professional. It was often necessary to differentiate the role from the physician-assistant position that was developing at Duke University and elsewhere.

The physician-assistant role is clearly a dependent one. No role for the physician-assistant exists without the doctor. Assisting the physician to accomplish his medical mission is the physician-assistant's "raison d'etre." Conversely, the mission of nursing is to help people to accomplish optimal wellness by assisting them to successfully adapt daily living patterns from "situationally derived needs."[19] Substituting for the physician is not a nursing role. Nor is the nurse's primary goal to save the physician's time; however, adjusting the functioning of both professionals to use wisely the talents and time of each must come about if people are to receive continuous, comprehensive, high-quality health care.

Differentiating the nurse with special competencies in a limited area, such as pediatrics, from the clinical specialist in nursing deserves mention. The clinical specialist serves to exemplify the profession's most talented clinician. She arrives at this level of clinical expertise through advanced preparation in formal graduate degree programs. The clinical specialist contributes to the advancement of the field through research and publication; exercises freedom and self-direction; assumes a position of power and authority through nursing competency in health-care systems; can function effectively as a consultant teacher or practitioner; appropriately assumes autonomy in her nursing role in team delivery of care; and develops colleagialities with other professionals in clinical and functional aspects of the health-care system. She should be qualified to offer leadership to talented nurses such as the pediatric nurse practitioners in furthering their clinical expertise and in helping them develop career patterns for continuing their education.

The future in well-child care offers many opportunities for all levels of practitioners of nursing if nurses will assume creative and dynamic leadership in developing their respective roles.

There is a growing belief among some professional nurses, particularly those in community health settings, that nursing's major contribution and autonomy in practice will be realized in the arena of high-level wellness[20] for society. With this direction, nursing's expanding role can be accomplished in adjusting daily living patterns in target populations in services where nurses are functioning currently, for example, school and college health services, occupational health services, outpatient departments, and physicians' offices. Other needs of certain groups, for example, geriatric patients, maternity, persons with stabilized chronic conditions, may be considered as the prerogative of nursing. The nurse can serve as the primary caretaker—not only to provide direct access to the system but also through and within the system.

Expanding the role of the nurse requires a thorough examination of other health team members' activities if efficient and effective use of the nation's scarce health manpower resources is to be realized. It also requires that health professionals do not evolve roles in isolation. Realignments of activities in practice will be needed if changes are to occur. Dialogue and discussion about these changes on interprofessional levels by individual practitioners and professional organizations must be initiated. Some efforts in this direction are now underway. Following the recent pronouncements by the American Medical Association and the American Academy of Pediatrics on the utilization of nurses and the reply of the American Nurses' Association condemning the American Medical Association's "unilateral action,"[21] organizational efforts to bring about understanding of the professional nurse's role will occur. Albeit progress to this point in time has been slow, the future looks bright.

After five years of intensive experience in evolving this role of the nurse in child care that emphasized wellness, a definition of the expanded role has evolved. It is one in "which the nurse performs increasingly complex acts in health care based upon a scientific background which permits increasing sophistication in her clinical judgments as advances in physical, biological, psychological and social sciences become significant to health care."[22]

Expressive and instrumental functions of the nurses are blended together beautifully into professional practice as the nurse supports and guides the mother in her efforts to competently care for her child and family. Blending of these functions allows certain segments of society to have direct access to the health-care system. Norris,[23] in discussing the physician as the gate keeper of the health-care system, challenges nurses to identify the points in the health-illness continuum where the nurse can claim direct access to the patient. The point and patterns of wellness in child care offer such an opportunity.

Increasing the productivity of current health manpower resources has not been fully explored, although heroic efforts are being made to increase numbers of different kinds of health workers primarily for care of the ill. The expanded role of the nurse is a way to utilize the strengths and increase productivity of the available worker and thereby influence the quality of health care. It offers hope to expand and accelerate the delivery of health services, stemming the tide of illness, but more importantly, redirecting the course of child care to wellness. It is an effort to find new solutions to the age-old problems.

References

1. Lee, Philip: Health and the city, a paper presented at the American Public Health Association Convention, Detroit, Mich., Nov. 12, 1968.
2. Falkner, Frank: Infant mortality—an urgent national problem, Children **17:**83-87, May-June, 1970.

3. Hunt, Eleanor: Infant mortality trends and maternal and infant care, Children 17:88-90, May-June, 1970.

4. Conference on Health Services for Children and Youth, March, 1969, part II, Amer. J. Public Health 60(suppl.):1-133, April, 1970.

5. Darley, Ward: American medicine and the inevitables in the future, J. A. M. A. 196:267, 1966.

6. Freeman, Ruth B.: The criterion of relevance, Amer. J. Public Health 57:1530, 1967.

7. Siegel, Earl, Dillehay, Ronald, and Fitzgerald, Carol J.: Role changes within the child health conference: attitudes and professional preparedness of public health nurses and physicians, Amer. J. Public Health 55:832-841, 1965.

8. Ford, Patricia Ann, Seacat, Milvoy S., and Silver, George A.: The relative roles of the public health nurse and the physician in prenatal and infant supervision, Amer. J. Public Health 56:1097-1103, 1966.

9. Non physician personnel in ambulatory child health care: a review, Chapel Hill, N. C., March, 1970, Health Services Research Center, University of North Carolina.

10. Ford, Loretta C., and Silver, Henry K.: The expanded role of the nurse in child care, Nurs. Outlook 15:43-45, Sept., 1967.

11. Schiff, Donald W., Fraser, Charles H., and Walters, Heather: The pediatric nurse practitioner in the office of pediatricians in private practice, Pediatrics 44:64, 1969.

12. Pediatric Nurse Practitioner Evaluation Project: Report I, Rural community health survey and community acceptance of the pediatric nurse practitioner, The Center for Action Research, Institute of Behavioral Sciences, 1968, University of Colorado (U.S.P.H.S. Grant No. PH108-68-76).

13. Stearly, Susan G.: Preliminary report on findings: study of physical assessment in pediatric nurse practitioner project, University of Colorado Institute of Behavioral Science, July, 1970 (unpublished).

14. Jackson, Jay: A conceptual and measurement model for norms and roles, Pacif. Sociolog. Rev. 9:35-47, Spring, 1966.

15. Hunter, Robert M.: Notes on findings: pediatric nurse practitioner study, Boulder, Colo., 1969, University of Colorado Institute of Behavioral Sciences (unpublished report).

16. Bellaire, J. M.: Paper presented at the Thirty-Eighth Annual Meeting of The American Academy of Pediatrics, Chicago, Ill., Oct. 23, 1969.

17. Andrews, Priscilla, Yankauer, Alfred, and Connelly, John P.: Changing the patterns of ambulatory pediatric caretaking: an action-oriented training program for nurses, Amer. J. Public Health 60:870-879, 1970.

18. Lewis, C. E.: Final report: dynamics of nursing in ambulatory care, Washington, D. C., 1968, United States Government Printing Office (U.S.P.H.S. Grant No. NU-00145).

19. Woodridge, Powhatan T., Skipper, J. K., and Leonard, R.: Behavioral science, social practice and the nursing profession, Cleveland, Ohio, 1968, Case Western Reserve University Press.

20. Dunn, Halbert L.: High level wellness, Arlington, Virginia, 1964, R. Beatty Co.

21. Nurse groups ask R.N.-M.D. dialogue; some get it, Amer. J. Nurs. 70:953-954, May, 1970.

22. Murchison, Irene, and Nichols, Thomas: Legal foundations of nursing practice, New York, 1970, The Macmillan Co.

23. Norris, Catherine M.: Direct access to the patient, Amer. J. Nurs. 70:1006-1010, May, 1970.

Chapter 15

A mother's ability to love her child

Margaret Sagar

Much has been written about maternal love and the effects on children who have or have not experienced their mother's love. But there are still many questions related to maternal-child love that nurses must answer. How can nurses assess maternal love? In fact, what is maternal love? How is it demonstrated by mothers? And how does one assess whether or not a child is experiencing love? A mother may be trying desperately to love her child, but the message may not be getting across to him.

In this chapter the problem of assessing mother-child love will be outlined and its relevance to nursing discussed. Then emphasis will be directed toward understanding mothers in relation to their ability to love their children and thereby to foster their children's ability to give love. A schema for recognizing problems will be advanced, and examples of situations and treatment methods that were tried will be outlined.

For the purposes of this chapter, Deutsch's definition of maternal love will be used. She defines maternal love as "the direct affective expression of the positive relationship to the child. . . . Its chief characteristic is tenderness."[1]

It is assumed that the presence or absence of maternal love is reflected in nearly everything that a mother does with and for her child and that it cannot be evaluated by how much time a mother spends actually demonstrating her love to her child. It is also assumed that the mother is the person who is responsible for the upbringing of the child and who provides "tenderness," whether she be a biological, adoptive, or foster mother. No mention will be made of those children who have no mother-figure.

The problem

Nurses working with well children tend to assume that since the child is well, the mother-child interaction is satisfactory. In describing the behavior of well children, nurses often include little more than isolated and dissected facts about the child's health, behavior, development, personality, and appearance. Descriptions of the mother and of her ability and effectiveness to perform the maternal role are often overlooked or, at best, are fragmented. The mother-child interaction process is not considered. No attempt is made to determine whether or not the mother is able to give love to her child, or whether or not the child is able to experience his mother's love. When the child is ill, the nurses' attentions are directed toward the illness, and they often miss the mother-child interaction process and its relevance to the situation.

Thus nurses' descriptions of a child often fail to incorporate the most crucial and significant factors affecting his future mental,[2] physical, and social health, that is, the significance of his mother and her ability to give him love and to have him experience it. This failure to describe mother-child interaction is partially due to nurses' unfamiliarity with descriptive terminology related to affection. Nursing research to develop meaningful, accurate, descriptive terminology and a conceptual framework related to the mother-child interaction process are sorely needed.

So the problems remain. How does one elicit whether a mother loves her child or a child loves his mother? How does one ascertain whether a child is experiencing the love given by his mother? How can one describe behavior related to the maternal-child interaction process associated with loving? If one discovers a problem, what nursing techniques can be employed to improve the bonds of love between a mother and her child?

The importance of knowing the mother

Since it is crucial that the child relate constantly and intensely to his mother during his earlier years, it is important that the nurse know a great deal about the mother. Even such simple facts as the time and place of her birth can be revealing.

For example, doctors, nurses, and a social worker in a well-child program were confronted by a mother whose 2-year-old child demonstrated great anxiety. He cried constantly, clung "like a limpet" to his mother, refused all contact and communication with others, made constant demands, and was constantly dissatisfied, fretful, and unhappy. The child neither slept nor ate well and was literally "a bundle of misery."

His mother knew little about her early childhood. She was Jewish and born in Hungary in 1944. She experienced immediate separation from her mother at birth because her mother had had to flee, and she had been hidden under an assumed name in an institution-like setting. She was reunited with her mother two years later.

This mother had experienced much deprivation, especially of love and attention. Not having received this love and attention at the time when she was so needful of it, and so vulnerable without it, she was unable to give love and attention to her child. It was not an innate part of her makeup. She was baffled and frustrated by her son's constant outrage and was helpless to deal with it.

We have come to recognize that the mother's conscious and unconscious memories of her childhood determine, in part at least, the way she cares for her own children. A dramatic example of this phenomenon is the battered child syndrome. A less dramatic but yet important example is the mother who, as a child, neither received nor felt any warmth of relationship with her own mother. She too tends to perpetuate this pattern. The ability to give and to receive love and affection appears to be learned, at least in part, from one's own mother and at an early age.[2] Thus nurses need to ask many questions of mothers. By whom was this mother reared? Where was she reared? Being raised by a spinster aunt is different from being raised by one's own mother. A teen-age mother is different from a middle-aged mother, a healthy mother is different from an ill mother, and a happily married mother is different from an unhappily married, separated, divorced, widowed, deserted, or unmarried mother. An educated mother is different from an uneducated mother; a mother with an occupation outside the home is different from the mother with no outside occupation. One can go on and on, size of family, order of children, health status of each family member, socioeconomic group, the role of the mother's father, education, and occupation patterns are all important factors.

Then one needs to ask how the mother feels about her experiences as a child. Which experiences produced pleasure, which ones were painful? How does this mother get along with her own mother now? Or if her mother is not living, with what thoughts and ideas has this mother been left?

One needs to know something about the attitudes toward children that existed in the mother's family. Were children considered to be bundles of uncontrolled impulses and aggressions to be coerced and controlled until they become adults? Were children merely small adults? Or were children innocent angels? Was childhood to be cherished or endured? Was a child's birth anticipated with joy, with fear and anxiety, with regret, or with downright anger? What parental needs were to be satisfied by having children?

One needs to know something about the patterns of affection that existed in the mother's family. Was affection demonstrated openly or was it not displayed at all? Were the parents fearful of "spoiling" the children by showing them affection, as if the children would come to demand unlimited amounts of affection and "gobble the parents up," or were the parents generous with their affection in anticipation of the children's becoming able to reciprocate? What were the predominating conversational tones? Were members of the family able to provide comfort, sympathy, reassurance, and encouragement when one of them was in need, or was one expected to stand alone, "take it like a man," "to buck up"?

Was one allowed to "be oneself" at home, to assume one's natural rhythm when possible, to regress at times, to "blow off steam," or was one expected to conform to a rigid formalized pattern?

One needs to know about the mother's special skills and interests, and the opportunities she has to indulge in them. In what ways does this mother achieve a sense of accomplishment, of self-worth? In what ways does she experience defeat and how does she handle it? An illustration may be helpful.

A mother who attended a pediatric clinic was a gifted artist, *had* won prizes for her paintings, and *had* received much recognition for her art works. Her husband was a gifted musician who earned their living teaching music and performing publicly. For this he received much recognition and achieved much satisfaction. However, the mother was caught up in the routines of her children, the family's somewhat limited budget, and her husband's long hours of practice and frequent public appearances. She had neither time nor opportunity to indulge in her "first love"— painting—and she was angry and frustrated.

The children reflected this situation. There was an excessive amount of sibling rivalry and much crying and general unhappiness. The oldest child bit a younger brother at every opportunity as well as any other child or adult who happened to be available.

This husband and wife were helped to recognize the wife's frustration and to plan for the wife's "escape" regularly through employment of a baby-sitter twice a week. The wife again experienced satisfaction and a feeling of self-worth. She became more sensitive to the needs of her children and spent what time she had with them more constructively and with more warmth in the relationship. The children's rivalry settled down to more normal proportions and the biting ceased.

One also needs to know the circumstances associated with a mother's selection of a husband, her marriage, and the circumstances associated with it. For example, it is important to know if the marriage was forced by a pregnancy, if the parents objected to the marriage, and the mother's age at the time of marriage.

One needs to discover how a particular mother thinks about mothering and motherhood. What, to her, is a "good" mother and what is a "bad" mother? For example, one frequently hears about "good" mothers who stay home with their children. This can sometimes be carried too far, and one finds mothers, especially with their first babies, who are loath to leave them for even a few hours, and yet they need this brief period of separation for diversion, for companionship with their husbands, and for renewing social contacts. One often sees these mothers tired, depressed, disillusioned with their new roles, and angry at the child who has caused their misery. Helping them to plan for a brief separation is often difficult, but once they have been separated from the child for this brief period and come back, they experience a renewal of energy and enthusiasm to meet the child's needs for love, care, and attention. In what ways was her own mother a "good" mother? In what ways was her own mother not a "good" mother? Would she prefer to be like her own mother, something like her, or not at all like her? What patterns of her own mother does she see in herself? Does this please or displease her?

Sometimes the only way one comes to recognize problems in mother-child affection is via one's own feelings. For example, does this child (or mother, or father, or family) generate positive feelings in me? Or does he make me feel hostile? Which factors in his personality do I like? Which ones do I dislike? What is there about the whole situation that produces these positive or negative feelings? Or if there has been a change of feeling tone, why has this happened? What new feelings are operating?

For example, a 2-year-old foster child had a visual problem and minimal cerebral palsy. She had no speech and was very hyperactive. She had been in a series of foster homes since birth and appeared to be deteriorating both physically and mentally. None of the foster parents felt any love for this child, and many damaging situations had occurred, such as forcing her to learn to climb stairs without her glasses. It was recommended that this child be placed in a foster home where children were given a great deal of affection. Both parents had limited educations, but they loved children and had much patience and understanding.

The child did well in this family until a year or so later when the foster mother began to express negative feelings about the child and planned to return her to the Children's Aid. However, she felt very guilty about her feelings. After a series of interviews, the author discovered that this mother's chief complaint was fatigue due to the death of her mother, her husband's being away on business, and the hyperactivity of the child.

It was arranged that someone outside this foster family would take the child to a nursery school two mornings a week. The foster family would not provide transportation nor be involved in the nursery school in order that the period of separation give them a well-defined "break." This arrangement was increased to three mornings a week as the child grew older, and she remains in this same home three years later. She has become a very lovable child who gets along well with other children and adults, and the bond of affection is deep between her and her foster parents.

Then one needs to ask questions about oneself as a nurse. Very importantly, why am I, the nurse, responding the way I am? Is my response appropriate to the situation? Am I identifying with this mother? Am I critical of her? Do I have difficulty being a loving person?

A schema for recognizing problems in mother-child love

Having looked at some factors affecting the mother's ability to love her child, one can then look at the interaction between the mother and her child. Some of the best observations can be done while the mother is alone with her child in the waiting room as well as in the home or during the interview. These observations might include:

1. Do this mother and child get any pleasure from each other's company? Do they look happy, smile, and talk pleasantly? Do they cooperate? Do they interact freely, move freely, and express themselves freely bodily and verbally?

2. Does the mother permit the child to have any physical contact with her? If so, is it rough or gentle? Is there any tenderness? Can she comfort him?

3. Do this mother and child trust one another? Is the mother reliable? Is the mother's inconsistency limited or wide-ranging, for all parents are inconsistent at times.

4. Can this mother and child reassure and encourage one another?

5. How much force and compulsion exists in their relationship? Is it appropriate? How are rage and anger handled between mother and child? Is the mother threatened by the child's hate, destruction, or threats? How does the mother handle her own negative feelings?

6. Does the mother promote independence and how? Does she have a sense of timing in developmental expectations and in introducing her child to his environment? Does she permit him any experimentation and under what circumstances? Does she permit the child to teach her something about his own rhythm? Can she accept this rhythm and use it to promote harmony and cooperation?

7. Can this mother use periods of normal regression (that is, hurts, fears, and grief) to reassure the child and to demonstrate her affection? Does she try to be understanding and to see the situation as the child sees it? Does she try to help the child cope with the situation at a level appropriate to his development?

8. Can the child play? Can he play alone and with others? Is he imaginative?[3]

Helping a mother to love her child

Once a problem in the expression of love between a mother and her child has been identified, the nurse must find some way of improving the situation. Some methods will be outlined, using specific cases as illustrations.

Case 1

Mrs. T is the wife of a student who is obtaining a doctorate in history. They have one son, 6 months old. When Mrs. T brings her son for regular well-child visits, the nurse notices:

1. Mrs. T seems unable to comfort her son when he becomes upset over minor episodes such as moving from one room to another.

2. Mrs. T is threatened and defensive when suggestions are made in response to her questions, yet she appears to have no solutions of her own.

3. Mrs. T does not seem able to accept praise or compliments, yet her behavior indicates she wants and needs them.

4. Mrs. T is lonely, yet she is unable to make friends and will not join in any groups.

5. Mrs. T refuses to leave her son with anyone for even an hour, although she is angry at him for imposing restrictions on her.

6. Mrs. T was adopted at 2½ years of age after living in foster homes. She describes her adopting mother as "cool, undemonstrative, refusing to set limits, much more intelligent than I."

The first step in the treatment process was the formation of a relationship with Mrs. T. Her primary problem appeared to be one of basic trust—she did not trust anyone, therefore she did not get involved with anyone. Great care was taken in making appointments for suitable times when neither Mrs. T nor the nurse would have to cancel or change them.

Mrs. T was reassured many times that the record kept of the visits was shared only by the nurse and the doctor and that she would be consulted before any other sharing of information took place.

Mrs. T was encouraged to do those things that she said she could do well, such as baking and providing stimulating materials for her child. The nurse then assumed the role of learner and encouraged Mrs. T to teach her some of her skills and exchange some ideas. Compliments and praise were given with care in an attempt to avoid "phoneyness." They were given when Mrs. T recognized she had done well and indicated that she wanted praise. In this area the nurse assumed the role of a mother by attempting to promote security and provide opportunity for achievement and by creating situations where Mrs. T achieved success and therefore merited praise. This is not an easy feat when the patient has a poor self-concept and feels unworthy of praise and of the nurse's care and attention. Patients such as Mrs. T introduce situations into the relationship, consciously and unconsciously, that give the nurse opportunities to "drop her"—which is what Mrs. T expected. Mrs. T was able to express this once—"My own (biological) mother 'dropped me' (that is, put me out for adoption). I guess that's why I expect everyone else to do so too."

Mrs. T was helped to verbalize some of her feelings concerning her adoption, which she had not done before. She was encouraged to ask her adoptive mother questions that she had not asked, but to which she wanted the answers. She was helped to compare and contrast her childhood with that of her son's, and she was helped to recognize the similarities and differences and what this could mean.

As Mrs. T got better (that is, came to terms with her own childhood experiences) and became more receptive to the nurse's attempts to help her care for her son, the nurse allowed the relationship to become as between friends. Making friends was the biggest problem to be overcome by Mrs. T, and the nurse assumed the role of "friend" to promote growth in this area. Chats on the phone, visits for coffee, exchanging recipes, etc. as one would do with friends, were implemented as a therapeutic measure, until finally Mrs. T was receptive to the friendly overtures from others. She was then encouraged to engage in relationships with other nurses in the clinic, who acted as "friendly nurses," and then Mrs. T began to move out and make friends in the community.

Once Mrs. T had developed enough trust to engage in a friendship relationship, she became more relaxed and "comfortable" and was beginning to be able to "give of herself" to her son. The final outcome was that Mrs. T became a more loving mother and was able to perform her mothering role more easily, and with greater satisfaction. Mrs. T also grew in maturity and self-confidence.

Case 2

Mrs. K is a mother with her first baby, just born. She told the nurse that her mother died when she was an infant and that she was raised by her father and some aunts. She stated that Mr. K's mother died when he too was an infant and he was raised by his father.

Mrs. K expressed great concern over every aspect related to child care. She appeared insecure and emotionally fragile. An assumption was made at the beginning with respect to Mrs. K, that is, that every step of the mothering process would have to be taught because it would not likely be innate. This turned out to be a correct assumption.

With respect to giving affection Mrs. K did not present the same problems as Mrs. T. Mrs. K did not have overwhelming needs for acceptance and affection for herself. When the activities were appropriate, Mrs. K was given direct demonstrations and then encouraged to practice rocking the baby, cuddling and nuzzling him, caressing, kissing, comforting, and singing to and talking to the baby. In other words, actions had to be "spelled out."

Gradually, Mrs. K began to observe other mothers and try out what she liked about what they did. She became so interested that she enrolled as a student in a preschool nursery education program to improve her skills as a mother.

Case 3

Mrs. B was a young mother of three children. She was often noted to be depressed and seemed disinterested in the children, although she said she would like to have more. The following information was obtained about Mrs. B:

1. Mrs. B's parents were divorced following a very stormy marriage. Mrs. B, at age 14, chose to live with her father after the divorce and does not know her mother's whereabouts. Her mother was an alcoholic.

2. Mrs. B's only sibling, a brother, committed suicide in prison at age 25. He was diagnosed as schizophrenic.

3. Mrs. B appeared happily married. Her husband was a successful graduate student who had attained considerable renown through his research. He spent regular periods of time with his family, and they all appeared to value this relationship.

4. The children were quiet, unable to play with the toys at the clinic, shy of other children, and did not attempt to touch their mother or speak to her.

5. Mrs. B was afraid to disagree in any way with her husband for fear that her marriage would become like her parents'.

She also said that her husband was kind, considerate, and not unreasonable.

This case was discussed between the nurse, doctor, and social worker because of its complexity. It was decided that Mr. and Mrs. B needed assistance in working through marital problems. They had to be helped to cope with Mrs. B's great insecurity concerning the stability of her marriage. Mr. B was encouraged to "draw his wife out" and to get her to express her feelings, including negative ones.

Once improvement occurred within the marriage and Mrs. B became more secure, her interaction with her children improved; she needed little assistance in expressing love and affection. She loved her children very much and it was gratifying to watch Mrs. B express this freely.

Case 4

Mrs. D was a foster mother who had recently received a 2-year-old girl, Lisa, to care for.

Lisa had been in two foster homes, and in both homes she was not accepted. Following this was a period of hospitalization because of "failure to thrive," that is, she appeared to stop gaining in height or weight. The investigations were negative, and adoption was tried but failed immediately. Now she was with Mrs. D. The following observations were made:

1. Lisa, at first docile and superficially affectionate, quickly became belligerent, destructive, and hateful. She rejected anyone's attempts to cuddle or fondle her, scorned praise, scowled, bit, fought, and had frequent and uncontrolled temper tantrums.

2. Mrs. D was frustrated, upset, unsure whether to love or to punish, and thwarted by the child no matter what she did. Mrs. D's natural urge was to hug and comfort Lisa who struggled until she got away.

Mrs. D was encouraged to verbalize her pent-up feelings about poor foster mothers, social workers, "terrible people who would do this to a child," and her frustration at being rejected by Lisa. Mrs. D was helped to explore what these experiences did to Lisa in terms of feeling wanted and being secure, and why she "didn't trust" and was "so superficial."

Discussion also centered around "how do you help Lisa feel secure," and the similarities and differences between discipline and punishment were explored. Mrs. D was encouraged to be as consistent and reasonable as she could, but she was to feel free to discipline Lisa when all else failed. However, discipline should not involve rejection of Lisa or deprivation because she had had too much of this. Banishment to another room to "cool off," and yet where she could still see Mrs. D, proved to be the best method.

Mrs. D was encouraged to curb her instinct to hug and comfort Lisa, to redirect this instinct to promoting activities Lisa enjoyed, and to help Lisa to verbalize feelings. Lisa was given a doll to hug and kiss and comfort. Gradually she began to want the same things for herself, and Mrs. D was encouraged to give hugs, kisses, and caresses when Lisa could tolerate it and only for as long as Lisa could tolerate it.

It was suggested to Mr. and Mrs. D that they plan regular outings with Lisa alone, and to indulge her on these occasions, that is, buy a ribbon for her hair, have a drink at a soda fountain, look at animals in the pet shop. The D's on their own got Lisa a kitten, which she treated kindly and with affection.

Mr. and Mrs. D were also encouraged to plan for outings and socializing without Lisa, as a method of handling their own feelings. The D's and Lisa became so attached that she was adopted by them a year later.

Summary

Some factors involving the giving and receiving of love between mothers and their children have been presented, and some suggestions for recognizing problems have been outlined.

The author has included some cases and techniques used to remedy the situations presented, but she recognizes that nursing research is needed in this area to develop a framework for nursing action to improve mother-child love.

References

1. Deutsch, H.: The psychology of women, vol. I. Motherhood, New York, 1945, Grune & Stratton, Inc.
2. Bowlby, J.: Child care and the growth of love, Harmondsworth, 1961, Penguin Books, Ltd.
3. Winnicott, D. W.: The child, the family, and the outside world, Harmondsworth, 1964, Penguin Books, Ltd.

Bibliography

Bowlby, J.: Attachment and loss, vol. 1, New York, 1969, Basic Books, Inc., Publishers.

Cahill, I. D.: Mutual withdrawal: the nurse and the low socioeconomic mother. In Bergersen, B. S., Anderson, E. H., Duffey, M., Lohr, M., and Rose, M. H.: Current concepts in clinical nursing, vol. 1, St. Louis, 1967, The C. V. Mosby Co.

Caplan, G.: Concepts of mental health and consultation: their application in Public Health Social Work, Washington, D. C., 1959, Children's Bureau, U. S. Department of Health, Education, and Welfare.

Levy, D.: Psychosomatic studies of some aspects of maternal behaviour, Psychosomatic Med. 4: 223-227, 1942.

Marshall, H. K., Kennell, J. H., Plumb, N., and Zuehlke, S.: Human maternal behaviour at the first contact with her young, Pediatrics 46:187-192, 1970.

Maternity nursing

With an introduction by
Edith H. Anderson

As the tempo of change quickens modern living, we look with relief to those seemingly unchanging features of life. At least childbearing has been the same through the ages. But is it? For as science has made remarkable advances, particularly in genetics and fetology, the "watch and wait" attitude that has been characteristic of maternity care has given way as the authors in this section illustrate.

To many it is a fundamental right of a woman to determine whether or not she will bear a child. Reflecting this attitude is the recent trend toward modification of state laws restricting abortions. As a result the increasing number of women admitted to hospitals for abortions challenges nursing service to respond to the special needs of these patients. Murphy and Jones describe the effects on a nursing service of a liberalized abortion law in one state. Their view that abortion patients have the characteristics of a subcultural group gives maternity nurses a framework with which to analyze the care of these patients.

Cahill points out problems that have resulted from a conflict of values among the staff who attend a woman who is having a therapeutic abortion. She indicates that we are expressing future shock as defined by Alvin Toffler in his recent book.

What determines the size of a newborn? Gilien carefully reviews the anthropological literature and tells of the relative significance of genetic and environmental factors, including maternal weight and smoking.

Assessing the condition of the fetus is becoming more accurate with the variety of instrumentation available. Strickland describes fetal assessment techniques and illustrates nursing intervention in a series of patient situations in which nurses display sensitivity to parent's burden of choice about the outcome of pregnancy when knowledge about the fetus is available.

Pain and labor have been closely associated through the ages. Goodwin reviews the historical association, the attempts to control pain, and the present state of knowledge about pain during labor. She describes psychoprophylaxis and evaluates its effectiveness in making labor a positive experience for the woman and her husband. The need of the woman in labor for support concerns Rich, too. Her research led her to investigate the interaction of the nurse and the woman in labor in terms of ego-supporting mechanisms.

The new mother's stay in the hospital after the birth of the baby is only a few days. To make the care of new mothers significant during the brief postpartum hospitalization, Tanner outlines and develops a nursing assessment that will assist nurses to use their contacts with new mothers effectively.

Should maternity patients continue to be cared for within the setting of a general hospital? Cameron takes a futuristic view of the question and proposes a design for a new facility for mothers and newborn infants that is more natural for the family, less expensive, and potentially more effective in making the expertise of maternity nurses available to families.

Motherhood is far from simple according to Bennett and Walker. In their view, today's young woman is caught in a dilemma as she tries to set a satisfactory lifestyle that includes being a good mother in our society. They suggest that maternity nurses embrace a liberalized view of motherhood and help women deal with their dilemma. They cite studies of different and acceptable styles of motherhood.

Traditional barriers to adoption are being broken down; in some states single women can now adopt children and babies of mixed racial background are being sought by couples. Concerned with couples who adopt children, Shelley Horton explores changing attitudes toward adoption and suggests an active role for nurses in assisting parents to be successful with their adoptive children.

Chapter 16

Nursing the therapeutic abortion patient

Juanita F. Murphy
Sharon M. Jones

Nursing, as one of society's institutions, is constantly undergoing change. Changes within nursing, as in other institutions, are the result of both internal and external factors. An internal factor that has affected nursing during the past decade is the introduction of clinical specialization. The passing of new laws is an external factor that modifies nursing to varying degrees. The purpose of this chapter is to describe some changes that have occurred in obstetrical-gynecological nursing as the result of a new, liberal therapeutic abortion law in one of the fifty United States.

History of abortions

The simple injunction "thou shalt not kill" has become a permanent part of our social and moral fabric. Contrary practices are considered to be heretical. Consistent with our societal values that place infinite importance on *life,* nursing is concerned with the protection and maintenance of life.

For nurses the questions of when life begins and when life is terminated are of recent importance. In nursing education and nursing practice, laws concerning the termination of life are considered primarily from a legal rather than from a moral or social perspective. Such laws are considered to be problems extraneous to nurses and their practice and are given peripheral treatment in lectures dealing with the legal aspects of nursing. Most nurses are totally unprepared to cope with the moral, social, and practical issues emanating from recent laws that liberalize therapeutic abortion practices.

Our civil laws and the canon law of the Roman Catholic Church concerning abortion are of rather recent vintage. Lader[1] maintains "prohibitions against abortion are essentially a product of Christian philosophy." Abortion practices were incorporated into the basic moral and legal framework of most societies prior to the Christian era. Lecky[2] states "the practice of abortion was one to which few persons in antiquity attached any deep feelings of condemnation" and describes this practice as "almost universal."

Aristotle viewed abortion as an appropriate form of population control. An extensive literature on abortive techniques was developed by the Greeks and Romans as well as by the Egyptians. Prior to the beginning of the Christian era, abortion was not subject to Roman law or social stigma. The termination of fetal life was not a violation of law or morality, since the fetus was not a human being and only at birth acquired a soul. Lader[1] notes that only the husband, whose control over the family was absolute, could order an abortion.

Authorities of Christian teachings tended to exert pressure toward change in two divergent directions concerning the solidly ingrained Roman custom of abortion. (1) With an emphasis on the emancipation of women, Roman women demanded abortions not only to control family size but also for personal and social reasons. According to Lader,[1] "the incidence of abortion was at its peak during Caesar's reign." (2) Christian doctrine was based on the principle that life itself was of divine origin. Conception was a divine act. Termination of fetal life at any point in development was branded as murder.

The question of when the fetus is imbued with a soul has remained a dilemma of the church. Most of the early theologians retained Aristotle's three stages of development of the soul in which there is a "vegetable soul" at conception, an "animal soul" as it becomes vivified, and a "rational soul" into which it develops ultimately. These three stages of the soul were accepted by the Roman customs and to some degree by the church authorities. Thus, abortion prior to animation was justifiable.

During the thirteenth century, church doctrine became enmeshed with English common law, and abortion was placed under civil law. The theological principle of soul beginning with animation was supported by the physiological principle that maintains life begins with "quickening," or first feelings of life. According to Lader,[1] "abortion before quickening was probably practiced with minor interference" for hundreds of years prior to the turn of the nineteenth century.

After numerous swings of the doctrinal pendulum, from abortion as justifiable before animation to abortion as murder at any point in fetal development, the church ended the debate in 1869 by the negative sanction of abortion from the moment of conception. This position is staunchly defended by most church authorities today. The steadfastness of the defense has created and continues to create an impact on the civil laws of our country.

Recent attempts to liberalize abortion laws

The legal termination of pregnancy is prohibited in almost every state. Yet beyond question abortions occur frequently, and most induced abortions are performed under conditions that defy medical and legal control. Even though the conditions under which illegal abortions are performed have improved, the risks associated with this practice have not been explicitly altered. For example, antibiotics, blood transfusions, and asepsis are not utilized readily by most illegal abortionists.

The scope and impact of the problem of illegal abortions in the United States are not known. In 1955 a committee was appointed to estimate the number of induced abortions (legal as well as illegal) performed annually. As a result of the committee's work, a range of 200,000 to 1,200,000 induced abortions was estimated.[3] Recent surveys have likewise been unsuccessful in determining the number of induced abortions because of respondents' unwillingness to divulge such personal information.

While data on legal abortions are more accessible than that on illegal abortions, a valid national figure is not available at this time. On the basis of reports submitted to the Commission on Professional and Hospital Activities during 1963 to 1968, a national figure of 8,000 therapeutic abortions annually was estimated, with a ratio of 2 per 100,000 live births.[3]

As a result of the commission's study and the work of other interested groups, several states have liberalized their legal statutes along the lines suggested in the Model Penal Code of the American Law Institute.[4] Approximately one year after enactment of new laws in Colorado and California, respectively, 1.2 and 1.1 pregnancies per 100 live births were terminated. Even with more sophisticated techniques for collecting survey data, little is known about the impact of legalization of abortions.

Beck, Newman, and Lewitt[3] offer a listing of major research areas where further knowledge concerning abortion is needed. One of these areas is that of the number of authorized medical abortions and their implications for public health. The paucity of nursing literature dealing with the nursing care of patients who have had either authorized medical abortions or illegal abortions is appalling.

The state law under consideration in this chapter was changed recently to provide therapeutic abortions after securing written justification and consent of three physicians who are licensed to practice surgery or medicine. This law differs somewhat from the more recent laws passed in the states of Hawaii and New York. New York law requires that a therapeutic abortion can be performed upon securing the agreement of one physician. Hawaii's law, in addition to such an agreement between the patient and one physician, stipulates a three-month residency requirement for the patient.

Soon after the passage of the law under consideration, the nursing staff in the Obstetrical and Gynecological Department of one of the larger hospitals in the state noted a definite increase in the number of patients coming into the department for the specific purpose of having a therapeutically induced abortion.

Changes in the obstetrical-gynecological wards

As a result of the new law, specific geographical and subcultural changes have occurred. The exact sequence in which these shifts have occurred cannot be described in detail, but some of the major changes will be recounted.

Prior to instituting the new abortion law, the nursing personnel assigned to the ward was already working to full capacity. On most occasions the geographical area assigned to the department was fully utilized in the treatment and care of gynecological-obstetrical patients. How could the existing nursing staff take care of more patients without an increase in personnel? And, how could the already crowded facilities be expanded to treat and care for a sizeable increase in patient population?

Money had not been budgeted to increase the number of nursing personnel, which meant that the same number of persons would do less for the regular obstetrical-gynecological patient population in order to do something for the additional patient population. This "something" was still ambiguously defined. As a result, the nursing care for both patient populations was lacking in depth.

The existing geographical area assigned to this department was not expanded. It consisted of three main areas: (1) an area for gynecological patients, (2) a labor and delivery suite, and (3) a postpartum area. Drastic but unplanned changes in room assignments occurred almost overnight to accommodate the increased patient load.

Geographical changes

One of the most pressing decisions to be made concerned where the dilatation and curettage (D and C) procedures would be performed. The initial decision was made to admit patients who were to undergo this procedure either to the gynecological or to the postpartum areas, depending on the availability of beds. These patients were prepared for surgery the evening of admission and taken on call to a specified delivery room the following morning. After the procedure was completed, the patients were returned to the initially assigned rooms on the ward. The patients usually were discharged the following morning.

Several problems became apparent as a result of this plan. The first obvious problem was the attempt to accommodate a drastic rise in patient population in a pavilion where beds already were being utilized to capacity. It had been decided previously that the number of patients for gynecological surgery would not be reduced. Yet it was almost impossible to add more beds to the already crowded pavilion.

The second problem concerned the assignment of therapeutic abortion (TAB) patients to the same rooms as either gynecological or postpartum patients. It was decided from the outset that TAB patients would not be assigned to rooms in which there were postpartum patients. The attempt to assign patients with similar problems, that is, D and C or hysterectomy, to specific areas became impossible mechanically. There were fewer difficulties in room assignments of patients having a TAB by means of a hysterectomy.

Third, the population on the postpartum ward could not be predicted. The problem became acute when the postpartum area was filled to capacity. Some scheduled TAB patients stayed in nearby motels the evening prior to surgery and were expected to arrive at the hospital at seven o'clock the following morning. After admission to the hospital some of them had to wait in chairs in halls or lounge areas on the ward until they were called to go to the surgical suite.

It became apparent that specific rooms on each area would be required for TAB patients. Two three-bed wards were set aside for TAB patients in the postpartum area and were expanded to four-bed wards.

Since additional nursing personnel were not assigned to the department, the use of one of the delivery rooms as a surgical suite for D and C patients was discontinued. The decision was made to send all TAB patients scheduled for a D and C to the regular operating area situated in a different section of the hospital.

Initially TAB patients undergoing dye or salt procedures (to be discussed later) remained on the wards until the onset of active labor. They were then transferred to the intensive care unit for labor and delivery. The actual abortion occurred in bed. If a D and C was deemed necessary by the attending physician following the abortion, it was performed in the specified delivery room. After stabilization of vital signs, these patients were transferred back to their previously assigned rooms. It was later decided that these patients should be assigned, at the outset, to the intensive care unit and would be discharged from this unit.

After analyzing the situation, it was decided that TAB patients would be admitted to the hospital early in the morning and assigned a bed in the obstetrical-gynecological pavilion. After the procedure, patients are transferred to the intensive care unit until vital signs have stabilized. They return to their initially assigned rooms after intensive care and remain there until discharged. Generally, they are discharged the same day of admission. This streamlined plan is feasible only for TAB patients undergoing the D and C procedure, not for patients undergoing any of the other three methods (hysterectomy, dye, or salt procedure). The space problem has become less acute by making the TAB patients more transient and by decreasing the length of hospitalization.

Cultural changes

Our society views the family as one of its most important institutions because society is dependent on the family for procreation of the species. Adding family members not only fulfills a societal obligation but also produces some personal satisfaction for the parents. Consistent with parental satisfaction derived from parenthood, the aura of the obstetrical ward is traditionally that of valuing the beginning of *life* and the fulfillment of bringing *life* into the world. In the past the maternity ward generally has been depicted as a happy place, especially if the baby is wanted. Nurses working with the new family unit have expressed a sense of personal satisfaction.

Thus it might be argued that the maternity ward of a hospital develops a culture that is somewhat different from the larger hospital culture. Normative behavior for the nurse tends to focus on the relationship between two patients (mother and baby). This symbiotic relationship between mother and baby is valued and supported. Modifications in the condition of either mother or baby are viewed as having immediate and definite repercussions on the other. Motherhood is a process with which most female nurses can relate on a personal basis. Finally, patients on the maternity ward are not generally viewed by nurses as sick. Procreation and parenthood are considered to be healthy.

What happens to this rather firmly entrenched set of values and norms when a set of antithetical values are present in the same situation? In a recent interview study of fertility in the United States, Westoff, Moore, and Ryder[5] report the following expressions of attitudes by some married women:

> I disapprove. I believe the child is alive from the time of conception and has a right to be born.
> I feel that in anything except extreme cases where the doctor has to save the mother, it's just plain murder.
> I feel that this is both wrong and foolish—because once life is evident, it is wrong to disrupt it for any reason and foolish because you can always manage with one more.

The values, attitudes, and norms of TAB patients and abortionists are sufficiently different from the traditional culture of the maternity ward so that a subculture, or counterculture, becomes analytically distinguishable. The meaning of "producing life," family, and parenthood is quite different in this subculture. Westoff, Moore, and Ryder[5] report these attitudes of proponents of the subculture.

> It's her business. I think if a woman doesn't want to have a baby, she shouldn't have to have it.
> It's up to the women and if they don't think it's wrong for them, neither do I.

Niswander, Klein, and Randall[6] suggest that the parent culture is progressively taking on the values, attitudes, and norms of the subculture. In their study of the therapeutic abortions done in two hospitals from 1943 to 1964, these researchers found that lay attitudes toward the abortion are becoming more liberal. Unmarried women, women under 20, and women of the Jewish faith accounted for an increasing percentage of the legal abortions, as did multiparous gravida and gravida afflicted with rubella in the first trimester.

While both lay and professional attitudes toward abortions are constantly becoming more liberal, the concepts of the culture and the subculture, or counterculture, have practical implications for nurses. Should the TAB patients be separated from other patients? Should nurses initiate birth-control teaching programs so that a repeat abortion might be eliminated? Should obstetrical nurses resign their jobs if their values are in conflict with those of their patients? Can nurses develop a supportive role when their patients' values differ from those which the nurses cherish?

In a nationwide survey of practicing physicians reported in *Modern Medicine* in 1967,[7] it was revealed that, on the basis of 40,089 returns, 86.9% physicians were in favor of more liberal therapeutic abortion laws. Psychiatrists were most in favor of liberalization, whereas obstetricians and gynecologists were least in favor of it. Specific conditions and the percentage of physicians who thought these indications should be legal included the following*:

Substantial risk of maternal death	76.5%
Pregnancy after rape or incest	75.1%
Direct, positive evidence of fetal abnormality	71.7%
Substantial risk to maternal physical health	69.7%
Possibility of fetal abnormality (rubella exposure, Rh incompatibility, inheritable disorders)	62.7%
Substantial risk to maternal mental health	60.6%
Substantial risk to maternal suicide	58.6%
Substantial risk to maternal emotional health	44.5%
Illegitimacy	29.1%
Socioeconomic reasons	26.6%
At the request of the pregnant woman for any reason	14.3%

To date the attitudes of nurses have not been surveyed. Perhaps as physicians' handmaidens they are not expected to have attitudes differing from physicians!

Description of the TAB procedures

Abortions are accomplished in the large hospital previously described through the following four procedures: (1) dilatation, suction, and curettage, (2) injection of a dye, (3) the salting technique, and (4) a hysterectomy. The first procedure is one with which most nurses are familiar, that is, dilation of the cervix and mechanical curettage of the products of conception from the endometrial lining of the uterine cavity. Presently the suction curettage tech-

---

*From Newsfeature: Mod. Med. 35:12-32, 1967.

nique is used most frequently. It is carried out under aseptic conditions after the patient is under general anesthesia.[8] The time involved in doing the procedure amounts to only a few minutes, but this procedure should be done before the fourteenth week of gestation.[3] After the first trimester, the dangers associated with the technique are greatly increased. Uterine perforation and hemorrhage are of great concern, as is the chance of infection.[8] In our survey of thirty patients, 47% of the total number of pregnancies were terminated by this means.

The second technique involves the injection of a specially prepared lactate dye [2-ethoxy-6,9-diaminoacridine] into the uterine cavity through a soft rubber No. 8 French catheter that has been threaded into the extraovular area of the uterine cavity via the cervical os.[9] As a result of the chemical or mechanical irritation the medication causes, the patient begins to "cramp" in twelve to twenty-four hours. At this point, intravenous fluids with varying amounts of an oxytocin are started according to the doctor's orders. The patient then enters a period of active labor and eventually expels the fetus. Analgesics and narcotics usually are given to help ease the patient's discomfort. This technique is used after the fourteenth week of pregnancy. Case studies from the literature reveal in rare instances that when the pregnancy is advanced far enough the fetus may be born alive but dies shortly thereafter.[9] It usually takes twenty-four hours, including an eight-hour observation period after the patient has aborted, to complete the process. Possible complications might occur from improper preparation of the dye. Symptoms to be noted are hyperpyrexia, chills, and headache. These symptoms develop simultaneously within a few hours after the injection. In the event of a reaction the dye is removed and symptoms disappear. If the dye injection does not produce labor within eight to twelve hours, the injection is repeated. On rare occasions, three dye injections are needed to produce the desired effects. Contrary to what might be expected, the risk of infection is not greater when a repeated injection is required. Our survey of thirty patients revealed that 20% of them underwent the dye procedure.

The "salting" technique involves the principle of amniocentesis. There is an equal replacement of amniotic fluid with hypertonic saline solution (not to exceed 20%) by means of a needle inserted into the amniotic cavity through the abdominal and uterine wall or through the vagina and uterine wall. The physiological processes that make this procedure effective are not understood completely. The procedure results in the death of the fetus in utero within a short time.[10] Manabe[9] states that it is reasonable to assume that some changes occur in the fetoplacental unit during the abortion process. He notes that the time involved may be from two to five days, which allows for resalting if necessary and an observation period before dismissal. This method is generally used after the sixteenth week of pregnancy. Drastic maternal complications from this technique recorded in the literature include cardiovascular shock, hypotension and apneic episodes, acute pulmonary edema, extensive hemolysis, cortical necroses of the kidney, and central nervous system disorders as well as maternal death.[10] According to the results of our survey, this procedure was used on 10% of thirty patients without complications. It has been found that patients whose pregnancy is less than twenty-four weeks and who have undergone the salting procedure have better results (fewer complications) if suction curettage is carried out after the abortion.

It should be noted that the D and C is the safest and simplest procedure.[11] Moreover, it requires a shorter period of hospitalization. It should also be noted,

however, that this procedure should be done before the twelfth week of pregnancy. One of the most obvious problems is terminating pregnancies by the twelfth week to be able to utilize this relatively safe and simple procedure. Some of the reasons for delay in termination of the pregnancy are (1) some women are not aware that they are pregnant even at twelve weeks, (2) some women do not accept the fact of pregnancy and tend to deny its existence, (3) some women are not informed about the opportunities to legally terminate the pregnancy, and (4) the time involved in arranging to have the procedure done often extends the pregnancy beyond twelve weeks. With regard to the latter, after the patient recognizes that she is pregnant there might be a time lapse before she can get a doctor's appointment to verify her pregnancy. After the pregnancy has been verified, there might be another time lapse before the consent of three physicians can be secured. After securing the consent of three physicians there is the possibility of a time lapse before the women can be admitted to the hospital. At the institution described above, the waiting list is long. Some patients obviously have to be turned away. The available facilities and personnel at the institution cannot meet contemporary demands.

The fourth technique involves an abdominal hysterectomy that results in permanent sterilization. The signing of sterilization papers by the patient and the husband is no longer required. Since this action constitutes major surgery, the hospital stay usually lasts about a week. Older multiparous patients usually select this procedure. In our survey, 23% of thirty patients chose this means.

Reactions of patients to the TAB procedure

What are some reactions by patients to these procedures? The following reaction of one patient was observed. When first seen in the intensive care unit the patient spoke in a normal tone. She joined the other three patients, their mothers, and friends, in asking questions about what could be anticipated. She seemed not to mind that the other patients knew she was to have a therapeutic abortion. Her specific questions were, "How long will the procedure take?" "Would medications be available for pain?" "What particular medications would be given?" "Who would be her attending physician?" "Was he a 'good' doctor?"

Later, in the admitting room an ever present, anxious tension on the part of this patient was easily observable. She displayed constant fidgeting with her hands and continuous, darting movements of her eyes. She watched every movement of the doctor. Realizing her anxiety, the observer moved to the patient's side and asked her nonthreatening questions. The patient began to talk. She became more relaxed and the constant movement of her hands and eyes ceased. Her incessant conversation related to her family and schooling at first. Later, she began expressing feelings, thoughts, and questions about her pregnancy, her present hospitalization, the procedure, and the whole abortion process itself. One of her most revealing statements was, "I'm scared . . . I told my mother so out in the waiting room . . . I didn't think I would be . . . but I really am . . . isn't that silly?"

Following the abortion procedure the patient was transferred to the postpartum area. Her demeanor changed entirely. The curtains were drawn around her bed. She talked quietly, almost in a whisper, and nervously. She kept glancing at the curtain behind which there was another patient. She recounted how scared she had been when she saw the catheter and syringe for the dye procedure. She related how much more afraid girls must be if they have had no contact with medical equipment. She talked about the entire process and related that it was "really different . . . really kind of a weird experience . . . not what I expected at all." She talked of future pregnancies, saying, "I do know one thing. I won't be nearly as scared when I have my first baby." She said she was "so glad it's over." Several times she stated how "thankful" she was that everything went well and that the procedure could be performed. During the conversation she mentioned that she had heard about "a friend of a friend of a friend" who might have helped her terminate the pregnancy. The third-removed friend was an illegal abortionist. She decided not to follow that route and by the time she was able to secure appropriate consent for a legal abortion it was beyond the twelfth week of pregnancy. One of her main concerns was the welfare of the other three patients she had been with in the intensive care unit. She told of how she had been the first to begin cramping. She related how "upset and nervous" the other three patients became because it seemed that the procedure was being prolonged for them.

Observations of another TAB patient admitted to the intensive care unit revealed the following. The patient displayed obvious nervousness, which became more intense as other patients asked questions. Her questions and responses were on a superficial level and she made many irrelevant comments, constantly referring to food and eating.

Postabortion, she continued with superficial, irrelevant conversation. When she asked about her former hospital roommates, she rarely mentioned the words "abortion," "therapeutic abortion," "labor," or "delivery." When conversation came to a close she tensely but laughingly remarked, "I hope I won't see you again." Her closing remarks seemed to imply that she hoped she would never have to return for a second abortion.

The reactions of these patients to their therapeutic abortions indicate that patients *do* want to talk about what is going to happen to them during hospitalization and that the TAB procedure itself is traumatic.

The patients

What are some sociodemographical characteristics of TAB patients? In an attempt to answer this question, information was gathered from thirty patients' charts. In general, patients who underwent the D and C procedure tended to be (1) pregnant less than fourteen weeks, (2) in their teens, (3) single, and (4) pregnant for the first time. Patients having the dye procedure tended to be (1) pregnant over fourteen weeks, (2) in their teens, (3) single, and (4) one-half of them were pregnant for the first time. Those patients having the "salting" technique tended to be (1) pregnant from seventeen to nineteen weeks, (2) in their twenties, (3) single, and (4) pregnant for the first time. Finally, those patients undergoing an abdominal hysterectomy tended to (1) vary in the length of their pregnancy but the majority were over fourteen weeks, (2) be in their twenties, (3) be married, separated, or divorced, and (4) be in a second or later pregnancy.

In addition, other sociodemographical characteristics were noted. It was found that of the thirty patients, 40% were residents of the state. Of this survey group, 90% were white and 10% Negro. Ten percent were Roman Catholic, 67% Protestant, and the remaining 23% indicated no religious preference. In terms of financial classification upon admission, 77% of the group were classified as being "private" patients either with or without insurance. Twenty-three percent were classified as indigent or "clinic" patients. In almost all cases the reason given for justification of the TAB was based on the patients' mental or emotional condition during the present pregnancy. Patients were expected to have letters from three physicians, usually one of whom was a psychiatrist. These letters generally stated that the present pregnancy represented a serious threat to the patient's life and mental health and contained the recom-

Table 3. Sociodemographical characteristics of thirty patients undergoing TAB

Procedure	Gestation period (weeks)	(patients)	Age (years)	(patients)	Marital status		Percent of first pregnancy
D and C 47%	10-11	4	14-19	8	Single	11	81%
	12-14	10	20-29	4	Married	3	
			30-39	2	Separated	0	
					Divorced	0	
Dye 20%	14-16	2	14-19	3	Single	5	50%
	17-19	4	20-29	2	Married	1	
			30-39	1	Separated	0	
					Divorced	0	
Salt 10%	17	1	14-19	0	Single	3	100%
	18	1	20-29	3	Married	0	
	19	1	30-39	0	Separated	0	
					Divorced	0	
Hysterectomy 23%	10	1	14-19	0	Single	0	0%
	12-14	1	20-29	6	Married	2	
	14-16	2	30-39	1	Separated	3	
	16-18	3			Divorced	2	

mendation that the pregnancy be terminated.

Stigma

A conceptual framework that could be used to analyze the behavior of TAB patients vis-a-vis nurses focuses on the concept of stigma. Goffman[12] defines stigma as "the situation of the individual who is disqualified from full social acceptance." In the context of interaction there are the stigmatized and the stigmatizers (normals). The stigmatized is reduced from a whole and usual person to a tainted, disoriented one and is deeply discredited in the process. During the periods of mixed contacts between stigmatized and stigmatizers, there is a tendency for uneasiness. In anticipation of mixed contacts, both parties attempt avoidance patterns. Lacking the salutary feedback of daily social intercourse with others, the stigmatized can become suspicious, depressed, hostile, anxious, and bewildered. Uncertainty arises when the stigmatized individual does not know in which category he will be placed, that is, normal or abnormal. In other words, he is uncertain as to what others think of him as an individual.

When the stigmatized individual is present among normals, he is likely to feel that he is nakedly exposed to invasions of privacy. The implications are that the stigmatized person feels that he can and will be approached by strangers at will. According to Goffman,[12] reactions by stigmatized persons to mixed social contacts take one of three routes: (1) cowering, (2) hostile bravado, or (3) vacillation between cowering and bravado. The stigmatized are perceived by normals as being either too shamefaced or too aggressive.

Because of our societal values toward the importance of life, individuals who violate these values by terminating life are stigmatized to varying degrees. If a teen-ager violates these values, her parents tend to feel that they, too, will be

stigmatized. In the hospital context the nurse is faced with a dilemma if she feels that abortion violates her values toward life. On the one hand, she is expected to give nursing care to patients regardless of age, race, creed, or religion. As mentioned before, the ethos of nursing is to maintain and preserve life. On the other hand, the nurse is expected to carry out the physician's order that, in the case of abortion, means helping to terminate life.

Expressions of the stigmatization of patients and the *real* dilemma of following contradictory mandates are found in verbalizations of nursing personnel. Some nurses have strong feelings about the entire situation, as indicated in the following remark made by a nurse.

> It's murder! When you get right down to it, that is all there is to it. It's downright murder.

Another nurse placed the burden of guilt upon the parents.

> I can't see it. Most of the girls are railroaded into the abortion by their parents. The girls don't want it. They would rather have the baby and give it up. But mama is the one who wants the abortion because of what all the townspeople will think.

While this is one nurse's perception of the situation, it should be noted that a number of unmarried women seeking abortion want to conceal their activities from their parents.

One nurse recognized the changes in her own feelings as a result of caring for TAB patients.

> You know, I used to really feel sad and sorry for the ladies who came in and were spontaneously aborting, especially those who wanted their babies. Now, I don't even feel that way. I can see it and I don't like what's happening to me. If working with these TAB's has done this to me, then I don't want to work with them any more. I'll get out.

One nurse said the following about the nurse who is routinely assigned to care for TAB patients.

I don't see how X does it, working with the TAB's all the time. She's had to work her own feelings through. I don't know if I could ever do it. . . . Well, maybe, I could. . . . No. I really don't know. She's very mature to be able to do it.

While some of the nurses seem to be able to work through their feelings toward TAB patients, on occasion, the nurse's negative feelings focus on one patient.

I can't work with that girl. I just can't. I'd lose my cool so fast. Now, other nurses can go in there and be so nice and sweet to her and care for her, I just can't.

Another nurse generalized her feelings toward all TAB patients.

Why do they all have to be so mean and nasty. They're all demanding as hell. They're bitchy. Why do they all have to be so damn bitchy!

Some nurses take the definite stance that the TAB patients should not even be on the obstetrical wards. One nurse presented it this way.

We shouldn't have to work with them if we don't believe in it. To me they are really committing a sin. It is not right to force me to work with those patients since I feel this strongly about them.

Pursuing the same idea, one nurse said:

We should have a separate ward for TAB's .because it is not good for them to be with new mothers. I do not think it is good for either of them. But I don't think we'd ever find enough nursing staff to work with just TAB patients. Besides, they would go crazy if they had to work with TAB patients all the time.

These verbalizations reflect many of the negative feelings of some of the nursing personnel who have been involved in the care of TAB patients. In the process of interacting with TAB patients, these negative feelings play a part in modifying the nursing care given TAB patients.

The above-mentioned dilemma has also affected the nursing education faculty who use these areas as a clinical laboratory for nursing students. The contemporary policy of student assignments excludes TAB patients in that there are "better learning experiences."

For the most part, nursing service personnel have attempted to solve some of the personnel problems by assigning one particular nurse to care for the TAB patients during the day. On the other shifts the regular nursing staff cares for all patients in the areas, including TAB patients. At present, no attempt is made to give follow-up nursing care after dismissal. Usually, before dismissal, a specified nurse gives information to each TAB patient regarding the various methods of contraception.

The future of obstetrical-gynecological nursing

The recent endorsement of abortion reform by the American Medical Association will undoubtedly enliven abortion reform in many of the states. How do medical institutions and personnel prepare for the liberalization of their state's abortion laws? It is expected that each state which liberalizes its abortion law will set up somewhat unique mechanisms for the enforcement of the law. For instance, when the abortion law was liberalized in Colorado in 1967, the Colorado Medical Society formulated guidelines that interpreted the law and suggested proper process and documentation.[13] The guidelines proposed that no physician was bound to carry out what the law allowed. The guidelines attempted to exclude out-of-state patients. The Colorado Psychiatric Society also formulated guidelines for careful psychiatric examination of all patients requesting TAB.

In 1968 the American Nurses' Association published a statement of intent to study state legislation on abortion.[14] The results of the intended study are not known at this time. As mentioned previously, nurses have reported in the literature only minimally their experiences with abortion patients. However, nurses no longer can hide ostrichlike from their responsibilities toward therapeutic abortion. Their responsibilities toward social reform must be relevant to contemporary society that includes liberalization of abortion laws.

Some leaders in social reform maintain that many of our welfare agencies dedicated to child care are dealing with the problem of unwanted children. The focus should be on the a priori conditions of unwanted children so that all children will have a fair chance for social and physical development.

From the above it is obvious that the efforts toward liberalization of abortion laws are becoming increasingly strengthened and solidified. The results of such liberalization should be obvious to nurses. Many nurses will, in fact, be caring for an increased number of patients undergoing TAB. Three main problems can be identified and dealt with by nurses before liberalized laws are put into effect in particular states or particular institutions. (Not all hospitals and, thus, not all maternity nurses will be contending with the problems.)

1. Where, in the hospital, will the abortion procedures be carried out and where will the patients be cared for? The description of how one hospital handles these problems should indicate that, if possible, existing facilities must be expanded to care for the increased patient load. It seems appropriate that nurses enter the decision-making process regarding facility arrangement.

2. What kind of nursing care is needed for TAB patients? Do they need more emotional-supportive care or more physical care? Do they need more information about the actual process of abortion or does such information serve to frighten some patients? Equally important, how can the psychological difficulties in approving abortions be handled by nurses who are oriented toward the preservation of life? Perhaps in-service programs could be inaugurated for dealing with such psychological difficulties of nurses. The services of a psychologist should be useful for overcoming some of the stigmatic aspects of nurses toward patients. The incorporation of midwives on the health team is another possibility.

3. How much follow-up nursing care do these patients need? In an analysis of 224 cases of TAB at Denver General Hospital,[13] forty patients had postoperative complications of hemorrhage, infection, uterine perforation, ileus, or clinical depression. Are these postoperative complications manifested during or after hospitalization? If follow-up nursing visits are carried out, can the privacy of the patient be protected? Should dissemination of information on contraception be a routine procedure during the patient's hospitalization, after hospitalization, or neither?

The nursing care of TAB patients is and will be increasingly a responsibility of many maternity nurses. If problems can be identified and explored and if there is an exchange of objective information, the nursing care of TAB patients can be improved. Clear and objective data are needed on which to base nursing judgments of TAB patients. To ignore the problems of TAB means to ignore the patients and the contemporary social changes that allow patients to be *therapeutically* aborted.

References

1. Lader, L.: Abortion, Boston, 1966, Beacon Press.
2. Lecky, W. E. H.: History of European morals from Augustus to Charlemagne, London, 1869, Longmans, Green, & Co.
3. Beck, M. B., Newman, S. H., and Lewitt, S.: Abortion: a national public and mental health problem—past, present, and proposed research, Amer. J. Public Health **59:** 2131-2143, 1969.
4. Abortion, Model Penal Code, 189-192, Philadelphia, 1962, American Law Institute.

5. Westoff, C. F., Moore, E. C., and Ryder, N. B.: The structure of attitudes toward abortion, Milbank Memorial Fund Quarterly **47:**11-37, 1969.
6. Niswander, K. R., Klein, M., and Randall, C. L.: Changing attitudes toward therapeutic abortion, J.A.M.A. **196:**124-127, 1966.
7. Newsfeature: Mod. Med. **35:**12-32, 1967.
8. Shafer, K. N., Sawyer, J. R., McCluskey, A. M., and Beck, E. L.: Medical-surgical nursing, St. Louis, 1967, The C. V. Mosby Co.
9. Manabe, Y.: Abortion in midpregnancy by extraovular instillation of Rivanol solution correlated with placental function, Amer. J. Obstet. Gynec. **103:**232-237, 1969.
10. Manabe, Y.: Danger of hypertonic-saline-induced abortion, J.A.M.A. **210:**2091, 1969.
11. Manabe, Y.: Artificial abortion at midpregnancy by mechanical stimulation of the uterus, Amer. J. Obstet. Gynec. **105:**132-146, 1969.
12. Goffman, E.: Stigma, Englewood Cliffs, N. J., 1963, Prentice-Hall, Inc.
13. Heller, A., and Whittington, H. G.: The Colorado story: Denver General Hospital experience with the change in the law on therapeutic abortion, Amer. J. Psychiat. **125:**121-128, 1968.
14. ANA Statements on Health and Social Issues. Statement to study state legislature on abortion, American Nurses' Association Subscription Service, No. 2, Sept., 1968.

Chapter *17*

Conflicts in values: staff attitudes toward therapeutic abortion

Imogene D. Cahill

Therapeutic abortions are not a new phenomenon, nor is the discomfiture accompanying them. However, recent legislation in some states has resulted in a sharp increase in the number of women considering, applying for, and being allowed to have legal abortions. There are active movements that will undoubtedly result in further liberalization of abortion laws. It is predicted that, eventually, all states will allow therapeutic abortions, and that, furthermore, they will provide for the procedure to be a matter between a woman and her physician rather than a decision of several physicians and restricted to such conditions as incest, rape, or the mental or physical well-being of the woman or her infant. The frequency is not only changing but the choice of having a child, once conceived, will become more and more that of the woman herself.

This extraordinary course of events is a result of social change of a complex nature. It can only be guessed what changes it, in turn, will bring. It is certain, however, that to those involved in the caretaking process, the change or the rapidity with which it occurs is causing more anguish, tension, and conflict than has any one thing that has ever happened in maternal and child care. In settings where abortions are being planned or performed in substantially larger numbers than ever before, there is a great deal of "acting out" of feelings that seems to indicate some difficulty in accepting this procedure or the woman having it. This is particularly noticeable when amniocentesis is done; that is, emptying the uterus after the twelfth week, usually by the injection of saline solution. In these cases the women are admitted to the maternity unit, heretofore a place focused on saving the lives of unborn fetuses.

A common type of behavior is avoidance. Everyone seems to be uncomfortable in the presence of the woman having the abortion. Contacts are as brief as possible and restricted to essential care. There is little or no information given as to what will happen or what is happening. There is no encouragement given or ventilation of feelings permitted. The woman might be placed in an isolated area of the ward. She may be assigned to the "lowest man on the totem pole."

There may be relief expressed when, because of overcrowding, the patient is moved to another unit. All of this might be done in a manner that is not overtly hostile, but certainly not one exuding warmth.

A "know-nothing" attitude may be found. A nurse who is proficient in watching mothers in labor may be strangely awkward in the presence of a woman who is expelling a 16- or 17-week fetus. Another nurse, familiar with postpartum care, may plead ignorance of the care needed for such a woman. It might never occur that she is a potential bleeder or might develop an infection. The physical care of a woman having a D and C during the first ten weeks of a pregnancy is minimal. However, she might get less attention than a woman having a D and C for a gynecological cause.

Another attitude that can be quite hurtful is the one an oversolicitous nurse might have. In the course of being what she considers understanding and helpful, she might pry into matters of no concern to her rather than allowing spontaneous ventilation—or no response at all.

Incredibly, sometimes behavior that is outright hostile is demonstrated and often by people not usually so angry. Women having had saline injections by amniocentesis in the second trimester may be allowed to labor alone and not be considered for medication on the basis that it will stop labor, even when delivery is imminent. Occasionally, one hears an overt expression to the effect that this "is what she deserves."

There may be interpersonal problems among the staff. Blaming occurs. One nurse may refer to another whom she does not like by saying, "She shouldn't be here. She doesn't approve of abortions." This may be true but it may also be projection. "She is a Catholic and hates to take care of abortion patients." This may also be true, but it may also be that this nurse

may not approve of abortions but does not perceive of this having anything to do with the way she cares for a patient. A student of mine reported that one nurse became hostile toward her every time she saw her spend an unusual amount of time with an abortion patient. "Rigidity" and "antiabortion" become synonymous epithets.

Nurses are not alone in their anxiety over abortions. Physicians can be ambivalent about the right of a woman to have one and can be angry and resentful of her at the same time. They can, and do, act out all of the same behaviors as nurses, and they carry more responsibility than do nurses for withholding medications. Sometimes they are more intense in their feelings, since they must perform the procedure. In one hospital the house staff who did the saline injections referred to the place where this procedure was carried out as the "murder room." Despite the vulgarity of such a term, one cannot help but feel compassion for those who are troubled enough to use it. Among physicians, too, there is resentment over the increased amount of time required to carry out abortion procedures, especially the amniocentesis. Young house staff complain of the time taken out of their training to care for these patients.

The examples given paint a bleaker picture than is necessary, of course, and were given to make a point. In no one setting would everyone act out these kinds of behaviors at the same time. Many positive examples could be included. Yet these examples are real and all occurred in agencies giving better than average care. Physicians, understandably enough, are often more perceptive of the nurses' shortcomings, in regard to their relationships with patients, than they are of their own. A psychiatrist stated at a recent conference on abortion, ". . . I keep a list of nurses whose reactions to patients I know. On the nursing floor and in the operating room there may be a few cold and hostile nurses, usually Roman Catholic, and the patient should be protected and isolated from these women during her short hospital stay."[2] At the same conference, another physician said, "Dr. ——, when differentiating between therapeutic and illegal abortions, was making a plea for the quality of abortion experience. If the ward nurse is against it, a woman may have a better experience with an illegal than a therapeutic abortion."[2]

We can only speculate about the reasons for the obvious conflicts and highly charged attitudes among personnel caring for women having therapeutic abortions. The most common reason given is a religious one. Everyone involved is familiar with the stand of the Roman Catholic Church regarding this issue. It is true that it has fought any liberalization of legislation regarding abortions. Its members are taught that human life begins at conception and destroying it is tantamount to murder. This doctrine is sometimes so strictly interpreted that even assisting in the procedure in any way is insupportable. If one accepts this point of view, the conflict is obvious and overwhelming. During the recent increase in abortions in Southern California, the clergy in one diocese announced from the pulpit that anyone participating in this procedure was in danger of excommunication. Needless to say, the reaction among Roman Catholic public health and hospital personnel was immediate and disturbed. A subsequent series of seminars helped ease the tension, and many were able to resolve the problem for themselves. However, at the same time, there was no such stirring of emotions in other dioceses having more liberal leadership. There is controversy even among the theologians of the church in this matter. Some, such as Donceel and Wassmer,[2] do not believe the fetus takes on human form until the time of quickening, and abortion for a serious cause is permissible up to that time.

Most liberal Roman Catholics, whether or not they accept their church's policy, believe it is their responsibility to give care to any patient, regardless of diagnosis or procedure. However, those who are conservative or ambivalent can cause tension in a patient care setting. Unfortunately, the liberal group is stereotyped with the conservative group and the liberal group becomes the scapegoat for the anxieties both groups seem to feel.

Joseph F. Fletcher, a Protestant theologian, states that it is impossible to speak of a Protestant viewpoint because it would be pluralistic, and he believes that historically there has been opposition to abortion in a vaguer, less defined way by Protestants as a "disregard of the 'sacredness' of life—a kind of vitalism." A few theologians, such as Bonhoffer and Barth, take the Roman Catholic position. The National Council of Churches advocates acceptance of abortion on the basis of health. The Baptists favor it on request during the first trimester. The Unitarian-Universalists leave the decision to the physicians and their patients. Most churches have remained silent, however. Fletcher believes that the Roman Catholic viewpoint of abortion as "murder" and the Protestant taboo have never been convincing, only inhibiting.[2]

Jewish and Muslim theologians have the most liberal points of view. It is interesting that Muslim women who have had abortions discuss it openly with their friends, something not found in Western cultures. Among primitive people it is widely accepted as a permissible procedure.

The attitudes of American society as a whole might be reflected in a survey done in New York concerning change in the state law on abortion, which allows abortion only if the mother's life is in danger. Ninety-eight percent of the Jews, 83% of the Protestants, and 72% of the Catholics favored change. This population was composed of forty-eight discernible subgroups and subcultures.[2]

Some scholars believe that the sanctions against abortion are associated with population control. Up to 1900 a growing population was favorable to mankind. Changing attitudes have come about, particularly recently, since the threat of a population explosion.

Another explanation of sanctions against therapeutic abortion is that of male chauvinism. According to this point of view, men associate pregnancy in a woman with male virility, and since the decision making about abortions is made by males, the restrictions are the result of their bias. The Women's Liberation Movement takes this position and their plea is to allow women to make this kind of a decision themselves.

A shibboleth of our society is motherhood. It is expected that every woman will be a mother and a good one. Any rejection of the role, or any phase of it, creates antipathy. Regardless of the cause of the taboos against abortion, this is probably inherent in all because it is so rooted in our culture. It probably accounts for the relative acceptance of abortion for reasons of disease or congenital malformation, rape or incest, etc., over that of "mental health of the mother." The latter can be, and often is, interpreted to include mild as well as severe aberrations in the mother's emotional well-being. The fact that a woman would seek to terminate a pregnancy if she is unmarried is understandable, if undesirable, but it is unthinkable that a married woman should seek to terminate a pregnancy, even if it means an unwanted child or parents unable to care for or love him, and the consequences of this to the child. Perhaps this feeling is behind the assumption that all women who have an abortion automatically feel guilty, when all that at least some feel is relief. Deutsch states, ". . . a motherly woman, who finds sufficient gratifications for her motherliness in her previously born children, reacts to the loss [through abortion] rationally, that is to say, without further

emotional complications."[2] The same author believes, however, that abortion often produces feelings of guilt. Scandinavian studies have been done that indicate that the majority of women do not harbor feelings of regret or develop emotional illness as a result of abortion.[3] However, more research needs to be done on this, since it certainly affects the kind of care that is desirable for a woman having this procedure. Certainly, the decision-making process for some is a difficult one and the depression and grief that apparently accompanies an abortion is real enough. However, how much of the accompanying life circumstances account for this? We really do not know.

It is true that it is difficult to shed the attitudes and values we learn during the enculturation process. In a changing world this can be painful. No matter how much we intellectually accept something, if it contradicts our basic values, it is bound to create conflict. If we grew up in a world with taboos against abortion, how can they be overcome?

Alvin Toffler, in his recent book *Future Shock*, suggests that rapid change, during which we cannot count on anything as a certainty, creates much the same traumatic phenomenon as culture shock, which is what is experienced in going into a strange culture.[4] Certainly, the rapidity with which we have had to deal with a sudden rise of such an emotionally charged idea new to our culture as abortions may well account for the difficulty in dealing with the problem.

What is needed, of course, is research. We need to know more about the meaning of therapeutic abortions to women who are having them, to their families, and to society at large, but we also need to know what is effective in giving them care. We cannot wait, however, so the only immediate solutions are innovative; for example, the identification of which nurses are effective in giving care to these women and then trying to discern what makes them so. Experimentation in counseling and information giving is essential, as is appropriate follow-up procedures. We might find out what is desirable in hospital room assignments. Do therapeutic abortion patients prefer to be alone, with another woman having an abortion, on a separate ward, or does this matter as long as the milieu is warm and supporting? Is sharing experiences in ward rounds or conferences an effective way of coping with conflicts associated with caring for women having abortions? Perhaps the most traumatic thing for everyone concerned is the expulsion of the fetus during the second trimester when it begins to look human or even takes a few breaths. How can this be handled? In some areas, group conferences and workshops are being tried. Certainly they should be effective in information sharing as well as tension reduction. Perhaps the one most effective thing that can be done is upgrading care of all the patients on maternity and gynecology units, and particularly the former.

It is unfortunate that in a service so fraught with emotionality, we so often find coldness or indifference.

In time the nurses and physicians giving care to women having therapeutic abortions may alter their attitudes and values as the culture gap that appears to have been created closes. If they cannot, there may be some modification in the numbers of abortions given or the method used, that is, amniocentesis. Eventually, equilibrium should be established. Meanwhile, we can hopefully provide the best possible care to the women concerned.

References

1. The right to abortion; a psychiatric view, Group for the Advancement of Psychiatry **7:** 203-227, 1969.
2. Hall, Robert E.: Abortion in a changing world, New York, 1970, Columbia University Press.
3. Shur, Edwin M.: Crimes without victims, Englewood Cliffs, N. J., 1965, Prentice-Hall, Inc.
4. Toffler, Alvin: Future shock, New York, 1969, Random House, Inc.

Chapter **18**

Determinants of birth weight

Nancy Ragsdale Gilien

"How much does the baby weigh?"

This is usually the *second* question asked of the doctor. Birth weight, in the opinion of the family, sums up the size and condition of the newborn infant. Their attitude is that a hefty baby will be vigorous, healthy, and sure to grow well.

Of course, such an opinion is generally correct. For most newborn infants, a weight near the average implies a good prognosis. In the United States the average is 3,300 grams for white infants and 3,130 for nonwhite infants.[1] A high birth weight, above 4,540 grams, or a low weight, below 2,500 grams, is associated with high morbidity and mortality.[2]

Birth weight, because it is an easy and reliable measure, is the parameter used most often to indicate size. Weight can be given too much importance as an indicator. Yet in a discussion of the factors influencing the size of the normal infant, weight is a useful and significant measure.

The questions this chapter will deal with are as follows: What are the determinants of size at birth? What is their relative importance? What is the relation of size to survival and health?

Determinants of size
Sex

In every population investigated, boys tend to weigh more on the average than do girls. Boys tend to be heavier at each gestational age[3-8] (Fig. 12). In a study of normal English babies, the gestation time for the boys was slightly shorter than that for girls: 280.7 days, on the average, versus 281.5 days for the girls. Yet the mean birth weight for boys was 7.35 pounds versus 7.13 pounds for girls. Boys are heavier on the average because they grow faster.[9]

Length of gestation

Analysis of duration of pregnancy is difficult due to the uncertainty of the time of fertilization. Conventionally, the first day of the last menstrual period is used to calculate the expected date of confinement. When this day is used, it is assumed that fertilization takes place on the average fourteen days later and gestation is considered 280 days. Studies show that approximately 65% of births fall within fifteen days of the expected date of confinement.[9]

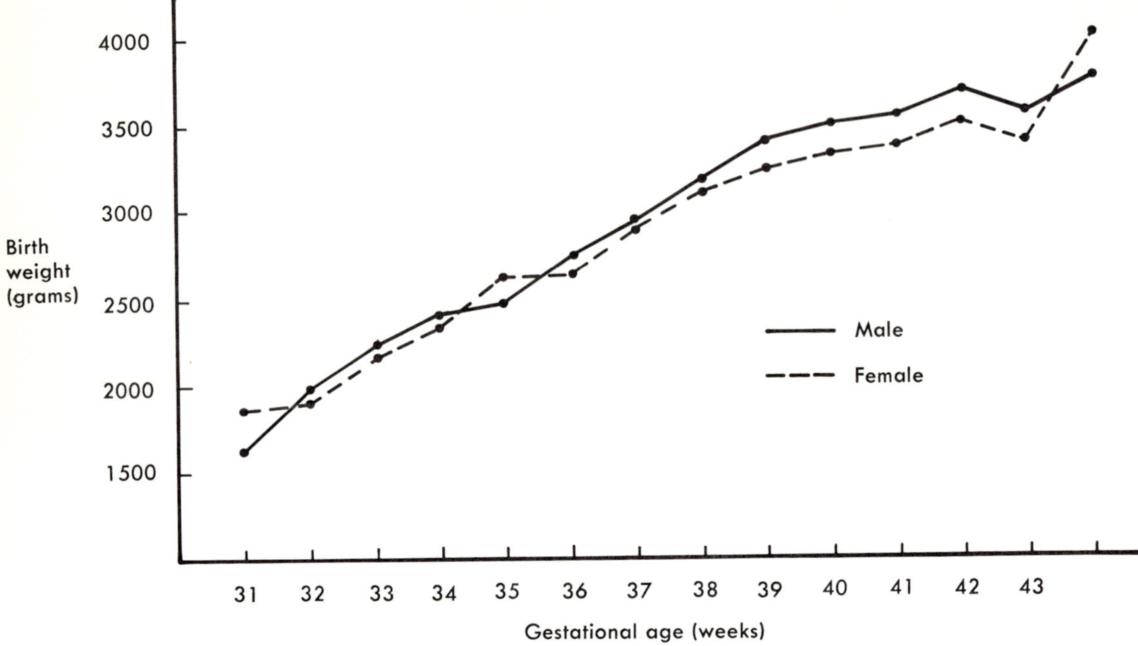

Fig. 12
Mean birth weight at each completed week of gestation for normal singleton infants of normal pregnancy. (From Love, E. J., and Kinch, R. A. H.: Amer. J. Obstet. Gynec. **91:**342-349, 1965.)

The relationship between birth weight and gestation time is complex. When over 23,000 live-born English babies were studied, it was found that the average birth weight rose with gestation time until about the fortieth week. After the fortieth week, the average birth weight did not rise as fast, and it dropped at the longest gestation periods.[10] Studies of Italian and Indian babies gave similar results. The close association of average birth weight with gestation time began to change at forty-one weeks in the Italian population and at thirty-six weeks in the Indian population.[4, 6]

When babies of birth weights under 2,500 grams were studied, it was found that 46% of the mothers had pregnancies of thirty-seven weeks or more.[11] Prolonged pregnancy was not associated with births of babies of 4,540 grams or more.[12]

When prolonged pregnancy, forty-two weeks or more, was the object of study, it was found that only 18% of the babies weighed 4,000 grams or more.[13]

Thus the length of gestation is related to birth weight. Yet the factor of rate of fetal growth is also an important influence.

Genetic factors

Birth weight is the result of both genetic and environmental factors. Probably many genes are involved in determining birth weight, since family studies do not show a pattern of transmission of weight typical of a single gene.[9, 14, 15] Although the exact genes involved are not known, some estimate of the genetic basis of the trait can be made by studying correlations, or similarities, between relatives.

It is assumed that similarity between relatives is a reflection of the percentage of genes they share. The child receives one half of his autosomes from each parent. So the child shares 50% of his autosomal genes with the mother and 50% with the father. On the average there is an overlap of 50% for any pair of siblings, except identical twins. Identical twins have 100% of their genes in common. First cousins have about 12% of their genes in common. The sharing of the genes on the sex chromosomes is more complicated and need not be discussed here. Studies of birth weight do not indicate that the genes on these chromosomes are involved.

Tests of resemblance in birth weights between relatives can be made.[16] Test values are usually expressed as values from 0 to 1. Values near 0.5 for first-degree relatives, except identical twins, 1.0 for identical twins, and 0.125 for first cousins support the hypothesis that relatives are similar in birth weight because they have genes alike. However, the values do not prove a genetic relationship. First studies were done on siblings. Test values near 0.540 supported equally well the hypothesis that siblings are alike because of a common maternal environment.[7, 17] Identical and nonidentical twins also have correlations like those of ordinary siblings.

Studies of half-siblings and cousins have helped clarify the problem. Half-siblings have about 25% of their genes alike. Half-siblings who have the same mother, however, are significantly more alike in birth weight than are half-siblings who have the same father.[15] Cousins whose mothers are sisters are more alike than cousins whose fathers are brothers, or when the father of one and the mother of the other are siblings.[18]

Full-siblings have been compared by birth order: firstborn with second, second-born with third, first with third etc. Birth weight similarities decrease the more siblings are separated by birth order. The increasing differences are due to the maternal age and parity factors.[7, 15]

From these results it is concluded that there is a maternal genetic factor that influences the weight at birth. In addition, there are maternal nongenetic factors, two of which are age and parity. Because the identical twin pairs are no more alike than nonidentical pairs, it is concluded that the maternal factors vastly outweigh the fetal genetic factors.[14, 15]

Inbreeding decreases birth weight slightly. Japanese offspring of cousins have an average weight of 3,075 grams as compared to 3,406 grams of children of unrelated parents.[15] Children of father-daughter or brother-sister incest have been noted to have lower than average birth weights.[19] However, the number of children is very few, and the influence of the inbreeding versus the influence of the related socioeconomic factors is difficult to assess.

Parental size

Height and weight are genetically determined to some degree, so the factor of parental size is in part a genetic factor influencing infant size.[14]

Most studies of size seem to show that the taller the woman, the heavier the baby.[3, 8, 20-22] Also, it is found that the total weight of twins rises with the height of the mother.[9, 10] However, in a study of a large number of Canadian women giving birth to live, single infants, it was found that weight is more important than is height in determining birth weight. When the weight of the mother was held constant, the correlation between maternal height and birth weight became insignificant. Taller women have heavier babies because of the increase in weight associated with greater height.[23]

Babies at the extreme of the weight distribution show maternal size effects. When babies 2,500 grams and under were studied, it was found that their mothers were not different in height from a group of women having babies of average weight. They were significantly lighter in weight.[11, 22, 24, 25]

The mothers of growth-accelerated babies (babies with unusually heavy birth weights for their gestational ages) were taller and heavier than was a control group. When their weights were adjusted for the weight of the fetal products (one and one-half times the weight of the fetus subtracted), there was a significant excess of obese mothers in the study group. On the average they were 18 pounds heavier.

The paternal size influence on birth weight is not clear. Some studies show that the father's height and weight bear some relation to birth weight.[27] Other studies show the opposite.[21]

Weight gain

There is no necessary relation between weight gain of the mother and birth weight: women who lose weight or who fail to gain during pregnancy can deliver babies of average birth weight.[22, 28, 29] Consequently, the literature on weight gain is often contradictory.

Some studies show no relation between amount or percentage of weight gained and birth weight.[22, 29, 30] Another study shows that the heavier the baby, the more the mother gained.[23] On the other hand, a study of heavy babies does not implicate excessive maternal weight gain.[12] Many women delivering prematures have not had an unusually low weight gain.[11, 25]

It may be said that the maternal weight gain is a weak index of both maternal nutrition and fetal growth, and that birth weight cannot be predicted from the weight gain alone.

Maternal age and parity

Studies controlled for maternal age and parity have been made on English, Chinese, Indian, and African populations.[6, 14, 17, 31-33] These studies are reasonably comparable, since they were done on live,

single births of babies surviving to at least the fifth day. The studies also separate the effects of age and parity in analysis of the data.

All the studies demonstrate that birth weight increases with parity up to the highest parities. At parities four and above the relationship is not so close.

For example, infants of Bantu women under 20 had a rise in mean birth weight from 6.21 pounds at zero parity to 6.75 pounds at parity four and over. Women from age 25 through 27 at zero parity had babies with a mean weight of 6.32 pounds. At parity four and over, the mean weight rose to 7.09 pounds. Over 30, the change in mean weight with parity was 6.85 to 6.83.[33] The difference in average weights between low- and high-parity births was usually less than a pound in any population studied, but the difference was significant.

The influence of increasing maternal age is not as clear. A study of over 36,000 American women, age 25 and over, having their first child, revealed a slight rise in mean birth weight with maternal age. Babies of women age 25 through 34 averaged 3,200 grams in weight. Babies of women over 35 averaged 3,100 grams. This difference of about 3½ ounces was not considered significant.[34] In the Bantu sample the first babies of women over 30 averaged 8 ounces more than those of the women under 20.

The average weight of English and Chinese babies dropped slightly with increasing maternal age.[17, 32] Indian babies' weights rose slightly with age. In one Indian group the average weight fell again at the oldest maternal ages.[35]

Parity has a definite and consistent influence on birth weight. Age has less influence. In English women there is a tendency for the average length of gestation to decrease as parity rises.[17] It may be that English babies of higher parity are heavier due to an increased rate of fetal growth. This relationship was not studied in the other populations mentioned.

Socioeconomic differences

The influence of general health, diet, housing, medical care, and the like is probably best approached through the study of social class differences. Presumably, the better favored groups economically are on the whole better favored on all the other factors mentioned.

Studies of class differences tend to show that average birth weight increases as the socioeconomic circumstances of the family improve.[4, 31, 36-38] A typical example is a study of all married primigravida in Aberdeen, Scotland, who delivered in the years 1949 through 1951. The group was divided into five social classes, based on the occupation of the husband. Women of classes I and II, the more favored, tended to be taller, and to have better physical health. They had the lowest stillbirth rates. Women of classes IV and V had the highest rate of stillbirths and of low-weight babies. However, within each social class the shorter women and the oldest and youngest had more babies of low birth weight.[36]

Studies of Indian babies also show that mean birth weight increases with rise in family income.[4, 37] When mortality rates were studied, it was noted that many babies of the poorer groups, although 2,500 grams or less, were mature babies from full-term pregnancies who did well. It was concluded that the definition of prematurity should be different for different social classes.[37]

Part of the influence of social class may be due to maternal size differences. In England and Scotland the higher class women were, on the average, larger and would tend to produce larger children.

Smoking and birth weight

Studies indicate that there is an association between low birth weight and smoking.[20, 39] Women who smoke five cigarettes or more daily have, on the average, shorter pregnancies and lighter babies.[39] In a study of total births, including stillbirths, it was found that women who smoked at least one cigarette daily had babies lighter on the average by 170 grams (6 ounces) than did nonsmokers.[20] In a study of women delivering full-term, live babies, it was found that the smokers (ten cigarettes or more daily) delivered babies on the average 396 grams (13.2 ounces) lighter than did a control group of mothers.[40] These findings suggest the weight difference is increased as the mothers smoke more. In one English study, large numbers made feasible a more de-

Table 4. Some racial and ethnic differences in mean birth weights

Source	Date	Group	Place	Mean weight (grams)
Karn and Penrose[17]	1951	English	England	3,294
Millis and Seng[32]	1954	Chinese	Singapore	3,027
Comas[5]	1966	Swedes	Sweden	3,520
		Chinese	South China	2,890
Adams and Niswander[3]	1968	Hopi	U. S. A.	3,401
		Chippewa		3,761
Kovar[1]	1968	"White"	U. S. A.	3,300
		"Nonwhite"		3,130
Simpkiss[33]	1968	Bantu	Africa	3,010
Madhavan[37]	1969	Indian	Andhra Pradesh	2,901

tailed analysis of the data. It was found that babies of smokers were lighter at each gestational age.[20]

Babies at the extremes of the weight distribution have been studied for the effects of maternal smoking. The mothers of babies of low birth weight have been found to smoke more than do mothers of babies of average weight.[25] Among mothers of very heavy babies, few smoking mothers were found.[15] Evidence indicates that smoking retards fetal growth and lowers birth weight.

Race

Different average birth weights for different populations have long been noted[5] (Table 4). Yet, assessment of the racial genetic factor is difficult. It is hard to control for all the known influences on birth weight except that of race.

Since infant size is related to maternal size and since adult stature is partially genetically determined, attempts have been made to relate average birth weight to average adult size. If there is a relation, then it is reasoned that part of the difference between population birth weights may be attributed to racial factors. Such a study of 14,000 American Indian babies, grouped by tribal affiliation, did show that the mean birth weight of each group varied with the mean height of the adults of the same group.[3] However, the heights of the adults were derived from the literature, and some information was old, scanty and based on small numbers. It would be of interest to repeat the study utilizing current heights and weights.

Racial differences in fetal growth rates have been noted. Some workers have found that Negro babies are lighter at each gestational age than are white babies.[20,41] In a comparison of white versus nonwhite, it was found that nonwhite babies weigh more than whites below the thirtieth week, and weigh less at 30 weeks

or more. Nonwhite babies seem to mature at lower weights and at shorter gestation times than do whites.[2]

Studies of Negro and Indian babies, as mentioned, indicate that in some populations, babies below 2,500 grams are mature at birth and do well as measured by perinatal or neonatal death rates.[2, 37, 38] One worker proposes that the World Health Organization criterion of 2,500 grams for the upper limit of immaturity is too high for Indian babies and this worker would reduce this criterion by 250 grams.[37]

More studies are needed to demonstrate racial differences in fetal growth. Indices of maturity at birth that do not depend upon weight but upon observations of color, edema, neurological signs, presence of body hair, and the like are being developed and should be used in studies of population differences.[42, 43]

Environmental factors

Little could be found to show that climate has obvious effects on birth weight. Chinese and Caucasian babies born in Singapore were compared with babies born in temporate areas of China and England. No significant differences in mean weights and growth were found between the babies born in Singapore and babies of the same race born in the homeland.[44]

Altitude *does* seem to depress birth weight. In Lake County, Colorado, at an altitude of 10,000 to 11,000 feet, babies averaged 2 655 grams as compared with 3,035 grams for babies born in Denver (5,000 feet).[45] A study of 145 Lake County babies revealed that they had the same pattern of gestation time as babies born at sea level, but the weight and head, chest, and length measures were reduced.[46]

Relative importance of birth weight determinants

A bewildering number of fetal, maternal, and environmental factors determine size at birth. Establishment of their relative importance has been attempted.

Data on more than 17,000 births and 7,000 stillbirths and neonatal deaths in Great Britain were analyzed according to the combined effect of certain maternal characteristics on birth weight. It was found that parity had a significant effect on birth weight, regardless of associated effects of maternal age, social class, height, presence or absence of preeclampsia, or smoking. Also, the effects of height, smoking, and preeclampsia were each significant after allowing for the effects of the other five factors. Neither maternal age nor social class significantly affected mean birth weight after allowance was made for the other factors.

The magnitude of the effect on birth weight of different combinations could be estimated. For example, the weight of a baby of a woman 65 inches tall, who does not smoke and who is having her second child, can be estimated to be 3,490 grams. This would be 485 grams more than would be expected in the baby of a mother who is 60 inches tall, who smokes, and who is having her first baby. Of course, such esti-

Table 5. Approximate partition of causes of variation of birth weight between hereditary and environmental causes*

	Percent
Maternal hereditary constitution	20
Fetal hereditary factors: sex	2
Fetal hereditary factors: remaining constitution	16
Maternal general health and nutrition	16
Maternal health during each particular pregnancy	8
Maternal parity	7
Maternal age	1
Unidentified intrauterine influence, posture, etc.	30

*From Penrose, L. S., editor: Recent advances in human genetics, London, 1961, J. & A. Churchill, p. 63.

mates apply only to the English population studied.[20]

An estimate of the relative importance of the genetic and environmental factors has been made[9] (Table 5). It is estimated that the total fetal factors, genetic and nongenetic, account for only 18% of the variation in birth weight of normal, western European children. The rest of the variation is due to factors operating through the mother. It is offered as a rough estimate that applies only to the population mentioned. Furthermore, relative importance of the various factors could differ in different populations or change under different circumstances, such as war or famine.

Birth weight and survival

Within any population there are different mortality and morbidity rates for babies of different birth weight groups.[2, 7, 37, 47] Babies at the extremes of the population distribution of birth weights are at a disadvantage. Relatively fewer of the heaviest and the lightest will survive to reproduce.[2, 12, 24, 26, 48] Natural selection, in this instance, acts to preserve the babies of average size.

According to selection theory the babies with weights near the average should have the best chance for survival. However, some studies show that the baby who is heavier than average has the best chance of survival to the fifth day, twenty-eighth day, or thirteenth month, depending on the study cited.[6, 17, 31, 47] In one study of English babies, duplicating one on the same population fifteen years earlier, it was found that the average birth weight had risen over a pound. The best weight for survival also rose and still remained *above* the mean.[49] It may be that the weight which gives the best chance for survival in infancy is not the same weight that gives the best chance of survival to the age of reproduction. Or, it may be that factors such as malnutrition reduce the numbers in the weight class which would make the mean weight and the optimal weight for survival the same. But at present, for hospital-born Indian, English, and Italian babies, the best chance of survival in the first month is associated with a birth weight *½ to 1 pound above the average.*

Summary

In conclusion, there is general agreement that maternal size, infant sex, parity, and maternal smoking have a significant effect on birth weight. The mother's constitution is of more influence than is the infant's genetic endowment. Maternal age and social class, after allowing for related factors, do not strongly affect birth weight.

Less clear-cut and requiring further study are the effects of paternal size, maternal weight gain, and race. Altitude may be an important factor affecting weight, but a tropical climate seems to have no influence.

The best chance of survival in the first days of life is associated with birth weight ½ to 1 pound above the mean.

References

1. Kovar, M. G.: Variations in birthweight: legitimate live births 1963, United States Public Health Service Pub. no. 1000, Washington, D. C., 1968, United States Public Health Service.
2. Erhardt, C. L., Joshi, J. B., Nelson, F. G., Kroll, B. H., and Weiner, L.: Influence of weight and gestation on perinatal and neonatal mortality by ethnic group, Amer. J. Public Health 54:1841, 1964.
3. Adams, M. S., and Niswander, J.: Birth weight of North American Indians, Hum. Biol. 40:226-234, 1968.
4. Banik, N. D. D., Krishna, R., Mane, S. I. S., and Raj, L.: A study of birthweight of Indian infants and its relation to sex, period of gestation, maternal age, parity, and socio-economic class, Indian J. Med. Res. 55:1378-1386, 1967.
5. Comas, J.: Manual de Antropología Física, Mexico City, 1966, Universidad Nacional Autónoma de Mexico.
6. Fraccaro, M.: A contribution to the study of birth weights based on an Italian sample, Ann. Hum. Genet. 20:282-297, 1956.
7. Karn, M. N., Lang-Brown, H., Mackenzie, H., and Penrose, L. S.: Birth weight, gestation time and survival in siblings, Ann. Eugen. 15:306-322, 1951.
8. Timonen, S., Votila, U., Kuusisto, P., Vara, P., and Lokki, O.: Effect of certain maternal fetal and geographical factors on the weight and length of the newborn and the duration of pregnancy, Ann. Chi. Gynaec. Penn. 55:196-213, 1966.
9. Penrose, L. S.: Genetics of growth and development of the fetus. In Penrose, L. S., editor: Recent advances in human genetics, London, 1961, J. & A. Churchill, Ltd.
10. McKeown, T., and Record, R. G.: Influence of body weight on reproductive function of women, J. Endocr. 15:410-422, 1957.
11. Terris, M., and Gold, E. M.: An epidemiological study of prematurity. II. Relation to prenatal care, birth interval, residential history and outcome of previous pregnancies, Amer. J. Obstet. Gynec. 103:371-379, 1969.
12. Sack, R. A.: The large infant, Amer. J. Obstet. Gynec. 104:195-204, 1969.
13. Beischer, N. A., Evans, J. H., and Townsend, L.: Studies in prolonged pregnancy. I. Incidence, Amer. J. Obstet. Gynec. 103:476-482, 1969.
14. Hunt, E. E., Jr.: Developmental genetics of man. In Falkner, F. editor: Human development, Philadelphia, 1966, W. B. Saunders Co.
15. Morton, N. E.: The inheritance of human birth weight, Ann. Hum. Genet. 20:125-134, 1955.
16. Churchill, E.: Statistical considerations. In Falkner, F., editor: Human development, London, 1966, W. B. Saunders Co.
17. Karn, M. N., and Penrose, L. S.: Birth weight and gestation time in relation to maternal age, parity, and infant survival, Ann. Eugen. 16:147, 1951.
18. Robson, E. B.: Birth weight in cousins, Ann. Hum. Genet. 19:262-268, 1955.
19. Adams, M. S., and Neel, J. V.: Children of incest, Pediatrics 40:55-62, 1957.
20. Butler, N. R., and Alberman, E. D., editors: Perinatal problems: second report of the 1958 British perinatal mortality survey, Edinburgh, 1969, E. & S. Livingstone, Ltd.
21. Caweley, R. H., McKeown, T., and Record, R. G.: Parental stature and birthweight, Amer. J. Hum. Genet. 6:448-456, 1954.
22. Kaltreider, D. F.: Effects of height and weight on pregnancy and the newborn,

Springfield, Ill., 1963, Charles C Thomas, Publisher.

23. Love, E. J., and Kinch, R. A. H.: Factors influencing birth weight in normal pregnancy, Amer. J. Obstet. Gynec. 91:342-349, 1965.

24. North, A. F., Jr.: Small-for-date neonates, Pediatrics 38:1013-1019, 1966.

25. Terris, M., and Gold, E. M.: An epidemiologic study of prematurity. I. Relation to smoking, heart volume, employment and physique, Amer. J. Obstet. Gynec. 103:358-70, 1969.

26. Ounsted, M.: Accelerated fetal growth, Develop. Med. Child. Neurol. 11:693-711, 1969.

27. McKeown, T., and Record, R. G.: Influence of prenatal environment and the correlation between birth weight and parental height, Amer. J. Hum. Genet. 6:457-463, 1954.

28. Eastman, N. J., and Jackson, E.: Weight relationships in pregnancy. I. The bearing of maternal weight gain and pre-pregnancy weight in full term pregnancies, Obstet. Gynec. Survey 23:1003, 1968.

29. McIlrow, A. L., and Rodway, H. E.: Weight changes during and after pregnancy with special reference to the early diagnosis of toxemia, J. Obstet. Gynec. Brit. Comm. 44: 221-244, 1937.

30. Klein, J.: Relationship of maternal weight gain to weight of infant, Amer. J. Obstet. Gynec. 52:574-580, 1946.

31. Jayant, K.: Birth weight and other factors in relation to infant survival. A study of an Indian sample, Ann. Hum. Genet. 27:261-267, 1964.

32. Millis, J., and Seng, You Poh: Effect of age and parity of the mother on birth weight of offspring, Ann. Hum. Genet. 19:58-73, 1954.

33. Simpkiss, M. J.: Birth weight, maternal age and parity among the African population of Uganda, Brit. J. Prev. Soc. Med. 22: 234-237, 1968.

34. Kane, S. H.: Advancing age and the primigravida, Obstet. Gynec. 29:409-414, 1967.

35. Namboodiri, N. K., and Balakrishnan, V.: On the effect of maternal age and parity on the birth weight of Indian offspring, Ann. Hum. Genet. 23:189-203, 1959.

36. Baird, D., and Illsley, R.: Environment and childbearing, Proc. Royal Soc. Med. 46:53-59, 1953.

37. Madhavan, S., and Taskar, A. D.: Birth weight of Indian babies born in hospitals, Indian J. Pediat. 36:193-204, 1969.

38. Ramiah, T. J., and Narasimhan, V. L.: Birth weight as a measure of prematurity and its relationship with certain maternal factors, Indian. J. Med. Res. 55:513-524, 1967.

39. Buncher, C. R.: Cigarette smoking and duration of pregnancy, Amer. J. Obstet. Gynec. 103:942-946, 1969.

40. Mulcahey, R., Murphy, J., and Martin, F.: Placental changes and maternal weight in smokers and non smokers, Amer. J. Obstet. Gynec. 106:703-704, 1970.

41. Clough, W. S.: The young primipara, Obstet. Gynec. 12:373-381, 1958.

42. Dubowitz, L. M. S., Dubowitz, V., and Goldberg, C.: Clinical assessment of the gestational age in the newborn infant, J. Ped. 77:1-10, 1970.

43. Farr, V., and Mitchell, R. G.: Estimate of gestational age in the newborn infant, Amer. J. Obstet. Gynec. 103:380-383, 1969.

44. Millis, J.: Effect of equatorial climate on birth weight and subsequent weight of infants, J. Trop. Pediat. 3:105-107, 1957.

45. Lichty, J. A., Ying, R. T., Bruns, P. D., and and Dyar, E.: Studies of babies born at high altitude, J. Dis. Child. 93:666, 1957.

46. Howard, R. C., Lichty, J. A., and Bruns, P. D.: Studies of babies born at high altitude. II. Measurement of birth weight, body length, and head-size, J. Dis. Child. 93: 670, 1957.

47. Connor, A., Bennett, C. G., and Louis, L. S. K.: Birth weight patterns by race in Hawaii, Hawaii Med. J. 16:626-632, 1957.

48. Baird, D.: Perinatal mortality, Lancet 1: 511-515, 1969.

49. Jayant, K.: Birth weight and survival: a hospital survey repeated after 15 years, Ann. Hum. Genet. 29:367-375, 1966.

Bibliography

Barker, D. J., and Record, R. G.: Relation of presence of disease to birth order and maternal age, Amer. J. Hum. Genet. 19:433-449, 1967.

Beischer, N. A., Brown, J. B., Smith, M. H., and Townsend, L.: Studies in prolonged pregnancy. II. Clinical results in urinary estriol excretion in prolonged pregnancy, Amer. J. Obstet. Gynec. 103:483-495, 1969.

Erhardt, C. L., Joshi, J. B., Nelson, F. G., Kroll, B. H., and Weiner, L.: Racial differences in weight-gestation patterns, Amer. J. Public Health 54:1841, 1964.

Hollingsworth, M. J.: Observations on the birth weights and survival of African babies, Ann. Hum. Genet. 28:291-300, 1965.

Kirk, D.: Patterns of survival and reproduction in the U. S.; implications for selection, Proc. Nat. Acad. Sci. U.S.A. 59:662-70, 1968.

Matsunaga, E.: Possible genetic consequences of family planning, J.A.M.A. **198**:533-540, 1966.

McKeown, T., and Gibson, J. R.: Observation on all births in Birmingham (23,970) 1947 II. Birthweight, Brit. J. Soc. Med. **5**:98-112, 1951.

Mulcahey, R.: Effect of age, parity and smoking on outcome of pregnancy, Amer. J. Obstet. Gynec. **101**:844-849, 1968.

Newcombe, H. B.: Screening for effects of maternal age and birth order in a register for handicapped children, Ann. Hum. Genet. **27**:367-382, 1964.

Newcombe, H. B.: Panel discussion on epidemiological studies, Second International Conference of Congenital Malformation of International Medical Congress, New York, 1964.

Newcombe, H. B., and Tavendale, O. G.: Maternal age and birth order correlations: problems of distinguishing mutational from environmental components, Mutat. Res. **1**:446-467, 1964.

Ounsted, M., and Onsted, C.: Maternal regulation of intrauterine growth, Nature **212**:995-997, 1966.

Pohlman, E.: Timing of first births: a review of effects, Eugen. Quart. **15**:252-63, 1968.

Roberts, D. F., and Tanner, R. E. S.: Effects of parity on birth weight and other variables in a Bantu sample, Brit. J. Prev. Soc. Med. **17**:209-215, 1963.

Robinson, D.: Precedents of fetal death, Amer. J. Obstet. Gynec. **97**:936-942, 1967.

Salber, E. J., and Bradshaw, E. S.: Birth weights of South African babies, Brit. J. Soc. Med. **5**:113-119, 1951.

Schull, W. J., and Neel, J. V.: Effects of inbreeding on Japanese children, New York, 1965, Harper & Row, Publishers.

Siegel, E.: Biological effects of family planning, J. Med. Educ. **44**(supp. 2):78-80, 1969.

Soumplis, A. C., and Lolis, D.: Elderly primiparae, analysis of 1574 cases, Int. Surg. **52**:340-344, 1969.

Talbert, G. B.: Effect of maternal age on reproductive capacity, Amer. J. Obstet. Gynec. **102**:451-477, 1968.

Chapter 19

Fetal assessment techniques: a challenge to the nurse practitioner

Marie D. Strickland

Modern obstetrics can be a far cry from the watchful waiting that used to characterize the nurse's or physician's time. In obstetrics, decisions frequently must be made with an immediacy that places a premium on the acquisition of accurate knowledge of the condition of the mother, her fetus, and its intrauterine environment during all the phases of pregnancy.

Most of our knowledge of the fetal effects of maternal diseases has been based on the retrospective observations of the neonate. Now, with the development of a variety of new laboratory and obstetrical techniques as well as electronic devices, fetal outcomes can be more reliably predicted. The prospect of being able to determine the point of maximum fetal embarrassment so that the pregnancy may be interrupted to offer the fetus a better chance of survival presents an exciting challenge to reduce fetal wastage.

Obstetrical practitioners in nursing and medicine need to become fully cognizant of the advances being made in the area of fetal assessment and to move these techniques from a research viewpoint to widespread utilization in daily obstetrical practice. New laboratory techniques are being developed and refined rapidly as more individuals in the related fields of physiology, embryology, genetics, biochemistry, and biophysics become more sophisticated in their querics as to the variables that influence fetal survival.

Hospitals are looking to automation, commonly referred to as "patient monitoring," to achieve greater efficiency and accuracy in aiding them to fulfill their responsibility of providing quality patient care. Consequently, if one considers the impact of an increasing birth rate and a shortage of an adequate number of prepared professional personnel, one can anticipate the development and widespread use of electronic monitoring instruments in maternity units.

It is also inevitable that in order to reduce prenatal morbidity and mortality, obstetrical techniques, such as the intrauterine transfusion, will continue to be developed and refined so that more reliable methods will be available not only to predict fetal outcomes, but also to alter them and all importantly to select the opportune time for intervention in a pregnancy to increase fetal salvage.

The purpose of this chapter is to identify through patient situations how some of the newly developed techniques aiding in fetal assessment may challenge the nurse practitioner.

The amniogram

All too often the arrival of an infant with unsuspected congenital malformations or a death in the delivery room is met with psychological distress not only by the parents but also by the medical and nursing staff. Now, when an obstetrical history or clinical observations arouse suspicions of an anomalous fetus, an amniogram can be performed. This technique can aid in the diagnosis of many congenital defects, thus aiding in the determination of the best method of delivery, and it can also offer the parents an opportunity to adjust to the tragic outcome of the pregnancy.

Mrs. A (gravida 3, para 1, living child 1) was being followed during her current pregnancy in the isoimmunology clinic because of a slight increase in her Rh titer. At thirty-three weeks of gestation, she appeared to be suffering from the discomforts accompanying polyhydramnios. Amniotic fluid drawn off showed a high bilirubin content. An amniogram was ordered. When the radiopaque contrast medium injected into the amniotic sac dispersed uniformly throughout the amniotic fluid permitting fetal soft tissue to be readily visible on x-ray film,[1] an anencephalic fetus was recognized. To support this diagnosis, the gastrointestinal tract was not visible, which indicated impairment in fetal swallowing, a common companion of anencephaly.

The decision was made not to tell Mrs. A of the anomaly, since there was nothing to be gained by increasing her burden at this time. She was informed that the fetus

was in serious jeopardy and that intervention with an intrauterine transfusion would not alter the situation. The decision was also made to wait a week or two to see if spontaneous labor occurred. If the patient's discomfort increased, an induction of labor would be scheduled. Within the week after the amniogram, she went into spontaneous labor, delivering a stillborn.

The immediate need of a patient at the time of receiving such news in a clinic atmosphere is a quiet private area where she may feel free to ask questions once there is conscious awareness of the implication of the diagnosis. Often there needs to be reinforcement of the diagnosis by repetition. Frequently the patient and her family need support and reassurance that the mother is not in jeopardy also.

A nursing care plan should be initiated antepartally. It should include an assessment of the patient's or couple's reaction to the predicted outcome. It should also include a statement as to how much the patient knows and understands and by whom she was informed. This information needs to accompany the patient to the inpatient service. Fear that they may make inappropriate comments may frequently cause the staff to avoid or neglect patients in these tragic situations. Staff members need to be ever mindful that while the dynamics of the grief and the mourning process are painful, they are a healthy emotional response and its early initiation can be most beneficial for the patient.

After the infant is born, the parents need to be informed of the anomaly and given an opportunity to see the infant if it is so desired. Frequently they need help with future family planning, for now the questions and concerns may center about the chances for having an unaffected healthy infant. An opportunity should be given the couple to consult a physician before they plan or attempt another pregnancy.

The amniocentesis

Refinement of the amniocentesis technique has made amniotic fluid available now for analysis as early as the first trimester of pregnancy. Concurrently, advances have been made in laboratories that not only permit the analysis of amniotic fluid for biochemical and immunological assays, but also permit cytological examination for an antenatal sex diagnosis or to determine the degree of fetal maturity or the existence of a possible genetic defect.[2] It is believed that the fetus' own environment (amniotic fluid) will provide the most direct information about fetal conditions.[3]

Although the amniocentesis technique itself has been refined, patients approach it with a variety of feelings and concerns. For some it offers hope and happiness and for others sadness and despair. Most patients raise the questions, "Will it hurt the baby?" and "How will I feel afterward?"

An explanation of the procedure and of its value in obtaining information about the fetus seems the primary step. A written permission by the patient needs to be obtained for the procedure. There is always an element of danger, usually minimal, to the mother and fetus during the procedure. It is essential that the patient void prior to the procedure so that urine is not drawn off mistakenly for amniotic fluid. The patient must be instructed to remain quiet during the procedure. Hands resting under their heads serve as a reminder not to move or to grab the drape. Anxiety can be somewhat reduced by not flourishing in front of the patient the long needle used to make the puncture. If the patient is instructed to close her eyes prior to the physician's making the needle entry, she usually only feels pressure on her abdomen.

The author found that by standing near the head of the examining table, the patients often spontaneously reached out to hold her hand. Touch and body proximity seemed to offer tremendous emotional support. This idea seemed to be further supported by the patient's opening her eyes and smiling. If the procedure takes a long time, words of encouragement need to be given. Some patients broke out into beads of perspiration and appeared grateful when their faces were wiped with a cold towel.

After the procedure the physician checked the fetal heart rate, and patients were permitted to rest until they felt recovered. If a patient felt faint, turning her on her left side usually enabled her to recover more rapidly.

The patients who were having immunological assays done on the amniotic specimens waited in the clinic until the initial examinations were completed. Then they were seen by the physician again so that the patient was informed of the laboratory results, the future management of her pregnancy, and frequently its ultimate outcome.

Nursing care plans were initiated on all these patients. The care plans can show the uniqueness of the patient's situation, her emotional status and feelings about the pregnancy, the findings of each visit, and plans for future management. An essential component here seems to be the need to provide a continuity of nursing care for these patients. The nurse needs to be relieved of the mechanics of running the clinic so that she is free to become involved with the patients. The author found these patients could not be rushed through the clinic procedure. They needed and wanted time to communicate with the professional staff.

Genetic problems

Mrs. B and her husband came to the obstetrical clinic for consultation. She was seeking an abortion of her twelve-week unwanted and unplanned pregnancy. She had one child with cystic fibrosis, and both she and her husband had been determined to be cystic fibrosis carriers. A little girl whom they had adopted had been diagnosed as being mentally retarded. Both parents wanted the pregnancy terminated if there was a positive diagnosis of cystic fibrosis.

Even though both parents understood that testing at this point in time would produce no conclusive evidence as to the condition of the fetus, they agreed to participate in the study. It was reviewed with them that there was a 25% chance of an unaffected and noncarrier child. The latter evidence would show on a tissue culture growth.

Amniotic fluid was drawn off for cytological study as well as tissue cultures. Several weeks passed, during which time there was no evidence of a fetus with cystic fibrosis in the tissue growth on the cultures. The physician reported to the couple that at this point in time there was no evidence of genetic disturbances in this fetus. Mrs. B and her husband became exuberant. "I can't believe it. I was so afraid I'd be crying when I left here. I was so sure I had to have an abortion," the mother glowed. The physician repeated several times that he could not with certainty exclude cystic fibrosis even with negative tests. The couple decided to carry the pregnancy through and returned to the care of her private physician.

Mrs. C, 29 years old (gravida 4, para 3), arrived at the obstetrical clinic with a request for termination of a twelve-week-old pregnancy. She gave a family history of Down's syndrome in one of her sibling's children and an obstetrical history of one child who was mentally retarded and had a congenital heart defect. Another child had congenitally dislocated hips. The patient stated she was under severe emotional stress because of this unwanted pregnancy. She and her husband wanted the pregnancy terminated regardless of the laboratory findings.

Both the patient and her husband were karyotyped and both showed normal chromosomes. Studies done on the amniotic fluid from this patient revealed normal tissue culture growth. There was no evidence of a fetus with Down's syndrome. When the laboratory findings were presented to the couple, they agreed to carry the pregnancy through and returned to the care of their private physician. In this situation the laboratory findings were able to reduce anxiety about their fear of the outcome of the pregnancy, and there was reduction of fetal wastage by an unnecessary abortion.

Although the role of the nurse is relatively new in the area of genetic counseling, nurses need to have knowledge of genetic deviations. Nurses need to be familiar with their patients' significant obstetrical and family histories and to be able to assess how patients and their families react to genetic problems within their family situation. Assessment should include family relationships, how much information family members have of the situation, and their coping ability in these emotionally laden and draining situations. The nurse can be the continuing figure; she is present at the initial consultation, examination, and follow-up meetings so that she knows what has been presented to the patient. The nurse may frequently act as an interpreter of the physician's findings to couples and certainly as a reinforcer of the findings. Experience has shown there must be repetition of the findings before understanding or acceptance can take place. And certainly nurses can give support to the patient's decision to terminate or carry through the pregnancy when it is based on laboratory findings. Future family planning for couples with genetic problems seems essential. The nurse's role in the area of genetic problems and counseling is just evolving; its horizon for expansion is unlimited if the nurse is so motivated.

Isoimmunological problems

Patients with isoimmunological problems frequently look to an amniocentesis as a sign of hope that they will be able to deliver an unaffected infant, after their previous attempts at motherhood have been thwarted or severely threatened by factors over which they had no control.

Mrs. D, an attractive, alert, 31-year-old woman (gravida 5, para 3, living child 1), arrived at the clinic in her twentieth week of gestation. Her obstetrical history revealed one spontaneous abortion and two erythroblastotic infants immunized to the D factor. She was accompanied by her husband and had come a long distance for evaluation as a candidate for an intrauterine transfusion. The fetal heart tones and fetal activity, which were good, prompted the couple to ask if this was a good sign. They were given assurance that these could be positive signs. The patient was given a routine physical during which she appeared annoyed and hostile. She became openly angry when she learned an amniocentesis would not be done on this visit. She demanded that it be done because that was why she had come. The physician explained patiently that amniotic fluid was drawn off only at times when the information it yielded would enable them to intervene with an intrauterine transfusion and that this is done nearer the viable age of the fetus. After written material was reviewed with Mrs. D regarding the problem of isoimmunology and its treatment, she responded angrily, "Why should I come in for talk only?" The physician told her that when she returned in three weeks an amniocentesis would be done.

Three weeks later, when Mrs. D arrived at the clinic, she stated "the pregnancy had gone sour." Fetal activity had diminished considerably. Her suspicions were confirmed by a high bilirubin content in the amniotic fluid that indicated a severely affected infant. The couple was given an opportunity to accept or reject an intrauterine transfusion (I.U.T.). Chances for a severely affected infant with possible brain damage if it survived were great despite the I.U.T. The overall outlook was poor. The patient rejected the offer of an I.U.T. In view of her poor obstetrical history and the outcome of this present pregnancy, the patient and her husband said that now they would direct their future hopes for enhancing their parenthood to the adoption of a child.

If only a superficial interpretation of this patient's behavior had been made, she most likely would have been categorized by the medical and nursing staff as an angry, hostile, demanding, and uncooperative patient and ultimately rejected by them. Instead, a closer scrutiny and understanding of this overt behavior of anger and hostility revealed an individual who believed that this was her last hope to enhance her motherhood with an unaffected infant. Recognition of this aspect enabled the staff to be patient with her, to determine what information she and her husband needed as to how the amniocentesis and I.U.T. are used, and to explain that it was not the panacea for all isoimmunological problems. For this patient the use of booklets and diagrams were not enough. For explanation, she needed time to ask poignant questions and to get meaningful answers.

Use of a continuing nurse figure was invaluable here. Because the nurse had been present at the initial visit, Mrs. D did not have to repeat her story. The nurse was able to arrange for the same physician to see the patient and to remind him of her previous reactions and feelings. The patient was given the opportunity to make her own decision about the I.U.T. The probability of success or failure was presented to aid her decision, and her decision was supported by both the physician and nurse. The couple also needed information and support regarding the planning of future pregnancies. She and her husband were encouraged to give more consideration to adoption.

Mrs. E, 29 years old (gravida 4, para 2, living child 1), wanted desperately to have another baby, even though she was sensitized to J, K, and D factors and her husband was probably homozygous to D factor. She was adamant that she wanted to see this baby, dead or alive, regardless of its condition when it was born. She had not seen her last baby, who died shortly after birth, and she did not "know how to remember it."

The patient agreed to an amniocentesis that revealed a high bilirubin content. An intrauterine transfusion was scheduled. By dates, the uterus was twenty-seven weeks, by size twenty-three weeks, when her first intrauterine transfusion was done with 45 ml. of the mother's washed packed red cells. An amniogram was done prior to the I.U.T. to outline the fetal gastrointestinal tract for placement of the red cells. Mrs. E's response to the sedation medication given prior to the I.U.T. was excellent. It is essential that the patient not cough, jump, or move quickly during the procedure. Mrs. E kept her arms up behind her head as a reminder not to move. Fluoroscopy was done prior to and during the I.U.T. to assure proper placement of the packed cells into the fetal gastrointestinal tract, a truly remarkable feat with such a small fetus. This mother, although heavily sedated, strained to see her infant on the fluoroscopy screen. After the I.U.T. the baby remained active and the fetal heart good. The mother was placed on ampicillin prophylactically. She continued to be optimistic about the outcome.

Three weeks later Mrs. E was readmitted because of an increasing titer, and a second I.U.T. was done with maternal washed packed red cells. After this procedure there was decreased fetal activity. The mother remained nonapprehensive about the outcome. She was discharged

with the plan to interrupt the pregnancy if an amniogram on her return clinic visit showed the fetus to be hydropic. Before that visit, her membranes ruptured prematurely and the patient went into spontaneous labor delivering a 1½-pound living infant. The mother's recovery was uneventful. The infant required nine exchange transfusions. His gain and growth have been slow but steady, and weeks later he was discharged to his parents. The parents have been informed repeatedly that the infant could be brain damaged. They seem to be unaware of the implication of the statement.

It was impossible to get the mother to be realistic about the outcome of the pregnancy at any time. Her wish fulfillment for a living infant had finally been achieved after eleven years and now she had an infant to mother and care for.

What was essential now was that follow-up care be planned for this infant, who would need to be assessed as to growth and development at regular periods. A visiting nurse referral was made to assess the home before discharge and subsequent visits after discharge would depend on the visiting nurse's recommendations.

The need for a family-planning discussion with the couple had a high priority, since succeeding pregnancies could only produce infants who could be more seriously compromised.

Nurse clinician

The author sees the obstetrical nurse clinician as a valuable asset in helping to provide care to patients with these special problems. The nurse clinician is not bound by space and time, making her more easily accessible to these patients. She can develop rapport with them prenatally as well as consult with clinic nurses and the staff on the inpatient service to keep them informed of the uniqueness of the patient's situation as well as changing events. By keeping careful informative individualistic notes on a patient's chart and by having staff or team conferences for those involved in that patient's care, a reduction of needless repetition for the patient as well as opportunity to provide better understanding and care for that patient can be achieved.

The nurse clinician can act as a liaison between the mother and the high-risk nursery where these infants are usually placed. She can keep not only the mother but also the staff informed of changes in the infant's condition so that they may know how to work, care for, and interact with the mother. As soon as the mother is able, the nurse clinician can arrange for her to see her infant and try to help her and her husband to view the situation realistically. This practitioner works closely not only with nursing staff but also with other disciplines involved in providing care to these patients. The nurse clinician can help these patients move through these life experiences with better professional help and understanding.

Electronic fetal monitoring

If perinatal wastage is to be reduced, the development of a variety of techniques to make objective evaluations of fetal well-being appears mandatory. Obstetrical practitioners have long used the observation of a fetal heart rate 30 seconds after a contraction ends as a reliable indicator of fetal well-being or jeopardy. This criterion yields too little information and can be misleading. It is the correlation of fetal heart rate to uterine contractions that is most informative.[4] Continuous recording of fetal heart rate and uterine contractions can give the obstetrician more accurate data on which he can base his decision whether or not to intervene.

Mrs. F, a primigravida at term, began a driving labor immediately after an amniotomy. The nurse observer, using the standard techniques of auscultation and palpation, reported a fluctuating fetal heart rate, and a uterus that did not relax completely, and only briefly, between contractions. Even though medicated, the patient continued to thrash about because of the intensity of her contractions, and the nurse found it difficult to make meaningful observations of her patient.

A portable monitoring machine was brought to the patient's bedside. Since the cervix was dilated and the membranes ruptured, an electrode could be placed on the fetal scalp to record fetal heart rate. A transducer was placed in the uterus at the same time so that contractions could be recorded simultaneously. On this machine audiovisual observations could be made of the fetal heart rate.

Consent was obtained from the patient when she and her husband were told that the machine would be used to "keep the baby under constant observation." The mother was also informed that her discomfort during its attachment would be no more than during a vaginal exam. The husband was interested in the monitoring device and would frequently glance at the recordings himself, after the physician had pointed out what datum was revealed by the machine. The husband seemed to be favorably impressed that a scientific instrument such as this had been developed that could aid in the care of his wife and unborn child.

The objective data remitted by the monitoring device about the fetal heart rate and contractions permitted the physician to make the decision that the patient could deliver vaginally rather than by his intervening with a cesarean section. The labor culminated in a normal spontaneous delivery of an 8½-pound living male with an Apgar score of 9 at 1 minute and 10 at 5 minutes. This supports the findings of some researchers that the number of first cesarean sections for fetal distress can be reduced significantly by the collection of objective monitoring data.[5]

Obstetrical nurse practitioners are well

aware of the difficulties they have encountered in observing a fetal heart rate that has a low intensity itself and that must be heard through intervening fluid and maternal tissues, heard within bowel sounds of the mother's abdomen, or is affected by gross movements of the fetus as well as by the activity of the uterus during the first and second stages of labor. Fluctuations in fetal heart rates have been demonstrated during a single uterine contraction that would not be detected by listening at the end of a contraction.

Uterine palpation can tell the nurse practitioner the frequency of contractions, but this usually only gives one a vague idea of contraction amplitude and the basal tonus of the uterine musculature between contractions. Uterine monitoring devices can be invaluable in diagnosing false from true labor or tetanic contractions, the precursor of premature separation of the placenta. Thus by gathering reliable data, the physician can be aided in making prompt and correct decisions as to the management of a course of labor.

In most hospitals monitoring devices are still considered a research instrument and, when used, evoke much staff curiosity so that there may be many interruptions at the patient's bedside. All too frequently the distractions caused by questions or explanations at the patient's bedside can increase, rather than decrease, her anxiety. Thus the nurse may need to intervene here, reminding those involved that discussion should be limited or held outside the room.

The nurse practitioner should become familiar with the use and value of the electronic devices, since they do produce information that has value for the management of the patient's care. However, the data must not be so esoteric that the nurse cannot rapidly assess, interpret, and adapt the meaning of the information to the immediate care of her patient.

On occasion the utilization of these devices may prove threatening to the patient. Thus she must be made to believe that they are for her benefit and that of her unborn child. Many hospitals are looking to the use of a multiple monitoring console so that several patients may be observed at one time. The nurse practitioner must not allow this type of device, which is most likely located away from the patients' bedside, to isolate them from these patients, leaving them anxious, lonely, and fearful. All too often nurses fail to recognize that many of the demands for attention made on them are often subconscious attempts on the part of their patients to assure themselves that the nurses are "out there" and are interested in them personally. Lesser and Keane found that all the women in their study vigorously stressed that the satisfactory handling of their various needs during labor depended primarily on how their need for a human presence throughout labor was fulfilled.[6]

The patient attached to a monitor must be made to feel at ease to decrease base line interference for the graphs. Because the most desirable position for the patient with these attachments is the recumbent position, the patient may experience a great deal of discomfort in maintaining the same position. Back care and some freedom to move periodically would add to her comfort. There may be some situations where it may be necessary to keep equipment, oscilloscopes, and graphs out of the patient's line of vision, not only because of complications which might increase the patient's anxiety, but also because some patients might believe the staff is more interested in the scientific instruments than in themselves.

As nurse practitioners, we should encourage the use of these devices because of what they can do better than we can do. Thus we can be freed not only to give physical care but also to offer emotional support, coaching, and, on occasion, just human companionship.

Implications for change
in nursing practice

Fetal medicine is only in its initial stage of development. New techniques are continually being developed and refined that will permit not only an accurate assessment and prediction of fetal outcome, but also development of techniques to alter the outcome.

Laboratory methods have been developed to predict the sex of an unborn child, and new techniques are being developed to assure the sex determination at the time of conception.

Researchers are trying to find answers to the following questions. What is the recipe for a man? Can the genetic formula be rewritten to prevent disease? Can undesirable genetic determinants be altered so that genetic defects are not promulgated?

Techniques are constantly being refined so that fetal defects may be diagnosed early. Investigators are already trying to develop and perfect techniques by which a damaged fetus may be removed from the uterus, repaired, and returned to its natural incubator, the uterus, for continued growth.

A whole new facet of fetal medicine will be the technique of transplantation, which is being contemplated in a variety of ways. Two possibilities are transplantation of the fetus from a hazardous uterine environment to another more healthy one and giving a woman, by transplantation, a uterus that is healthier than her own, which would permit her to provide an environment that is more conducive to the growth of a healthy fetus.

What are the implications for nursing practice? The obstetrical nurse practitioner must keep abreast of the changes being brought about by medical science. As these techniques move from the laboratory animal to the patient, the nurse must be an integral part of the health team.

The nurse practitioner must not feel threatened by changes brought about by the use of these assessment techniques. Rather she should be alert and receptive to the ways in which they will enable her to give better care to her patients.

Nurses need to have knowledge of these techniques because information will have to be shared with patients and their husbands, and information that couples already have will need to be clarified and reinforced. As these techniques become an integral part of daily obstetrical practice, nurses need to be aware of conflicts that may arise in the individuals who agree to them. The role of the nurse practitioner in fetal medicine is not clearly defined. It will evolve only as strongly as we accept its challenge.

Summary

Many individuals still consider developments in the area of fetal medicine mainly from a research point of view. This chapter attempted to show the practical use of some of the fetal assessment techniques now available and how they may influence nursing practice.

The value of these techniques certainly rests in their ability to assess the fetal environment by collecting reliable data, which then better enables the clinician to manage the course of the pregnancy. As new techniques are developed and made available in daily obstetrical care, the nurse practitioner must be alert to their challenge, that is, how they influence or alter nursing practice so that we may deliver better health care to mothers and their unborn infants.

References

1. Queenan, John T., and Gadow, Enrique, C.: Amniography for the detection of congenital malformations, Obstet. Gynec. 4:468, 1970.
2. Fuchs, Fritz, and Cedarquist, Lars L.: Antenatal diagnosis of sex and congenital diseases, Clin. Obstet. Gynec. 13:169, 1970.
3. Fuchs, Fritz, and Cedarquist, Lars L.: Diag-

nosis of amniotic fluid analysis, Clin. Obstet. Gynec. **13**:182, 1970.

4. Cerevka, Joseph, Scheffs, J. S., and Vasicka, A.: Shape of uterine contractions (intra-amniotic pressure) and corresponding fetal heart rate, Obstet. Gynec. **5**:695-703, 1970.

5. Paul, Richard H., and Hon, Edward H.: A clinical fetal monitor, Obstet. Gynec. **2**:161-169, 1970.

6. Lesser, Marion S., and Keane, Vera R.: Nurse-patient relationships in a hospital maternity service, St. Louis, 1956, The C. V. Mosby Co.

Bibliography

Adamsons, Karlis, editor: Diagnosis and treatment of fetal disorders, New York, 1968, Springer-Verlag, Inc.

Barnes, Allan C.: Intra-uterine development, Philadelphia, 1968, Lea & Febiger.

Charles, Allen G., and Friedman, E. A.: Rh iso-immunization and erythroblastosis fetalis, New York, 1969, Appleton-Century-Crofts.

Frank, Sister Charles Marie: Spirit of nursing in a scientific age, Hosp. Progr. **45**:130-138, 1964.

Fuchs, Fritz, and Cedarquist, Lars L.: Antenatal sex determination: a historical review, Clin. Obstet. Gynec. **13**:159-177, 1970.

Fuchs, Fritz, and Cedarquist, Lars L.: Recent advances in antenatal diagnosis by amniotic fluid analysis, Clin. Obstet. Gynec. **13**:178-201, 1970.

Gregg, S., and Hutchinson, D.: The fetal transfusion survivor, J.A.M.A. **209**:1059-1062, 1969.

Hasselmeyer, Eileen G.: Indices of fetal welfare. In Bergensen, B. S., Anderson, E., Duffey, M., Lohr, M., and Rose, M. H., editors: Current concepts in clinical nursing, vol. 2, St. Louis, 1969, The C. V. Mosby Co.

Hirschhorn, K.: Anmiocentesis, enzyme tests aid in genetic counseling, Hosp. Med. **5**:77, 1969.

Kellar, R. J.: Modern trends in obstetrics, New York, 1969, Appleton-Century-Crofts.

Queenan, John T.: Modern management of the Rh problem, New York, 1967, Harper & Row, Publishers.

Saling, Erich: Fetal and neonatal hypoxia, Baltimore, 1968, The Williams & Wilkins Co.

Wade, Maclyn, Ogden, J. A., and David, C. D.: Criteria for intrauterine fetal transfusion, Obstet. Gynec. **2**:156-160, 1969.

Chapter 20

How does the patient use the nurse during labor?

Olive J. Rich

The question posed in the title of this chapter seems to be "backward." There must have been a printer's mistake! How does the patient *use* the nurse? That is not the way it is! What kind of nurse would submit to an uneasy and disorienting status of allowing the patient to use her? The focus of the question is inverted in relation to the frequently voiced questions about nursing care. What are the goals of nursing care for this patient? What are the immediate and long-term objectives? What is the nursing care plan that is to be coordinated and implemented? These are often heard queries and clichés about nursing care. The emphasis of the question—how does the patient use the nurse during the process of labor—is on the patient and how the patient sees her needs at this time and in this unique situation. The emphasis is not on the nurse's perception of the patient's needs nor is it on the superimposition of a plan of care.

The question suggests that if a warm, accepting, knowledgeable, skillful nurse is available to the patient during labor, the patient will engage this nurse in a dynamic and creative process of nursing care. This was the approach utilized in a study of the verbal behaviors of nineteen multiparous patients who were having normal, active labor processes. Two major insights have evolved from the study in relation to the patient's utilization of the nurse:

1. The patient utilizes the nurse for ego orientation in relation to inner processes and outer procedures in a changing time perspective.

2. The patient utilizes the nurse as a source of ego strength, a reservoir from which she can borrow during the temporary crisis period of labor.

Utilization of the nurse for spatiotemporal reality orientation

The laboring woman who enters the hospital undergoes some rather sudden changes: she loses her self-image as projected in her clothing when she doffs dress and dons hospital gown. She increasingly loses mobility as she trades shoes for hospital bed. She has already lost her field-

familiar environment and some of the people who are significant to her. Her ego integrity is also challenged by the unrelenting inner stimuli of the process of labor—a process over which she has minimal control. These losses, changes, and inner powers tend to disrupt ego structures and to place the laboring woman in a vulnerable position.

In the presently enlightened day of maternity care, this vulnerable patient is too frequently left alone. The identification band on her wrist and the intercommunication box at her head are only tenuous ties with "who she is" and "what is happening to her." Fragmented, uncoordinated nursing measures performed *on* her by a large number of different nursing personnel can leave her with a relative sense of isolation, that is, no one person really knows her or knows all of what is happening to her. She cannot "grasp" the time and concern of one person long enough to establish a trusting relationship.

Another form of sensory isolation experienced by the laboring woman is an outright "abandonment," except for the times when routine nursing tasks need to be performed. A form of abandonment and isolation seems to occur especially when the patient is in early labor and is "doing nothing"; when the patient engages in hostile, aggressive, and screaming behaviors during labor; and when "somebody," particularly the husband, is with her. In relation to this latter situation, it is asserted that the husband is primarily relating to his wife in the role of husband. Despite his acquisition of some knowledge and skills from attending expectant parents' classes, he is no pseudonurse. His wife should not be deprived of *nursing* care.

If the patient is so isolated, she has limited ties with reality Laboratory studies of sensory deprivation[1] suggest that the perceptual system may replace normal sensory input with hallucinations. The cognitive system elects to do constructive

thinking, but isolation disrupts cognitive concentration and fantasy takes over. Abandonment of the patient to hallucination and fantasy may result in experiences more devastating and frightening to her than are any reality-oriented experiences. One would hope that most women in labor are not isolated and abandoned to such an hallucinatory-fantasy extent.

The laboring patient needs nursing care not only to reduce the negative effects of isolation, but to assist in the accomplishment of her mental and physical work. There is a new and strange external environment in which she must locate herself—new physical surroundings, new people, and new procedures. There is a newness of the inner experience of labor because it never exactly "fits" her prior knowledge or experience. The laboring patient works hard at trying to understand herself at this time and in this situation.

The available and continuing presence of a caring-accepting-knowledgeable-skillful nurse allows her to work at understanding herself. Almost none of the patient's verbalizations can be classified as social chitchat (less than 3%). The patient is primarily occupied with giving and seeking information. She offers information so that she can be known (67% of verbalizations), and she seeks information for self-orientation (16%).

Samples of the patient's search for information about process and procedure include: "Why did he do that?" (Doctor does amniotomy and leaves.) "What was that . . . what did she give me?" (Nurse gives analgesic and leaves.) "Could I have something to drink?" "I hope this doesn't mean I'll have a difficult birth." (Rupture of membranes twenty-four hours previously.) "What's two . . . uh . . . what does one mean?" "Why do I get a pain in my thigh here during a contraction?" "Do these contractions harm the baby?" "What's this paracervical . . . when do they give it?"

None of this is idle chatter; these verbal productions represent a serious searching of the environment for information that is highly pertinent to the patient's orientation to the routines and sanctions of this hospital and staff, to the therapeutic procedures that have been or might be performed in her behalf, and to the function and performance of her body in the task of labor.

Examples of her search for temporal orientation include: "What time is it?" "How much longer before we get this over?" "Oh, is it only eleven o'clock? . . . I have a long day ahead of me!"

An available and concerned nurse can provide a wide range of information about physiological processes and therapeutic measures. Such information, available when the *patient* needs it, is significant in tying the patient to a reality orientation instead of a fantasy world. The patient's husband cannot provide such information from a stance of authoritative knowledge and experience. How can the patient accomplish this important work of ongoing ego orientation to process, place, and procedure if she is left in relative isolation and is deprived of nursing care?

Utilization of the nurse as source of ego strength

The majority of women who present themselves in labor are healthy, well-integrated personalities. They are suddenly faced with a telescoped and condensed crisis experience that has a natural, physiological onset and termination. The woman approaching labor faces one of her more important life test-tasks. The "chips are down'" and there is "no way out" of the process of labor. Can her body function adequately to produce the baby? Can she manage the associated pain and discomfort in such a manner that she can respect herself rather than feel ashamed? Can she produce a whole, healthy baby instead of a mental or physi-

cal reject? She faces one of life's comprehensive tests; she wants to succeed and she knows no one else can do it for her.

The best that the professionals have to offer is an alignment with her in her situation as helping, therapeutic persons. The professionals can stand by, try to understand, alleviate some of the pain, and give care and comfort. This is all that most patients want and need during this finite stress situation.

The nurse is in a unique position to lend the ego strength when the patient needs it because of her availability to the patient. The doctor is sporadically available and usually only at critical times. He brings expertise in obstetrical knowledge and skill at these crucial times. However, he is not usually available for orienting and ego-lending work. The husband, even if he is allowed to be present, cannot tolerate remaining with his wife during an extended period of stress.

The person with whom the patient interacts most frequently for the accomplishment of her mental seeking and sorting is the available nurse. Table 6 presents data that show the percentage of patient interaction with hospital and nonhospital personnel. Although fifteen of the nineteen husbands were with their wives in varying amounts of time during labor, the overwhelming percentage of verbal interaction was with the nurse-researcher (75%). The nurse was the continuing and available person to the patient over a period of time

Table 6. The specific other of verbal interactions during labor by percentage

Person	Percentage
Nurse-researcher	75
Nurse-other	04
Doctor	09
Hospital-other	02
Husband	08
Visitor-other	02
Total	100

for the ego strength she needed. Neither the doctor nor the husband were consistently utilized by the patient in her verbal-cognitive work.

"Potential availability" of the nurse is the selected term rather than "availability" because the difference between the terms is dependent on the knowledge, belief, and commitment of the nurse. If she has minimal commitment to the personal ministrations of nursing that can be employed to relieve pain and discomfort, she will not be available to the patient. If she has a significant commitment to this belief, she will find ways to be maximally available to the patient.

The nurse is also in a unique position to lend ego strength because she possesses the personal skills for providing bodily care and comfort. The personal ministrations of rubbing a back, giving sacral pressure, offering ice chips, wiping .a warm, perspiring brow, and changing soiled linens are in themselves physically comforting measures. These personal ministrations, sensitively selected and timed according to the patient's needs, also communicate the nurse's message: "I care enough to give you time, comfort, and a bit of myself as I stand by to assist you in your task. I will not run away . . . I will not abandon you." This is a lending of ego strength by the nurse to the patient so that she can proudly report to her husband, "I only screamed three times this time!" (During the first labor she screamed for four to five hours.) The following vignette of nurse-patient interaction illustrates one patient's response to ego-lending through personal caring ministrations:

The nurse gives a back rub and also applies sacral pressure during a contraction.
Patient: That feels good . . . I'll get so dependent on those back rubs . . . I don't know if I could do without them.
Patient: The pressure sure helps. I push my body against your hand . . . it helps a lot. I wish I'd known about that the last time. I didn't know what to do.

Patient: Don't leave me!

Patient: How come I'm so lucky to have you? Does everyone have someone?

Nurse: No, I'm afraid not.

Patient: It makes so much difference. It's half physical support and half moral support, I guess. Even though your husband's with you . . . he's not the same as a nurse.

This patient summarizes what the alignment of the helping person meant to her in the process she was undergoing and managing. The back rubs and sacral pressure felt good, but it was not merely the back rubs upon which she was dependent. Through the caring hands she perceived a transfer of ego strength or "moral support" to the extent that she did not want the nurse to leave her. This was an important ingredient of care from the *nurse.* The husband of this particular patient had attended classes with her; he was attentive to her during labor by his presence, his timing of contractions, and his applying of sacral pressure. She needed him as husband and she needed the nurse as possessor and giver of professional knowledge and skills.

The nurse's lending of ego so that the laboring woman can accomplish her task has many immediate effects during the crisis of labor. However, if the patient can be helped to accomplish her goals with a residue of respect and dignity for herself, she can also move toward a developing maturity and feminine identity. The joy in accomplishment that is connected with the gratifying experience of childbearing is in part related to the mastery of fear and pain.[2] Such mastery is a maturational process.

Kestenberg[3] suggests that the menarche is an "organizing trauma" for the adolescent girl. It is a trigger mechanism for differentiating the reality of the menstrual experience from the fantasy about it. Prior knowledge and anticipation can now be compared with the actual experience. She suggests that such a relief through mastery promotes ego organization.

One might reflect on the possibility of the labor experience as another "organizing trauma" in the life of a woman. The mastering of fear and pain promotes ego organization and ego identity. The following nurse-patient interaction occurred two weeks postpartum with a primipara who had expressed much concern that she not "cry like a baby" during labor:

Nurse: You know, I wonder if some of the things that have happened to you in the past weeks are making you think about things in a different way.

Patient: You mean I'm going through a change of life?

Nurse: Some changes, anyhow. Being pregnant, bearing a child . . . the responsibility of rearing a child . . . this all may affect how you're looking at things.

Patient: You mean I'm growing up? Maybe that's it . . . I'm growing up! I've been a child for many years . . . whatever I wanted, I got. My family all expects me to act like a child. I do have a quick temper, and when someone crosses me, I let 'em have it. Like when I was in labor . . . having the baby . . . my family thought I'd scream and kick and fight . . . but I didn't . . . I think I did pretty good.

Nurse: You did a good job.

This patient sensed a developing maturity that she was trying to understand. It became explicit when she cognitively verbalized "I'm going through a change of life" . . . "I'm growing up" . . . "I did pretty good." She had an ego-lending nurse during labor; she did not need to cry and she could affirm her management of labor in retrospect with "I did pretty good."

From the nurse's point of view

The kind of nursing in which the available nurse responds to the laboring patient's needs in a creative manner involves an extension of self that is energy depleting for the nurse. The nurse who remains with the patient experiences some of the disorienting "sameness" and isolation as does the patient in a slowly progressing labor. The nurse needs much control to manage the hostility expressed by the patient. She needs to be able to manage her own frustration when she has utilized all of her knowledge and skills and the patient cries out, "Why don't you *do* something!?"

However, the response of the patient to such nursing care is the nurse's ego input and stimulus for continuing the care of *this* patient . . . and the next . . . and the next. The feedback from the patient is sometimes immediately rewarding and ego gratifying to the nurse. It is frequently expressed by the patient during the early recovery hours after the birth of the baby. "Thank you for coming in and *staying* a while." "I can never thank you enough for staying with me." Positive feedback will not always be verbalized by the patient. The experience of her sense of accomplishment and fulfillment is shared by the nurse who has had a continuing assist in helping her to achieve her goals.

The individual nurse needs the support of her peer-colleagues and the sanction of the hierarchical nursing structure if she is to successfully engage in the creative nursing process that allows the laboring patient to utilize the nurse according to her needs. The patient needs and deserves this kind of nursing care; the nurse should not bargain for anything less than the opportunity to be fully professional in her practice of nursing.

References

1. Solomon, Philip, editor: Sensory deprivation: a symposium held at Harvard Medical School, Cambridge, Mass., 1961, Harvard University Press.
2. Deutsch, Helene: Psychology of women, vol. 2, New York, 1944, Grune & Stratton, Inc.
3. Kestenberg, Judith: Menarche. In Lorand, Sandor, editor: Adolescents: a psychoanalytic approach to problems and therapy, New York, 1961, Paul B. Hoeber, Inc.

Chapter 21

Psychoprophylaxis in childbirth

Beatrice Goodwin

The history of pain in childbirth is recorded in mythology and in the written and unwritten epics surrounding childbirth in ancient and modern times. Stories of excruciating ordeals involved in "confinement" (which is in itself rather negative in connotation) have been the heritage of women for many years. An intrinsic part of attitudes toward pain in childbirth has been the existing views of the nature of man and more specifically, what properly constitutes woman's "lot in life." Inherent in efforts to eliminate or to reduce the pain of childbirth has been a philosophical concept of pain and its "utility" in life.

Historical manuscripts from the earliest civilizations describe pain as concomitant with childbirth and provide some intriguing descriptions of early analgesia. Early Chinese history notes the use of opiates and soporific potions in childbirth. A primitive approach to pharmacological amnesia is said to have occurred when Helen of Troy learned from the Egyptian Polydamna how to prepare herbal remedies that banished sorrow from the memory.[1] According to mythology, when the hero Rustam, son of Zal and Rudabah, was being born, an eagle dropped a remedy onto the bed of the parturient that made possible painless childbirth.[1] Painless childbirth was considered an even more astounding feat for those of royal blood or for those who bore heroes, since such infants were perceived (and depicted in bas-relief) as amazingly large.

Superfecundation figured in Greek mythology in an unusual story of the suffering of childbirth. The goddess Actemia abhorred the suffering of childbirth that her mother had endured and sought to avoid a similar experience. She asked Zeus to safeguard her virginity. Perhaps forgetting her concern with avoiding pregnancy, Actemia seduced Endymion and was "punished" for her previous prudery by the birth of fifty daughters—all at one time.[1]

At the height of the Egyptian, Greek, and Roman civilizations, much attention was given to the care of the childbearing woman. With the decline of these civilizations, care of women deteriorated markedly. For thirteen centuries the practices developed by the Greeks were lost. Neglect was the dominant feature of care in childbirth.

The Judaeo-Christian heritage described in Genesis 3:16, "in sorrow shalt thou bring forth children," has had much influence on attitudes toward childbearing. Today some scholars believe the word *sorrow* was mistranslated and should have been instead, *labor.* However, what was considered fulfillment of the biblical prophetic curse was described in many of the books of the Old Testament. The prophet Isaiah drew graphic analogies between distress and childbirth. The prophet Jeremiah refers more frequently to "sorrow" than any of the other Biblical writers. Typical of the allusions is ". . . anguish and sorrows have taken her, as a woman in travail" (Jeremiah 49:24).

The medieval Christians viewed childbirth as the result of a carnal sin and thus appropriately "sorrowful." To support the expiative character of childbirth, treatment rendered was typified by indifference. Indeed, the medieval woman fared worse than did women in primitive cultures. The spread of disease, filth, and "urbanization" all combined to effect a new high in infant and maternal mortality. Despite religious fervor, little value was placed on human life. Thus, concern that led to the development of intrauterine baptismal syringes did not manifest itself in attempts to save the lives of mothers and infants.

In the sixteenth century witches were brought to trial for attempting to eliminate the pains of labor by charms and other means.[2] (Interestingly, one of the techniques employed by the alleged witches was mesmeric in nature—a sword was held before the patient, who was instructed to look at it steadily.) As late as 1591 Lady MacLayne died at the stake shortly after the birth of her twin infants. She was charged with employing a midwife to provide her with "a certain medicine for the relief of pain in childbirth contrary to Divine Law and in contempt of the crown."[1]

Three centuries later the punitive attitude toward those who would "tamper with" pain in childbirth was graphically illustrated in an 1847 issue of the *Edinburgh Medical and Surgical Journal.*

> Pain during operations is, in the majority of cases, even desirable: its prevention or annihilation is, for the most part, hazardous to the patient. In the lying-in chamber nothing is more true than this: pain is the mother's safety, its absence her destruction. Yet there are those bold enough to administer the vapor of Ether, even at this critical juncture, forgetting it has been ordered that 'in sorrow shall she bring forth.'[3]

While the prevailing view of pain in childbirth focused on its inevitability and its desirability, Mesmer had left an impact on a number of women and their attendants. Mesmer, whose popularity necessitated the use of mass hypnotism, was followed by James Braid who coined the word hypnotism. After observing the use of hypnosis in labor, Braid concluded the hypnotic state the women were in was subjective and resulted from intense concentration on the part of the patient, involving the whole of the nervous system. Thus he asserted the hypnotist had no supernatural powers and that nothing emanated from the hypnotist, no power or emotion (magnetic or otherwise). There were some objections to hypnosis from religious factions who thought it not right for one person to surrender his will to another.

The failure of hypnotism to thrive as an analgesic or anesthetic technique in folk and scientific medicine is reflected in the enthusiasm with which hypnotism was abandoned in favor of pharmacological pain relief. In 1848 the tide of public opinion abhorring attempts to eliminate pain of childbirth was dramatically mitigated. It was then Sir John Snow used chloroform in caring for Queen Victoria during labor and delivery. Such sanction by royalty apparently paved the way for tolerance of and even demand for a means of amnesia and total analgesia in labor and delivery.

The fervor with which new analgesic agents were identified and utilized in lying-in hospitals reached what was probably the pinnacle of obstetric usage in the early 1900s when "twilight sleep" was first used. This method, using morphine sulfate and scopolamine, was introduced in Germany and rapidly spread to other parts of the world. "Twilight sleep" seemed to capture the unqualified endorsement of many women as well as physicians. Gradually, a wise variety of drugs replaced "twilight sleep" in the pharmacological repertoire of the obstetrician. As maternal and perinatal morbidity and mortality associated with factors such as hemorrhage and infection declined, there concurrently developed an increasing sophistication in evaluating the effects of drugs on the fetus and neonate. Concern for the safety of the child became marked and probably had some effect in establishing the climate into which the seeds of interest in nonpharmacological means of controlling or eliminating the pain of childbirth were planted and have grown.

It was in this climate of concern for the safety of the baby that the rationale of Grantly Dick Read found many supporters among obstetricians and nurses as well as the lay public. On the basis of clinical observations, Dr. Read came to the conclusion that ". . . there was no law in nature and no design that could justify the pain of childbirth."[2] Even more adamantly Read argues, "The physiological perfection of the human body knows no greater paradox than pain in normal parturition."[2] Read postulated a triadic fear-tension-pain cycle and aimed his method of natural childbirth at interruption of this cycle. Thus he believed by means of an educational program the woman could be taught what to expect in childbirth and could be helped to dispel erroneous ideas regarding childbirth. Essential components of the Read method were (1) techniques taught the mother prenatally to foster relaxation during labor and (2) the presence of a supportive obstetrician to help her maintain a state of quiet and calm.

While the fervor with which the Read method was greeted in some areas of this country seemed to produce a "natural childbirth" era, one has only to look at present obstetrical practice to see that such is not the case. Prior to and concurrent with the Read method, there was interest in other aspects of nonpharmacological relief of pain. Thus we see again the thread of hypnosis rewoven into the fabric of obstetrical pain relief. Interest in hypnosis has been growing in Russia since the late nineteenth century, and its use in obstetrics was begun there in the early twentieth century. After World War I interest in and use of hypnosis increased rapidly. Platanov, founder of the Kharkov School of Psychotherapy, suggested the possibility of a mass application of hypno-suggestive methods of obstetrical analgesia. Chertok, among others, credits Platanov with laying the first foundations of the practical application of hypnosis in obstetrics. Platanov pioneered in this "hypnosuggestive analgesia." His theoretical interpretations of hypnosis were based on pavlovian principles. A Kiev obstetrician, Nicolaiev, developed an interesting application of hypnosis by using posthypnotic suggestion for delivery of the patient.[5] Parenthetically, it is interesting to note posthypnotic suggestion has been used by some obstetricians in this country in an effort to avoid the patient's difficulty in voiding in the early postpartal period.

In 1951 the French obstetrician Ferdinand Lamaze visited the Union of Soviet Socialist Republics and observed the use of the technique now called psychoprophylaxis. Impressed with the efficacy of the method, Lamaze returned to France and began using psychoprophylaxis for all patients delivered at the hospital that he directed. In 1955 Dr. Lamaze gave an address on his method to the International

Congress of Gynecology and Obstetrics. In 1956 Pope Pius XII sanctioned the use of psychoprophylaxis by Roman Catholics. Lamaze's first book on psychoprophylaxis was published in France in 1956. Two years later the book appeared in Great Britain with the title *Painless Childbirth.*[6] In that same year, Pierre Vellay's major work *Childbirth Without Pain*[7] was also published in Great Britain.

In 1959 the first major introduction of psychoprophylaxis came to the United States. In this country the method is more popularly known as the Lamaze method. A young American woman, Marjorie Karmel, had delivered her first child in Paris as a patient of Dr. Lamaze. Having returned to America and wishing to use psychoprophylaxis for her second delivery, Mrs. Karmel had great difficulty finding personnel to help her in this venture. Her book *Thank You, Dr. Lamaze*[8] was published in 1959 in an effort to proselytize the lay public. A year later Mrs. Karmel was co-founder of the American Society for Psychoprophylaxis in Obstetrics (ASPO) that brought together lay people, doctors, nurses, and physiotherapists who were advocates of psychoprophylaxis. ASPO now has chapters in fourteen cities.[9]

There are no statistical data concerning the frequency with which psychoprophylaxis is used in the United States as a technique of childbirth. The focal point of psychoprophylaxis activity in this country has been and continues to be New York City. A New York obstetrician, Dr. Irwin Chabon, made a major contribution to the literature on psychoprophylaxis in the United States. His book *Awake and Aware: Participating in Childbirth Through Psychoprophylaxis*[10] explains psychoprophylaxis as it has been modified by practitioners in the United States.

There has been a tendency among many writers to "lump" nonpharmacological approaches to relief of pain in childbirth in a single category, natural childbirth. Such classification belies some basic differences between the theoretical formulations underlying the Read method and psychoprophylaxis. Perhaps the most basic difference between the two methods is in their view of pain in childbirth. As mentioned above, Read believed normal parturition should be painless. At the time Read became vocal regarding his ideas (early 1930s) those who sought to discredit him scornfully referred to natural childbirth as analogous to women who delivered their babies during a brief interlude from work in the fields. That such women seemed to have little pain was not considered by Read critics as possibly supporting Read's position. Rather the implication was that such delivery was barbaric and was evaluated with the righteous indignation of ethnocentrism.

Read classified deliveries into three groups. First is normal or natural childbirth which he believed *could* account for 95% of all deliveries.[2] Second is average or cultural labor in which the woman is physiologically and mechanically well-equipped but not prepared for natural childbirth. Third is abnormal or surgical delivery. Read believed the cultural conditioning resulting in the triadic fear-tension-pain cycle accounted for pain in uncomplicated childbirth. He stated, "All nociceptors are specific, that is to say, they react to only one form of pain stimulation. It follows thus that the only pain stimulus that the uterus can record is excessive tension or actual tearing of tissues."[2] Read asks why if, as Wolfe believes, structure is adapted to function, the uterus has not made such an adaptation.[2] Quite simply, Read held that childbirth is a physiological process and that physiological processes are not painful. There is, then, according to Read, no reason aside from learned responses or abnormalities for pain in childbirth.

Psychoprophylaxis theory, on the other hand, concerns itself not so much with the theoretical question of the presence or absence of pain in childbirth but with the *interpretation* of painful stimuli. Thus it is seen by advocates of psychoprophylaxis that a painful stimulus is interpreted as pain only in the cortex. Mediation of pain is then seen subject to cortical control. It is in this mediation that pavlovian principles assume paramount importance. A conditioned reflex response to uterine contractions is advocated as a means of either shutting out or sublimating painful sensations.

Thus the explanation of pain in childbirth that is basic to psychoprophylaxis holds pain to be the result of irritation of specific pain receptors found in all tissues and organs which would, of course, include the uterus, genitalia, and perineum. Pain impulses are believed transmitted through "the spinal thalamic tract [which] is the main but not the only pathway of pain impulses which then are transmitted through Gower's tract, the medulla, the pons varolii, the cerebral peduncles and the thalmus to the superior parietal lobes of the cortex."[5] According to pavlovian physiology, pain is sensation, but only in the cortex is the pain stimulus converted into a sensation. Hersilie states as one of the objectives of psychoprophylaxis ". . . the total suppression of all painful sensation in the course of childbirth. But this is not the suppression of the sensation itself. It is the painful characteristics of the sensation—in other words the uterine contraction is perceptible but it is not painful."[5] Buxton characterizes and loosely translates Hersilie's remark as the quintessence of the childbirth without pain philosophy. Buxton comments: "When is pain not a pain? Answer: when it is a sensation."[5]

Having proposed pain as contingent on cortical interpretation, psychoprophylaxis advocates have logically concerned themselves with control of that interpretation. A leading psychoprophylaxis authority, Nicol-

aiev, believes transmission of pain sensation may be similar in all cases. "Properly trained" women do not suffer pain, he proposes, because of a high pain perception threshold related to a special dynamic state of the higher levels of their central nervous system. It is proposed such women have ". . . well equilibrated processes of stimulation and inhibition with a normal undisturbed relation between the cortex and the subcortex."[5] Psychoprophylaxis theory views nervous activity as very similar to the feedback mechanism of cybernetics. That is, nervous activity is in general a state of reciprocal induction-stimulation and inhibition. There is an inverse relationship between stimulation and inhibition, it is thought. Relatively stronger inhibition prevents wider cortical spread.[5] Psychoprophylaxis training can, it is believed, result in stronger inhibition of pain impulses.

How is such training effected? In both the Read and psychoprophylaxis methods, attention is given to providing the pregnant woman with factual information about pregnancy and labor and delivery. Velvovsky[11] states as two of the objectives of the pedagogical part of psychoprophylaxis training the following.

1. To eliminate the negative emotions of the pregnant woman and the excessive orienting reactions of the parturient woman by explaining and disproving the erroneous ideas of and attitudes to labour and by instilling appropriate, scientifically-substantiated views and conceptions of labour. The woman should become familiar with the atmosphere of the maternity home and the special medical equipment of the labour room.

2. To acquaint the woman with all of the basic phenomena of labour so as to impress on her the fact that these phenomena are normal; deprived of the elements of surprise they will not frighten her.*

Although the literature implies that misinformation and unhealthy attitudes of the

---

*From Velvovsky, I., Ploticher, V., and Shugom, E.: Painless childbirth through psychoprophylaxis: lectures for obstetricians, Moscow, 1960, Foreign Language Publishing House.

woman are dealt with simultaneously in prenatal education, a critique of the design, "curricula," and modus operandi of both traditional prenatal classes and psychoprophylaxis fails to reveal specifically how this is done. In essence there seems to be little difference between Read and psychoprophylaxis in the techniques of prenatal education, except in those aspects that deal with the role of the woman and her husband in labor and delivery.

However, there is a distinct difference in the way Read and psychoprophylaxis theorists view the mediating effects of prenatal education in their respective programs. Both schools would agree negative, learned, culturally determined attitudes and misinformation regarding childbirth are attacked in their training programs. The psychoprophylaxis school refers to this process as "verbal asepsis." It is interesting to note that in the early writings of Read and of the first proponents of psychoprophylaxis, allusions are made not only to dispelling fear and ignorance, but also to creating a climate of "joyful expectation." Pregnancy and childbirth are highly romanticized and described with ecstatic adjectives. While references are still made, in both Read and modified Read programs as well as psychoprophylaxis training, there seems to be a diminution (perhaps a healthy one) in the glowing adjectival pronouncements of the childbearing and childbirth experience.

The verbal asepsis of psychoprophylaxis is considered to be achieved by means of a pavlovian second signaling system.[11] In this context, one might translate this into a simple method in which language is used. Thus the technique of psychoprophylaxis in this matter is not uniquely different from other forms of prenatal education.

It is in the *activity* of the woman and her husband in labor and delivery that psychoprophylaxis is notably different from other psychophysical methods of pain prevention or relief. Activity is a prime ingredient of psychoprophylaxis. According to psychoprophylaxis theory, activity is designed to break the usual pattern of uterine contraction → stimulation of uterine receptors → sensory nerve impulses to the brain → cortical excitation → interpretation of pain → signals to subcortical area → effectors (pain perception, moaning, etc.).[10] Chabon[10] presents a succinct summary of the way in which psychoprophylaxis conditioning is believed to function.

. . . it is possible to evolve an indifferent, conditioned response to the uterine contraction, a response mediated by higher centers and therefore finer and more delicate than the coarse lower-center response commonly seen. Second, the cortical mechanisms of excitation and inhibition can be utilized as well. If the cortical center of excitation required to mediate the conditioned response is made stronger than the cortical center of excitation aroused by the uterine contractions, inhibition of the uterine signal occurs. In fact, if the conditioned response occurs slightly before the uterine contraction actually takes place, it can prevent the very formation of the cortical center of excitation in response to the contraction.*

Exercises are an integral part of psychoprophylaxis training. As might by expected, the exercises are of graduated complexity. They require increasing attention, or in pavlovian terms, increasing intensity of cortical excitation for their performance. Chabon[10] says of the exercises:

Being specific and directed toward the performance of highly integrated motor activity, there is no generalized subcortical inhibition, such as might affect labor. The subcortical motor responses are confined, and labor can progress unaffected.*

The format of psychoprophylaxis courses in this country is generally standardized. This is probably largely attributable to the efforts of the American Society for Psychoprophylaxis in Obstetrics (ASPO). ASPO has an active program of teacher

---

*From Chabon, I.: Awake and aware: participating in childbirth through psychoprophylaxis, New York, 1966, The Delacorte Press.

training and certification. The course is generally begun by the woman eight weeks before the expected delivery. Since the technique relies upon conditioning, a greater possibility of deconditioning occurs if the course is begun earlier in pregnancy. If it is necessary for the woman to begin classes earlier, a "refresher" course or session may be given to help maintain motivation for daily practicing of exercises.

The course is divided into six sessions, usually given at one-week intervals. In other countries a monitrice trains the pregnant woman and cares for her in labor. In this country, husbands are strongly urged to attend the course. Husbands then fill the monitrice role as well as add the special dimension of care which only a husband can provide the woman in labor.

The reader may at this point ask how a conditioned reflex to uterine contractions can be established in the absence of such (detectable) contractions. It is here the "second signaling system" comes into play. The woman is taught to respond to the verbal stimulus "contraction!" The advantage of having a monitrice or husband to give verbal signals for conditioning purposes is obvious.

Briefly, the content of psychoprophylaxis training in this country can be summarized as follows:

Class. I. General introduction—physiology of pregnancy and labor and delivery.

Class II. Exercises.

A. Concentration-relaxation exercises—learning to contract one or two groups of muscles while keeping other muscle groups relaxed.

B. Body-building exercises—general conditioning exercises not specifically designed for use as such in labor and delivery such as tailorsit and leg lifting while in supine position.

Class III. Respiration exercises.

A. "The cleansing breath"—deep inhalation then complete exhalation (to precede and follow each breathing exercise each time it is done).

B. Breathing for early labor—slow, deliberate rhythmic chest breathing, inhaling through the nose, exhaling through the mouth; six to nine breaths per minute. A rule of thumb often sug-

gested to women is not to start breathing exercises as long as they can walk or talk through a contraction.

C. Effleurage to accompany breathing exercises—with fingertips resting lightly on the skin, the woman is taught to stroke the abdomen in a rhythmic, circular massage. This activity falls into the category of counterirritants.

D. Breathing for well-established labor—rapid, shallow breathing (panting); breathing is to be kept as superficial as possible, almost in the throat. Pacing of the breathing is designed to match the increment-acme-decrement characteristic of the uterine contraction.

Class IV. Breathing for latter phase of first stage of labor—pant-blow; rapid, shallow breathing (panting) is combined with regularly occuring forceful exhalations (blowing). Four to eight panting breaths are followed by forcible exhalation through pursed lips.

Class V. Preparation for delivery. In the second stage of labor, the woman is advised to take two cleansing breaths. Then she is to take a third deep breath, lift and hold her legs, elbows out, head raised. Then while holding her breath, the woman is to bear down, using upper abdominal muscles and keeping pelvic floor muscles relaxed. The patient's position while pushing can be made more comfortable by use of pillows to support the head or by support from the nurse or husband. It should also be noted the half-sitting position is a departure from traditional American delivery room technique. There may be physiological advantages in increasing intraabdominal pressure.

Class VI. Review of exercises, what to bring to the hospital, and, often, a kind of "testimonial" from parents or husbands who have used psychoprophylaxis.[12]

It can be seen from the preparation given in psychoprophylaxis courses that the role of both husband and wife is a very active one in labor and delivery. The role of the husband is a particularly striking contrast to that of the Read method. Rather than being limited to an expectant waiting for news of his wife and baby, the husband participating in psychoprophylaxis works actively to help his wife maintain conditioned responses in labor. In a culture that traditionally has provided a role in childbirth antithetical to the couvade, the introduction of a *participant* role for the father is in itself worthy of note. For the woman in labor rather than emphasis on calm and relaxation (some have labeled it passivity) proposed by Read, the psychoprophylaxis mother is alert and quite active. It has been suggested that psychoprophylaxis strengthens the dyadic husband-wife relationship. However, this is yet to be demonstrated by objective research data and has come only from clinical impressions.

The criticisms of psychoprophylaxis have been numerous. Such criticisms range from one easily discounted as ethnocentric, that is, "I couldn't use it because it's a communistic technique," to those that have not been satisfactorily explored regarding the physiological effects on the fetus of the various breathing techniques used. Some obstetricians claim we are "deluding" ourselves if we believe the psychoprophylaxis patient is not suffering. These men insist pharmacological agents should be used no matter what the woman says.

Perhaps the most pervasive characterization of psychoprophylaxis is that it attracts a "certain type" of woman. It has been suggested that women who seek the course want to "be the obstetrician." Others believe women who want their husbands with them in labor and delivery simply want to punish them. Various other adjectives ranging from "neurotic" to the "phallic-aggressive castrating type"[13] have been used to describe psychoprophylaxis users. Unfortunately, there has been much greater interest in labeling than in studying psychoprophylaxis, its theoretical base, and its users. The American studies to date, for example, Tanzer,[14] have failed to substantiate negative differences between those who choose psychoprophylaxis and those who do not. Lapidus demonstrated a difference in cognitive control between women who chose preparation for childbirth and those women who did not. The preparation group showed more reliance on their own active participation in childbirth as a means of mastery and coping in stress.[4]

One of the difficulties in assessing the effectiveness of psychoprophylaxis for many types of women in this country is its being limited almost exclusively to upper socioeconomic classes. Few lower-class women know about psychoprophylaxis and even fewer can afford the classes for which fees are charged. According to the literature, psychoprophylaxis has "worked" for all socioeconomic levels in other countries.

There are many questions raised regarding psychoprophylaxis as it is and has been practiced. Perhaps the most important question is what is the essential ingredient in psychoprophylaxis? Is it truly the conditioned response? Or is it perhaps the comfort of *active* and continuing support in labor by another person?

What are the disadvantages of a prenatal educational program that begins as late as the third trimester? Although the state of prenatal education in this country may make this seem a dry, academic question, one must consider needs prior to the third trimester. Would a general prenatal program given earlier in pregnancy *enhance* psychoprophylaxis training? Another issue in courses that follow a rigidly set format is the possible diminution of group therapeutic benefits. Should psychoprophylaxis training be combined with group discussion techniques to listen to and deal with what parents have told and are telling us?

Although there are no statistics regarding the use of psychoprophylaxis in this country, clinical observations have demonstrated that the method does work for many women and for many types of labor and delivery, including the use of forceps and episiotomy. Thus far objective evidence does not allow us to stereotype the psychoprophylaxis user or her obstetrician. The literature does not reveal statements of any obstetricians who will not use analgesia or anesthesia for the psychoprophylaxis patient if her status indicates such use. The discomfort that many nurses and obstetricians feel with alert patients and their husbands in labor and delivery makes one wonder whether or not the "team" is reluctant to relinquish control of the delivery process to the parturient couple.

The fact that psychoprophylaxis subjects have reported positive experiences in labor and delivery suggests support of the ideas of Helene Deutsch.[15] Activity in childbirth and early exposure to the infant for both mother and father may have positive effects on the promotion of family unity.

All programs of childbirth preparation—and there are myriad varieties—report successes. It has been observed that even unprepared women seem to respond to more serene room or suite mates in labor. The question of suggestibility and desire to please thus arises. If, as it certainly seems, all programs have merit, it would seem appropriate to examine the various techniques of preparation. Can we identify the salient feature or features of the programs? Can we demonstrate that psychoprophylaxis is more effective for more women than the Read method? Should Read be abandoned completely? Are all (or none) the exercises taught necessary? Can breathing techniques be adapted to what can be learned about physiological effects on the fetus? What effect does having to "fight for" the right to use psychoprophylaxis (as many couples now must) have upon that family's working relationship with the health team?

Despite the fact that many couples experience pregnancy, labor, and delivery, we have an inadequate base of information for directing them to or teaching them about the kind of childbirth technique that is most appropriate for them. Only with a substantial ·contribution to the dearth of research in this area can we function with intelligence in meeting the health needs of the childbearing couple.

References

1. Cleland, John G. P., and Hingson, Robert A.: History of pain relief during childbirth. In Lull, Clifford B., and Hingson, Robert A., editors: Control of pain in childbirth, Philadelphia, 1948, J. B. Lippincott Co.
2. Read, Grantly Dick: Childbirth without fear, ed. 2, New York, 1953, Harper & Brothers.
3. Seaman, Bernard: Man against pain, New York, 1962, Chilton Book Co.
4. Lapidus, Leah B.: The relation between cognitive control and reactions to stress: a study of mastery in the anticipatory phase of childbirth, unpublished doctoral dissertation, New York, 1968, New York University.
5. Buxton, C. Lee.: A study of psychophysical methods for relief of childbirth pain, Philadelphia, 1962, W. B. Saunders Co.
6. Lamaze, Ferdinand: Painless childbirth: psychoprophylactic method, translated by L. R. Celestin, London, 1958, Burke Publishing Co., Ltd.
7. Vellay, Pierre: Childbirth without pain, translated by Denise Lloyd, New York, 1960, E. P. Dutton & Co., Inc.
8. Karmel, Marjorie: Thank you, Dr. Lamaze, Philadelphia, 1959, J. B. Lippincott Co.
9. ASPO News: 8:No. 1, March, 1970.
10. Chabon, Irwin: Awake and aware: participating in childbirth through psychoprophylaxis, New York, 1966, The Delacorte Press.
11. Velvovsky, I., Ploticher, V., and Shugom, E.: Painless childbirth through psychoprophylaxis: lectures for obstetricians, Moscow, 1960, Foreign Languages Publishing House.
12. Bing, Elisabeth D.: Six practical lessons for an easier childbirth, New York, 1967, Grosset & Dunlap, Inc.
13. Horowitz, Mardi J., and Horowitz, Nancy F.: Psychological effects of education for childbirth, Psychosomatics 8:196-202, 1967.
14. Tanzer, Deborah R. W.: The psychology of pregnancy and childbirth: an investigation of natural childbirth, unpublished doctoral dissertation, Waltham, Mass., 1967, Brandeis University.
15. Deutsch, Helene: The psychology of women: a psychoanalytic interpretation, vol. 2, New York, 1945, Grune & Stratton, Inc.

Bibliography

Bauman, Bernice C.: Personality characteristics of women who elect a program of educated childbirth as compared to those who do not elect such a program, unpublished doctoral dissertation, New York, 1960, Columbia University.

Bing, Elisabeth D.: The adventure of birth, New York, 1970, Simon & Schuster, Inc.

Chertok, L.: Psychosomatic methods of preparation for childbirth, Amer. J. Obstet. Gynec. 98:698-707, 1967.

Chertok, L.: Relaxation and psychosomatic methods of preparation for childbirth, Amer. J. Obstet. Gynec. 82:262-267, 1961.

Chertok, L.: Theories of psychoprophylaxis in obstetrics: prophylaxis or therapy, Amer. J. Psychiat. 119:1152-1159, 1963.

Fielding, Waldo: The childbirth challenge: Commonsense versus "natural" methods, New York, 1962, The Viking Press, Inc.

Fijalkowski, Wlodzimierz: Current trends in psychoprophylaxis of pregnancy and labor, Pol. Med. J. 8:768-775, 1969.

Fijalkowski, Wlodzimierz: New ways of psychophysical preparation for childbirth, Amer. J. Obstet. Gynec. 92:1018-1022, 1965.

Pavlov, Ivan P.: Conditioned reflexes, New York, 1960, Dover Publications, Inc.

Prescott, Frederick: The control of pain, London, 1964, English Universities Press, Ltd.

Read, Grantly Dick: Revelation of childbirth, London, 1943, William Heinemann, Ltd.

Read, Grantly Dick: Natural childbirth, London, 1933, William Heinemann, Ltd.

Vellay, Pierre: Childbirth with confidence, translated by Elliot E. Philipp, New York, 1969, E. P. Dutton & Co., Inc.

Chapter 22

Assessing the needs of new mothers in a postpartum unit

Leonide M. Tanner

Professional nursing care for the postpartum patient encompasses far more than the "routine" or "custodial" type of physically oriented care that has long been the norm on most hospital units. The critical importance of this early period for optimal development of the mother-child relationship and the necessity of sensitive and perceptive care by professional practitioners have been emphasized in recent nursing literature.[1, 3] A thorough understanding of the processes that occur during the early postpartal period, of behaviors arising from these, and of the maturational aspects of developing motherliness is essential if the nurse is to be alert to the special needs of new mothers.[4-7]

Another essential aspect of professional maternity care is the utilization by the nurse of an organized, preplanned approach for the identification of patient needs or problems and for taking action to meet or alleviate these. This is the process by which nursing care above and beyond physical monitoring and maintenance is carried out. Suggestions for an approach tailored to the unique circumstances of the new mother on the hospital postpartum unit will be described in this chapter.

Initial assessment from external data

When the nurse on a postpartum unit receives a patient on the unit directly from the delivery room, she has available several sources of information that might provide cues to special needs or problems of the new mother. From the chart the nurse has information regarding the patient's gravida/para, age, marital status, complications of pregnancy, and history of labor and delivery as well as the condition of the infant. Any of these may indicate a possible problem or need, as in the following examples:

A 17-year-old primipara who has been married for five months may need much help in realizing and accepting the demands of motherhood, in working through her feelings about becoming pregnant, in adjusting to her role as wife and the loss of other adolescent roles, in restructuring her relationships with her parents, and in learning skills necessary for infant care.

A woman who is gravida 4, para 1, has probably had a quite traumatic obstetrical history, and may be apprehensive about the condition of the baby she has just carried to term. She may need much opportunity to explore her baby, nursing support in doing this, and accurate, detailed information about the baby's behavior and progress in the nursery. Additionally, she may be struggling with problems in her self-concept in the areas of femininity and as a productive, adequate person.

A woman who experienced unexpected complications during labor and delivery may have needs in the areas of the condition of the baby, understanding and integrating her experience, questions regarding the cause and its implications for her behavior and self-concept, and perhaps to grieve the loss of having a normal, perfect childbirth experience.

The nurse also has the physician and delivery room nurses as sources of information about the patient's problems and concerns. The doctor may know about the patient's home situation, special fears during pregnancy, or any problems encountered that might become acute after the baby is born. The delivery room nurses may have data about the husband-wife relationship, how the mother copes with stress, and any concerns or fears mentioned during the critical labor period that might carry over postpartally.

This type of external data, although frequently useful in anticipating a problem, actually provides only a clue or indication that needs follow-up by the nurse in actual communication with the patient. Any external indicator of a possible problem should be discussed with the patient to determine existence of a problem, its extensiveness, and whether or not it is amenable to nursing intervention. Reliance on techniques of good communication is essential in exploring and intervening in sensitive or vulnerable problem areas.[8, 9]

Special needs of new mothers—areas for nursing assessment and intervention

In addition to possible problems indicated by external data, there are many common areas of concern expressed by new mothers. Although all of these will not be relevant for each patient, comprehensive and truly professional nursing care should include exploration of all areas to determine whether a need or problem exists and intervention by the nurse in the area of need identified. The nurse again will rely on communication skills and the therapeutic use of herself and her knowledge in both assessment and provision of nursing care. These common areas of concern, and some suggestions for nursing intervention, are given below.

The labor experience

Labor is often one of life's most demanding experiences for a woman. It is also the culmination of pregnancy, a definite breaking-off point that signifies far-reaching change. Some authors believe that how a woman experiences her labor affects how she will be able to mother her baby, at least initially.[4] Labor is undoubtedly a significant factor in the mother-child relationship. Additionally, labor is a critical life-experience that must become a part of the woman's personality and attitudes as it is integrated into the psyche. During the early postpartal phase the woman has a need to relive her labor in great detail. She must understand the sequence of events and identify her behavior. This reliving serves two purposes: (1) to finalize the pregnancy and bring into focus the reality of the separation of mother and infant and (2) to integrate this experience into the woman's life pattern, to incorporate it as a part of her. Much of the reliving of labor is done with the woman's roommate, husband, and friends. However, problematic aspects call for intervention on the part of the nurse, such as gaps in memory, vaguely understood events, contradictory information, and traumatic episodes. Here the nurse can be invaluable in obtaining and providing needed information, clarifying misunderstandings, and providing an accepting relationship in which to work through the troublesome or traumatic aspects of labor.

The "taking-in" need

Pregnancy and labor are psychodynamically "putting-out" types of experiences. During pregnancy the woman nurtures and provides for her fetus with the stores of her own body. Her body "gives to" the fetus and he "takes" what he needs, even to the woman's disadvantage. Labor is a tremendously demanding experience. Both physically and emotionally the woman expends a great amount of energy. Afterward she is exhausted and depleted. In addition, she must "put out" from the inner depths of her body the fetus that has been a part of her for nine months. This is viewed as "losing" a part of the self, both physically and psychologically.[10] It is certainly no surprise that women need "input" after these experiences. The first several days after delivery the postpartum woman has a marked need to "take-in." This is shown in her need for sleep and rest, for food, for comfort, and for solicitous attention. She seeks to restore the equilibrium of mind and body, especially in view of the demands that motherhood will soon be placing upon her.[11] The nurse must be alert to this need for restitution, and should try to facilitate satisfaction in all the above-mentioned areas. Various ways to accomplish this are getting extra nourishment, making special efforts to secure food the mother likes, assuring periods of rest, keeping the environment relaxing and conducive to sensory comfort, showing concern for the woman as an individual, and enhancing comfort through relief of pain from episiotomy, hemorrhoid, and afterpain.

The need to identify and examine the infant

During pregnancy women have many fantasies that concern the appearance and characteristics of the baby. They worry about abnormalities. After the baby is born, women have a compulsive need to look their baby over and to see that he is whole and complete and has everything he is supposed to. They also must know that all his functions are normal, that he can cry, wet, have a bowel movement, open his eyes, and move all his limbs.[6] This process of looking the baby over also serves the purpose of allowing the woman to identify this infant as a new and unique individual. She has to develop a relationship with him that is different from all other relationships.[10] To do this, she explores his likenesses and differences, trying to discover whom he looks like and whom he does not, which characteristics resemble which people in the family, and what is unique to this baby. The end result of this process is that the mother is able to see this baby as a separate and distinct new person with whom she has a different and unique relationship.

The nurse can encourage and facilitate this process. First she can assure that the baby is available to the mother for reasonably long periods of time. Then she can encourage examination of the baby, offering herself as support during the initial phases. The new mother's anxiety may be so high that she is afraid to look over the baby because she might discover something wrong. The nurse can be a supportive presence who in effect says "Go ahead, I'll help you cope with whatever you discover." Many questions will be asked, and the nurse should realistically reassure the mother without negating or belittling her feelings of concern or anxiety.

The importance of the new mother's examination of her baby cannot be overemphasized. This means freedom to completely unwrap the baby and undress him and to touch him all over, which has tremendous implications for some nurseries' policies.

The need for success in early mothering tasks

The inexperienced or apprehensive new mother needs much help in achieving confidence in her ability to mother successfully. Fears of inadequacy, which are quite common, create a great need to successfully carry out early mothering tasks.[4] This often centers around feeding, usually the first task given her by the nursery staff. The mother may be so anxious to get the baby to take the bottle or breast that she cannot perceive any of the baby's own needs, that is, that he is sleepy or not hungry, that he is in an awkward position which interferes with feeding, or that he is wet. The nurse can help the mother recognize these other factors and assist her to be successful with hints about how to feed and burp, change diapers, etc. Reinforcement when she has used good technique and gentle explanation of ineffective behaviors also enhance success. Broad reassurances or flippant cheerfulness, such as "You'll catch on in time" or "Don't worry, everyone learns eventually," are of no help when each small task seems to be insurmountable. The nurse also does the mother a disservice when she "demonstrates the right way" and so deftly performs exactly the task the mother has been struggling so hard to do. The key here is to help the mother achieve success by using the nurse's knowledge to assist the mother as the mother actually does the task.

The need for control and dependability of her own body

Far-reaching changes have occurred in the woman's body and it may have been unpredictable during pregnancy and labor. Now she has the serious task of motherhood ahead of her, and she needs to be assured that her body will be reliable, that it will function as it did before, and that she will have control over her body. During the early postpartum period, the woman is concerned about body functions.[11] She needs to be able to void and control voiding, she must ambulate without undue discomfort and without feeling weak, she needs episiotomy and hemorrhoid pain relief so these do not interfere with mothering tasks, and she needs to successfully have a bowel movement, to be able to eat and sleep well, and to generally "feel well." Another real concern is body appearance, and it is often important to the woman to regain her figure. She may ask the nurse about losing weight, exercises to regain muscle tone, and skin care to get rid of wrinkles, flabbiness, and even striae. The nurse can be of much assistance in all these areas by providing needed information and assistance in regulating body functions and by developing a plan of action to regain desired body appearance.

The need for preparation for going home

Homecoming with a new baby is an event for which a mother (and her family) cannot be too well prepared. Even the smoothest hospital course is not predictive of a trouble-free first few weeks at home. Actually, the major adjustments that are just initiated in the hospital will occur during the first several weeks at home, and this can be a very trying time for all involved. The new mother returns to the home in the still early phases of recovery from the demanding process of labor and delivery. Her body is not back to par, and her emotions are still in a state of upheaval. She encounters her "postpartum blues" as massive hormonal changes combine with the psychic "letdown" after delivery and with the demands of the baby and home environment.[11] The reality of caring for this completely egocentric and unsocialized little person often comes as a surprise after the best preparation. The baby is not yet in a routine for eating and sleeping and is erratic in behavior. The overwhelming responsibility for twenty-four-hour care often has tremendous impact on the parents. Demands from family and friends are felt as visiting is frequent. The mother tries to readjust her roles and to function well in all, but she finds this nearly impossible. She simply cannot care for the baby, keep up the house, do cooking and laundry, socialize with family and friends, and be attentive to her husband to the satisfaction of all and without feeling completely depleted.

Ideally, the public health nurse or hospital liaison nurse should visit the new mother in the first week at home to assist her in dealing with these numerous stresses. Practically speaking, however, the new mother is often completely out of touch with health workers between discharge from the hospital and her baby's first visit to the pediatrician (around two weeks), or her six-week postpartal checkup. Thus a great responsibility rests upon hospital nurses to help prepare the new mother as well as possible for going home. The areas that seem important to cover are as follows:

1. Skills needed for infant care—bathing, dressing, formula preparation or breast care, infant behavior, and prevention of illness
2. Rest—the need for much rest and sleep, avoidance of overactivity or trying to do all the housework, and giving the body time to recover
3. Visitors—setting limits on visitors, not oversocializing for the sake of both mother and baby
4. Help at home—if possible, at least part-time help that relieves the mother for a few hours (for example, a friend, relative, or paid help)
5. Reorganization of family roles—the changes that can be expected with the addition of a new member to the family, sharing of role tasks, and attention to the husband and other children
6. Self-care—the attention that the mother's body needs to fully recover, bathing and dress, exercise and activities, and intercourse
7. Postpartum blues—anticipation and understanding of swings in an emotional state, and what can be done to alleviate depression
8. Where to get help during this time—community resources that provide much assistance and special help with certain problems, what is available, and how to get this help

Family planning

The desire to control conception and plan one's family is more and more prevalent among today's childbearing couples. The nurse has a definite responsibility in contraception counseling, as a part of her shared function with all health professions to promote health and well-being. The new mother often needs information about family planning and she needs it now, not in six weeks when she might be pregnant again. The nurse should assess her patient's interest in family planning; then if interest is expressed, explain interim contraceptive measures for the first six weeks and familiarize the patient with various more effective later methods. She can refer the woman to her physician or a local family planning service, advising her about the procedure for setting up an appointment for contraception counseling.

An organized nursing approach

With the growing emphasis in nursing upon use of care plans, each postpartum unit might want to adapt various aspects of this suggested approach to meet the focus of its particular care plan format. The approach includes the following:

1. Initial assessment interview—within a few hours of the newly delivered woman's arrival on the unit, a preliminary assessment is made covering physical needs, the labor experience, and any potential problems identified from external

data. Immediate needs regarding information can be met at this time.

2. Exploration of areas of common concern—this should be ongoing, but begin no later than the first postpartum day. An assessment list, with specific areas that can be checked as to presence or absence of needs or problems, provides a basic tool to assure consistency among staff. Further verbal exploration of problematic areas, with intervention as indicated, can be concurrently carried out. Areas of concern important to cover at this time are the taking-in need, need to identify and examine the infant, success in mothering tasks, and control and dependability of her body.

3. Nursing care plan—once assessment has been carried out, the needs or problems identified can be developed into a nursing care plan with notation of intervention carried out and with suggestions for additional approaches.

4. Later assessment and care—the mother's concerns may fluctuate as different needs are uppermost at different times, and she may not be receptive to intervention in family planning or preparation for going home before she has adequately explored her baby or talked over her labor. Thus continuous reassessment is necessary, with alterations in the care plan as one need recedes and another gains prominence. Well before discharge, however, assessment of needs and provision of necessary information and referrals regarding family planning and preparation for going home should be carried out.

This approach presupposes the postpartum nursing staff's delineation of professional nursing care includes assisting the new mother, and her husband, to obtain maximum benefit from her brief hospital stay by facilitation of working through and integrating this critical life experience, assistance in mastering the many tasks (both physiological and behavioral) inherent in the postdelivery and early mothering processes, and provision of necessary learning to anticipate and prepare for homecoming.

References

1. Adams, Martha: Early concerns of primigravida mothers regarding infant care activities, Nurs. Res. **12:**72-77, Spring, 1963.
2. Bowlby, John: Maternal care and mental health, Geneva, 1952, World Health Organization.
3. Henning, Emilie, Martoglio, Gilda, Quita, Maria, Reinbrecht, Janet, and Strickland, Marie: A dynamic appraisal of the puerperium. In Lytle, Nancy A., editor: Maternal health nursing, Dubuque, Iowa, 1968, Wm. C. Brown Co.
4. Rubin, Reva: Basic maternal behavior, Nurs. Outlook **9:**683-686, 1961.
5. Rubin, Reva: Puerperal changes, Nurs. Outlook **9:**753-755, 1961.
6. Rubin, Reva: Maternal touch, Nurs. Outlook **11:**829-831, 1963.
7. Newton, Niles, and Newton, Michael: Mothers' reactions to their newborn babies, J.A.M.A. **181:**206-210, 1962.
8. Hays, J. S., and Larson, K.: Interacting with patients, New York, 1965, The Macmillan Co.
9. Kron, Thora: Communication in nursing, Philadelphia, 1967, W. B. Saunders Co.
10. Bibring, G. L., Dwyer, T. F., Huntington, D. S., and Valenstein, A. F.: A study of the psychological processes in pregnancy and of the earliest mother-child relationship, Psychoanal. Stud. Child **16:**113-121, 1961.
11. Fitzpatrick, E., Eastman, N., and Reeder, S.: Maternity nursing, New York, 1966, J. B. Lippincott Co.

Chapter 23

A design for a new maternity care system

Joyce Cameron

The professional nurse has a vital role to play in maternal and newborn health care (1) in the articulation and implementation of her professional maternal and newborn nursing practice and (2) in the design, development, and implementation of a health-care system that will meet the needs of the childbearing family at a reasonable cost.

The present chapter is a discussion of these areas of responsibility as they relate to the hospital postpartum and newborn period of the normal mother and baby. The discussion is focused on the problem of providing an adequate quality of health care at a reasonable cost in the United States today and its relevance to nursing, the needs of the postpartum family, a proposed framework for a health-care system for childbearing families, and suggested approaches to the implementation of concepts basic to effective clinical practice within such a system.

Problem

During recent years rising hospital costs and shortages of prepared nursing and medical personnel have been of grave con-

cern to both professionals and the public. Despite the expenditure of large sums of money and much effort, it is readily apparent that we are in the middle of a health crisis of national proportions. The nature of this crisis has been well discussed in the literature and the following excerpts from a recent conference, The Health of Americans, sponsored by the American Assembly are illustrative.[1]

This crisis is manifested by inadequate services, which are themselves fragmented, inefficient, inequitably distributed, and uncoordinated.

Steeply rising costs and inaccessibility of care have created widespread dissatisfaction with the delivery of personal health services. The delivery system itself cannot much longer withstand assaults from over-demand, under-supply, and disorganization. Unchanged, it will break down.

Health personnel are in short supply, inefficiently used, maldistributed and specialized without regard to priority of need. Health facilities [are] . . . uneconomically utilized, and often poorly managed. Health costs are inequitably distributed, rising faster than other costs, and are catastrophic for many.*

---

*From Jones, Boisfeullet, editor: The health of Americans, Englewood Cliffs, N. J., 1970, Prentice-Hall, Inc.

The conference participants made the following recommendations[1]:

1. Access to adequate health care for all in the United States must be recognized as a basic right.

2. The nation's health strategy must now emphasize health maintenance through preventive medicine, health education, and environmental management, in addition to treatment.

3. It is an urgent national priority to fashion comprehensive health services systems available to all people. These systems must include

    a. Emphasis on provision of primary care. . . . This must provide for professional supervision of a full continuum of services for individuals and families—a concern for the whole man in his environment and not just a part of the body or a category of disease.

    b. Incentive to encourage more efficient arrangements as a way of containing costs.*

Maternity care accounts for a large percentage of the health-care services given in this country. Hospitalization for deliveries accounts for a higher percentage of hospital discharges than does any other condition. In 1965 this amounted to 3.8 million or 15.4% of all hospital discharges.[2]

Maternity units have been established in the acute hospital setting to provide adequate medical care in the event of complications. However, 80% of the pregnant women deliver without untoward incident and have a normal postpartum course.

Placement of maternity care in an acute facility, although beneficial to many women, has had a number of unfortunate results.

1. *Normal maternity patients have had to bear the cost of care equally with acutely ill patients, despite the fact that they use fewer services.* A recent news release[3] stated that the average cost per day for hospitalization in the United States was $64 with the estimate that it could go as high as $100 a day in the next few years. One might conceivably justify this expenditure if all childbearing women were receiving a high-quality service in relation to their maternity experience. However, these services frequently fail to be responsive to the needs of the normal, newly delivered mother and infant.

2. *Methods of care developed for the proportionately few acutely ill women have gradually been applied to most maternity patients, resulting in an approach to childbearing as a pathological rather than a physiological event.* In recent years there has been a gradual trend toward viewing childbirth as a normal physiological function. This is evidenced by preparation-for-childbirth programs, supportive care in labor, minimal use of medication when appropriate, a general policy of noninterference as long as progress is normal, and programs of postpartum care geared to teaching and support. Despite this trend, there are still many professionals who view these practices as unnecessary and even undesirable and who feel that obstetrical and newborn services should function similarly to other units in the hospital for acutely ill patients.

3. *Health personnel have focused their attention on crisis care and on maintenance activities, neglecting the teaching and support that is needed during this significant developmental period of life.* The normal mother and baby frequently receive perfunctory care when both sick and well patients are cared for on the same unit. Nursing care activities on all too many postpartum and newborn units have focused on carrying out the routines of bathing, cleaning, and feeding with little or no time allotted to helping the new mother with the developmental tasks of the postpartum period. Teaching and support activities have been often viewed as the "frill" of postpartum care, to be carried out when the staff has the time and the inclination, rather than as a primary nursing role.

4. *Members of the family unit have*

---

*From Jones, Boisfeullet, editor: The health of Americans, Englewood Cliffs, N. J., 1970, Prentice-Hall, Inc.

been separated from each other. Fear of infection, overcrowded facilities, concern for the mother's rest and the baby's well-being, a belief that family should not be involved in the hospital maternity experience, and the desire to maintain control have all contributed to the development of the concept that it is "better" for family members to have limited access to the mother and infant and in some instances to be banned entirely. Even the mother herself is often permitted only limited access to her newborn infant and then under rigidly controlled circumstances. The results are the separation of the mother from resources of strength and support during a critical period in her life and the creation of unnecessary stress within the family unit. Although the above-mentioned policies have been relaxed in many areas, the concept of total family involvement is still more of an idea than a reality, despite evidence that it can be highly beneficial to all concerned.

Paradoxically, an American woman who voluntarily registers for care in the typical modern maternity unit would never willingly check into a hotel for a two- to five-day period if she realized that she would (1) be assigned to a room with three strange women; (2) be confined to that room or a small section of an adjoining corridor; (3) share a bathroom and shower facility with her roommates and perhaps others; (4) have her privacy infringed upon by strangers who enter and leave her room at will; (5) be served a limited selection of foods at a predetermined time not of her own choosing; (6) need to request all water and other beverages and wait for someone to find the time to bring them to her, often lukewarm rather than cold or hot; (7) be requested to carry out daily hygiene activities when it is convenient to others but not necessarily to herself; (8) have those nearest and dearest to her restricted from seeing her, or at most allowed in for a brief visit once or twice a day; (9) receive her visitors in a room crowded with other people; and last but not least (10) fail to receive the kind of assistance for which she came in the first place. The price of the above in the average hospital today is three times that of a first-class hotel.

A return to the care of women in their homes, where acute facilities would not be readily available should they be needed, is not proposed nor is a total self-care unit advocated in which professional personnel are not constantly present. Rather, a complete redesign of the system of postpartum and newborn care is proposed, with the implementation of a new role for the professional nurse within that system, a role long advocated but only rarely and incompletely practiced.

Relevance to nursing

The professional nurse is the obvious primary provider of care during the puerperium not only because of her potential for constant availability to the mother, but also because of the nature of the needs for help that newly delivered mothers experience, which can best be met through direct nursing care. Unfortunately in many instances nurses have relegated responsibility for direct care to nonprofessionals and have instead assumed managerial functions. This is slowly changing, however, with the increased use of nurse specialists as providers of primary care and with the increased number of programs designed to encourage all professional nurses to assume more direct-care activities. A critical look is being taken at the nature of professional nursing activities and the appropriate role of the nurse in maternal and newborn care. Many nurses are eager to assume or regain their position as providers of primary care, but they are handicapped in doing so by the systems currently in practice.

The professional nurse is in a unique position to play a major role in designing a new health-care system. Because of her focus of practice and knowledge concerning the consumer's needs and desires, she is able to articulate and implement the objectives of care during the puerperium, to delineate those aspects of the system appropriate to nursing, and to indicate areas where supportive services can be developed and maintained. A critical concept in systems design is that the planning, implementation, and operation of a system be geared to meet well-defined objectives. Without these objectives the system cannot function effectively. Since it must be designed to contribute to the achievement of maternal and newborn care objectives, the nurse must be actively involved in its development and maintenance.

Realistically the nurse cannot administer the desired professional services that are needed by the postpartum family within presently existing systems of care. Martha Pitel[4] states:

Hospitals for the future should be built for the maintenance of health and prevention of illness as well as for the care of the sick.

Because she is most aware of the many services necessary for the proper therapeutic plan for the patient, the nurse should be involved in the overall planning of the health complex. As the "keeper" of the patient care units, she should participate in the detailed planning of the units from the very onset of discussion. As a team member or prime initiator, her involvement in design and structural research is crucial to the improvement of patient care. With the knowledge and experience she has gained through interaction with patients, the nurse can be a most significant contributor and colleague of the architect. She may well help to humanize the hospital environment and alter the structure to better meet the patient's needs.*

Proposed system

An innovative system is proposed in which presently known principles of optimum individual welfare, effective health

____

*From Pitel, M.: A nurse's view, Hospitals **43:** 67-68, 1969.

care, environmental influences, and sound business management are synthesized and utilized in meeting clearly defined objectives of health care for normal childbearing women and their families. The major characteristics of the service would be a physical environment and program of care focused on providing a safe, satisfying childbearing experience directed toward promotion of maximum health for the participants at a cost much less than currently obtainable.

The objectives of the system are as follows:

1. Recognized standards of safety and quality medical care are maintained.

2. Normal physiological processes of childbearing and neonatal adjustment are fostered and supported.

3. The program of care is directed toward developing the ability of the participants to become increasingly independent in meeting their own health needs.

4. Adequate evaluation of mothers and neonates is carried out to ensure identification of (a) deviations from the normal and (b) problems and needs for help experienced by the mother and her family.

5. Teaching and support by competent practitioners is designed to (a) develop increased skill in the participants' abilities to identify and meet their own health needs, (b) develop sound health practices, (c) promote adequate mothering and fathering behavior, and (d) strengthen and support the family unit.

6. The cost per day would be much less than in the acute hospital facility.

All components of the system would be considered in the development of a maternity service that would meet the above objectives. These components are (1) the family, (2) the physical environment, (3) the supportive services, (4) the cost of care, and (5) the health professionals and the program of care. Although each component will be discussed briefly, the major emphasis will be on the clinical practice of the professional nurse during the puerperium as a major contributor to the health professionals and the program of care component.

The family

The needs and desires of the childbearing family should form the basis for the development of the health-care system and be the primary focus of professional nursing practice. What are the needs of the normal postpartum woman and her family?

For the purpose of this chapter the definitions of need given by Marion Lesser and Vera Keane[5] and Ernestine Wiedenbach[6] are used.

. . . any subjective desire or want on the part of a woman in childbirth, which when met, contributes to her physical, mental or emotional ease during the experience. This desire may be conscious and stated directly, or revealed indirectly. Conversely, when these needs are unmet, the result is a varying degree of discomfort and/or dissatisfaction.*

Anything the individual requires to maintain or sustain himself comfortably or capably in his situation.†

The following are identified as commonly recurring needs for all postpartum families although the extent to which each may present a personal need for help varies with individuals. They may also be considered the developmental tasks of the puerperium.

1. *Ability to cope comfortably and capably with the physical, physiological, and psychological changes and adjustments of the postpartum period.* Reva Rubin in a classic article, "Puerperal Change,"[7] states:

The puerperium is a complex state of the childbearing experience, during which the physical and psychological work of gestation and delivery becomes final. And, during this stage, a new role, with a complete set of new tasks is begun—before the previous work is quite finished. What is past and what is future combine to form the composite present of the puerperium. Intuitively, peoples throughout the ages have recognized the unique complexity of the puerperium by providing for the parturient the sanctuary of the lying-in period. . . .*

The nurse is in a strategic position to help the mother understand the changes taking place in her body and how she can best care for herself. She can help her anticipate potential troublesome experiences, handle them more effectively if they occur, and perhaps avoid them altogether.

2. *Initiation of effective parent-infant relationships.* The whole area of the development of mothering and fathering behavior is a vast one and much is being written on the subject. Most authorities agree that opportunity for interaction with the infant at the earliest possible point is basic to the optimum development of effective relationships. Touching, holding, feeding, bathing, and diapering are all simple activities that meet certain basic needs of the infant. They further serve as a means by which affective relationships can be developed between parent and child. Astute observations of parents with their newborns usually reveal highly significant information regarding the particular developmental state of the parental role and can be one indicator of problem areas.

3. *Development of comfort and capability in giving care to their newborn infant.* The postpartum hospital stay has great potential for assisting parents to become more comfortable with and confident in their ability to give care to their infant. In a relaxed environment free from other distractions and with the assistance of sensitive, well-qualified professional nurses who are able to give individualized

---

*From Lesser, M., and Keane, V.: Nurse-patient relationships in a hospital maternity service, St. Louis, 1956, The C. V. Mosby Co.

†From Wiedenbach, E.: Clinical nursing; a helping art, New York, 1964, Springer Publishing Co.

*From Rubin, R.: Puerperal change, Nurs. Outlook 9:753-755, 1961.

support and teaching, parents may learn much about their infant's needs and responses and may try out new procedures before being responsible on their own. Even experienced mothers appreciate the opportunity to ask questions, validate their information and skills, and receive assurance that they are functioning competently.

4. *Initiation and development of new roles within the family.* One of the major tasks of the puerperium is the identification and development of the new role of each member of the family whether the baby is a first child or an additional child to the family unit. Support or assistance in this developmental task can be an important part of postpartum care. Opportunities are eagerly sought by parents to discuss how they feel about their experiences and their fears and anxieties concerning the future and to use the professional person as a sounding board for possible approaches to integrating the new child into the family.

One area that has received little attention in hospital maternity units in this country is the need of the older siblings to become acquainted with and to accept the new baby and at the same time to be assured that they remain important and beloved in the eyes of their parents.

The puerperal woman has the right to expect (a) professional services from well-qualified, caring individuals who give preparation and teaching relative to caring for herself and her infant, prompt identification and treatment of deviations from normal progress, and support or assistance in strengthening and maintaining the family unit; (b) ready availability and access to significant persons who care about her; and (c) an environment conducive to accomplishing the developmental tasks of the puerperium in surroundings that are clean, comfortable, and esthetically pleasing, with ready availability of support services for physical hygiene and nutrition, and

with protection from infection resulting from the environment in which care is given.

Physical environment

To separate the sick from the well and to provide the optimum care required by both, a family-centered maternity unit would be developed as a part of the present hospital complex, adjacent to but physically separated from the acute hospital facility. Known high-risk mothers and infants would be admitted directly to the acute facility and all of the usual services would be available to them. Only essentially normal women would be admitted to the proposed maternity unit that would contain a labor and delivery area and postpartum modules, each designed for twenty mothers and their infants. The number of modules would depend on the population served. The labor and delivery area of this facility would be a "swing" unit in which mothers and babies could be transferred into one of the postpartum modules after delivery or, if unexpected problems develop, into the acute facility at any time.

The physical environment would be esthetically pleasing and create a relaxed, homelike atmosphere as well as facilitate the delivery of professional and supportive services. Some features which might be included in the unit are as follows:

1. Circular construction with patient rooms opening out into an enclosed outer lounge-corridor where family members, including young children, could visit the mother
2. Individual, self-contained patient rooms and bathrooms
3. Patient rooms opening onto an inner area with a pleasant lounge accessible to the garden area, community eating area, and the nursery
4. Colors, carpeting, and materials creating a pleasant, light environment
5. Bed constructed to swing in against

one wall under shelves forming a couch during the day and a double bed at night (husband permitted to spend the night with his wife if he wishes)

6. Small kitchenette with facilities for preparing light snacks as desired; ice water and juice dispensing machines readily accessible

Supportive services

Supportive services are defined as all those nonpatient or limited-patient contact activities essential to the comfort and well-being of the patient and to the maintenance of an environment in which the program of care can be effectively carried out. Supportive services are divided into the following areas: (1) central service and purchasing, (2) food service, (3) housekeeping, (4) engineering and maintenance, (5) unit secretaries and records, (6) laboratories, and (7) volunteer services. They would be readily available to both the patient and the professional staff and designed for rapid and economical delivery.

Concepts basic to the system design are as follows:

1. Nursing and supportive services would be separated to achieve greater economy of function and to enable the nurse to make maximum use of her time and professional preparation.

2. The professionally prepared practitioner would provide direct patient care services and nonprofessionally prepared individuals supportive services.

3. Each of the supportive areas would be designed to be as automated as possible with systems designed for maximum efficiency and economy.

4. All supportive areas must have as their primary goal the contribution to the achievement of the objectives of the unit.

5. The physical design of the unit would facilitate the efficient and economical delivery of supportive services.

Cost of care

The cost of providing care should be much lower than that now obtained in the acute hospital facility. An administrator of supportive services would be appointed to coordinate and direct the activities, including budgetary, of each of the supportive areas as they relate to the maternity unit. He would utilize services that could be provided at the least expense. Careful cost accounting would give an accurate assessment of the nature of the expenses incurred in the system.

Although the nursing staffing pattern would involve employing mostly professional personnel at higher salaries, the increased utilization of professional preparation would result in an increased quality of care at a lower cost. The present numerous levels of personnel would not be necessary because of the design of the supportive system.

Health professionals and program of care
The professional nurse in the puerperium

Care of the normal postpartum family should have as its primary objective preventive health services that will enable the family to become increasingly independent in effectively meeting their own health needs. To achieve this goal the professional nurse should devote full time and energy to those individuals needing her unique services. Although the present discussion relates primarily to nursing within the framework of a new proposed system, many of the facets presented are at present being carried out to some degree in hospitals throughout the country and more can be adapted to existing systems. The maternity nurse may ask herself to what extent these practices are found in her own hospital and what barriers exist to prevent her from utilizing the full range of her professional preparation.

Assessment

Physical, physiological, and psychological changes and adjustments occur at a rapid rate during the puerperium. Daily assessment of these changes, with intermittent and periodic evaluation as needed throughout the day, should form the basis for professional nursing care. Morning rounds to evaluate the status of breasts, abdomen, fundus, perineum, anus, lochia, and legs could provide the nurse with an opportunity not only to determine normal progress and possible deviations but also to teach the mother about the changes taking place. Involving the mother in her own evaluation results in earlier reporting of problems if they occur, since she will be more aware of untoward changes.

The nurse could help the mother understand the normal changes taking place within her body and what she could do to best facilitate these changes. For example, checking the proper fit of the brassiere and discussing the importance of proper breast alignment for comfort and prevention of stress to tissues could be carried out simultaneously with evaluation of the breasts. Teaching postpartum exercises appropriate to the early puerperium follows easily when the mother is helped to feel the diastasis of the rectus muscles. Feeling the changed position and consistency of the fundus before and after voiding demonstrates vividly the importance of keeping the bladder empty. Knowing the expected color and amount of lochia for her postpartum day would enable the mother to notify the nurse immediately should a problem occur. Most mothers appreciate knowing how their perineal area is healing, particularly if they are feeling discomfort and wonder if all is normal. Simple comfort measures, which the mother can use herself, might be taught, such as the perineal tightening exercise, proper cleansing, use of the shower or portable sitz bath, or the application of the heat lamp or analgesic spray.

Skilled listening, observation, and questioning on the part of the nurse might reveal problems and concerns that the mother may be experiencing. Identification of specific needs for help early in the day would allow the nurse to plan with the mother regarding the kind of help desired and required. Periodic observation and questioning would enable her to assess problem areas that might arise. The many aspects of baby care, questions or concerns regarding breast or formula feeding, resumption of usual activities, and integration of the new child into the existing family structure are areas of concern to many mothers.

The mother could be taught how to carry out many aspects of her own physical evaluation and record it on a specially designed sheet kept in her room. Such items as temperature, pulse, breasts, fundus, lochia, and special discomforts could be assessed and then discussed with the nurse when she makes her morning rounds. In this way the mother herself would become more knowledgeable and capable in relation to her own care.

Teaching

Teaching of the postpartum family might be carried out individually, in small group discussions or demonstrations, and by specially prepared audiovisual media. The mother and father could take advantage of a variety of teaching approaches suitable to their needs and interests. Simple skills or procedures could be viewed and reviewed at any time by utilization of the videotape or sound and slide programs available on the maternity unit. Some of the subject areas viewed might include the taking of the mother's own and the baby's temperatures, postpartum exercises, physical assessment of her own body changes or newborn characteristics, formula or breast feeding, and bathing and diapering her infant.

Individualized instruction and demonstration might be focused on specific questions and concerns, the clarification of information, and the validation of correct carrying-out of procedures. Short group discussion sessions for parents might be held several times a day to provide opportunity for parents to share experiences, clarify misconceptions, receive group support and validation, and, under the skilled direction of the nurse, explore their new role and how to cope comfortably and capably with the demands inherent in it.

A successful teaching program would ensure that each couple would leave the hospital secure in their ability to meet their own and their infant's needs and comfortable in the knowledge of where to obtain additional help should this be desired.

Support

The professional nurse would be constantly available to parents for any assistance they might need. Since she would be freed from all routine tasks associated with maintaining the unit, her total time and energies would be available to the families.

Visiting hours would be determined by the parents. Family members would be welcomed and appropriately included in the program of care. Husbands might plan to attend group or individual teaching sessions. Children could visit their mother and the new baby in the designated area outside her room.

Self-care

The physical environment would enable the mother to meet her basic care needs by herself or with minimal assistance. Individual patient rooms stocked with all necessary equipment and supplies and with a bathroom adjacent would enable her to carry out basic hygiene whenever desired without outside assistance. Food and beverages would be readily available. The baby crib on wheels could be moved from the nursery to the mother's room, lounge area, or garden.

True individualization would be possible. The pace and rhythm of the day would be set by the mother. Supplies, materials, and professional assistance needed would be readily available. For example, a mother who has had inadequate sleep during the night could sleep in the morning as long as she liked and still have a hot breakfast when she awakened. She could take a shower at 3 P.M. instead of 9 A.M. She could have her baby with her almost constantly or spend only a little time with him on any given day. The staff would accept these decisions and the mother's right to make them.

Staffing

Staffing patterns would be quite different because of the rearrangement of responsibilities in the new system. Instead of the multiple levels of nursing personnel now involved in care of the postpartum woman, direct care would be given only by professional nurses. On a module unit of twenty normal mothers and babies the day and evening shift would each be staffed by two professional nurses, preferably one a clinical specialist; the night shift would have one nurse. The nursery would be staffed by two nurse aides each shift.

The professional nurse would be responsible for carrying out basic assessment of both the mother and infant according to standardized criteria and methods. She would be responsible for individual teaching of mothers regarding their own care and that of their infants. She would be expected to be supportive and to function in a manner that would potentiate the capabilities of both the mother and father. She would be responsible for identifying problem areas and for referring to the clinical specialist those problems beyond her capability. She would be expected to base her care on an individualized assessment and to evaluate the results of her teaching and support.

The clinical specialist would carry out all the functions of the professional nurse enumerated above. In addition she would be responsible for the total assessment of each mother and baby and for group teaching. She would report all untoward findings to the physician and coordinate the efforts of other members of the health team. She would act in a liaison capacity to the community and, in particular, to the nurses who might be seeing the family in their home setting. If needed, she might make selected home visits with the nurse in the community. She would handle all problems referred to her by the nursing staff.

The nursery aide would be a nonprofessional person responsible for routine care of the babies in the nursery similar to that given by the mothers. This would include admitting babies from the delivery area, bottle feeding, diapering, bathing, and recording basic information regarding the infants' condition and behavior according to standardized criteria and methods. She would be directly responsible to the clinical specialist to whom she would report all problems. She would not be responsible for cleaning and stocking the nursery, which would be done by the supportive services.

The clinical nursing director would be responsible for the overall administration of the unit. Although the administrative functions of providing for supportive services would be under the direction of a nonprofessional director, this individual would be responsible to the clinical nursing director for maintaining a supportive system compatible with the philosophy and objectives of the unit. All changes in the supportive system would be approved by her, and she would have authority to initiate change in conjunction with the the supportive services administrator.

Conclusion

An adequate amount of high-quality professional nursing care can only be provided childbearing women when there is maximum utilization of present resources. Currently professional nurses are spending large segments of their time in nonprofessional activities while lesser prepared persons are expected to assume direct patient care. An analysis of the nature of the needs of the postpartum family indicates that these needs can be readily met by professionally prepared nurses who are freed from supervisory and unit maintenance responsibilities. A new system designed to provide rapid economical delivery of supportive services in an environment conducive to achieving defined objectives will provide high-quality care at a reasonable cost. Focus on preventive health teaching and care will result in healthier families who, in turn, will need fewer acute health services with their attending drain on personal and material resources.

References

1. Jones, Boisfeullet, editor: The health of Americans, Englewood Cliffs, N. J., 1970, Prentice-Hall, Inc.
2. National Center for Health Statistics: Hospital discharges and length of stay: short stay hospitals, U. S., July, 1963-June, 1964, Series 10, No. 30, Washington, D. C., 1966, U. S. Government Printing Office.
3. Editorial: Cutting hospital costs, Salt Lake City, Utah, Feb. 23, 1970, Deseret News.
4. Pitel, Martha: A nurse's view, Hospitals 43: 67-68, 1969.
5. Lesser, Marian, and Keane, Vera: Nurse-patient relationships in a hospital maternity service, St. Louis, 1956, The C. V. Mosby Co.
6. Wiedenbach, Ernestine: Clinical nursing; A helping art, New York, 1964, Springer Publishing Co.
7. Rubin, Reva: Puerperal change, Nurs. Outlook 9:753-755, 1961.

Chapter *24*

The double bind of motherhood

Margaret Bennett
Lorraine Walker

In the light of the recent resurgence of the movement for women's liberation, it seems both timely and prudent for the nursing profession to examine some of its practices, particularly in the area of maternity nursing. Hence, this chapter has been written with the intent of focusing on some current sociocultural conflicts associated with the mother role and the implications of these conflicts for the practice of a more relevant and socially aware style of maternity nursing. First, some of the conflicting values besetting women in their sex-linked roles within families will be described. Then a variety of proposals for dealing with these value conflicts will be set forth and examined. Concurrently, some implications for the practice of nursing will be drawn.

Women who find themselves in the role of mother are placed into what seems to be an implicit cultural double bind (that is, a situation in which there are strong, conflicting options). On the one hand, they are urged to practice our society's traditional values built into the notion of a "good mother": forbearance, self-sacrifice, selflessness, being sole custodian of their children's needs, and being ever present. On the other hand, such people as Betty Friedan[1] have vocalized the frustration and lack of personal fulfillment experienced by mothers because of a conflicting set of values oriented toward finding fulfillment in some productive activity outside the home. This latter set of values would have women opt for liberation from the personally stunting and inhibiting world of home and family and move into some personally satisfying area of occupational interest.

The inherently conflicting values in these two role options leave a mother in a resulting double bind. If she opts for fulfillment in some personally satisfying activity in addition to motherhood itself, she automatically conforms to the image of the "bad mother" based on the traditional conception of motherhood. Thus, although some career interest may have stimulated her intellect and provided more economic security, this liberation is accompanied by a sense of guilt for failing to live up to traditional values of motherhood. In turn, the mother who follows the traditional pattern of sole preoccupation with home and family feels that she is isolated within the narrow and immediate concerns of managing a household and child tending.

Militants in either camp may feel no sense of inadequacy when compared against the other standard; however, for the majority of women who have internalized values from both camps, the conflicts seem inevitable. It is to this problem area that maternity nursing needs to give its attention if it is to provide a socially relevant nursing practice.

Several courses of action are open to the nursing profession, and specifically to maternity nurses, for dealing with the conflict between these two role models, that is, the traditional mother notion and the liberated notion.

The first and most revolutionary alternative is to work toward the reconstruction of the various values and patterns of motherhood and child care, working toward a new pattern that would include a fractionalization of child care responsibilities among several individuals. This would include the development of new social roles and institutions, for example, state or privately controlled child care centers, which would share, or in some cases supersede, the responsibilities of child care with the traditional home setting.

In proposing this revolutionary alternative to the nursing profession, it is necessary to recognize that the mother role has not evolved in isolation within our society. When exploring the mother role one must explore the reciprocal nature of roles. It is the relationship of the family system within the larger social system that is important. Just to examine the family system and the roles therein is futile because that system has been influenced and shaped by the larger society. The larger society's values and expectations of the role members within the family have great psychological influence on the family system. The conflict that can result has a potent bearing on the pattern of interrelationships of fam-

ily members. Hence, at the outset it is necessary to recognize that the revolutionary alternative requires dealing not only with individual family relationships, but also requires that nursing as a profession confront the value systems at work within the larger society. Thus it seems imperative that nursing organizations, not just individual nurses, actively work toward revolutionizing conceptions of motherhood. Particularly, in a profession whose members are predominantly women it is perhaps doubly expedient. In line with this recommendation it seems obligatory that the state and national nursing organizations take stands on matters that would facilitate the reconstruction of roles and values connected with motherhood, for example, supporting the development of adequate child care centers.

In working out a reconstruction of the present system of values and role expectations of mothers in our society, it is helpful to be cognizant of other patterns of the mother role and child care. In other cultures the amount of time that mothers are responsible for children appears to be dependent on the availability of alternate caretakers for children. The alternate caretaker includes such family members as an older brother and sister, aunt, uncle, grandparents, or in the less complex patrilineal societies, the powerful mother's brother who acts as the nurturing caretaker, while the biological father acts as the disciplinary caretaker.[2, 3] It is the social system of the society that will define the mother's role in caretaking and that of the other kin. A particular society may value parent-centered socialization over relative-centered socialization; this is directly related to whether or not families are nuclear or extended. For example, the mothers of Tarong, Philippines, offer a different life-style from our society, and thus the mother's role is drastically different.[4] The group sociability makes child care a group project. There one finds the verbalized expression, "We all take care of our children." According to Minturn and Lambert,[4] this is no exaggeration, since no mother feels that she has the total responsibility for her children's care. The mother is expected to keep the baby close by her approximately six months after birth, although neighbors are close at hand when needed and may actually nurse the infant for the mother.

Although 50% of the Tarong mothers usually take care of infants, 83% of the mothers report that their infants are sometimes cared for by an adult other than the parents. . . . Whereas 50% of the Tarong sample usually care for infants, only 21% usually care for older children.*

These facts represent a real shift of the caretaking responsibilities from the mother to the father, older siblings, and other adults as the infant advances to young childhood. When this Filipino sample of mothers was compared with mothers from areas in New England, Mexico, Okinawa, India, and Africa, it was found that the Tarong, Philippines, sample ranked first in the proportion of time that nonparental adults take care of children.[4] Grandmothers and aunts are the usual nonparental caretakers. When a child is weaned he is encouraged and stimulated to adopt a sibling, aunt, or grandmother as a partial replacement or supplement to his mother.

Within the Tarong group, fathers assume many household tasks without loss of social status. There appears to be a general philosophy of nurture, comfortable dependence, and emotional stability. The community is one of cooperativeness where the obligation to help one's kin or neighbor is highly regarded. The group seems to function as did certain American groups when men would gather to raise a barn or house while the women would have a communal kitchen to feed their men and tend all the younger children.

The Tarong life-style centers around interdependency for both emotional companionship and for the provision of the physical necessities of life. Within the Tarong group, household tasks were not assigned according to sex. Sexual identity did not appear to be linked to what household functions one performed. Fathers may do cooking, housekeeping, and washing, and young male children are taught these tasks. Young girls are taught household tasks as well as carrying water, gathering wood, feeding or watering animals, and helping in the fields. The social system and the roles, the values and philosophy therein are quite different from the following example of a New England mother.

When studying a group of mothers in Orchard Town, New England,[4] it was found that they highly valued the mother's caretaker role and were convinced that no one else could adequately substitute for the mother. Because of this belief, this group rejected alternate caretakers even when they were available. The investigators also found a high degree of maternal emotional instability that they believed was in part due to the large amount of time spent in charge of their children. Independence, which is highly valued within this New England group, is congruent with parent-centered socialization of children.

In summary, the Tarong group and the New England group show the wide divergence that may exist in the way the mother role is defined within a society and the manner in which the caring of children is handled. The significance of these examples is this: there appears to be no one "naturally right" pattern of motherhood and child care. The "rightness" of a pattern would seem to be its ability to fit harmoniously into the culture of the society in which it occurs and to do so in a way that does not result in undesirable effects on those who must take on the pattern or be affected by it.

---

*From Minturn, L., and Lambert, W. W.: Mothers of six cultures, New York, 1964, John Wiley & Sons, Inc., p. 211.

As one of the helping professions which deals with mothers and families, nursing is in a position to either foster or inhibit the reconstruction of our society's notions of how the mother role might best be carried out and how children might best be cared for. While it is not the intention of this chapter to lay out a specific revolutionary program for the mother role and child care, it does seem appropriate to make several observations: (1) there is nothing innate about the way the mother role has been traditionally defined within our society; (2) there is nothing "unnatural" about the sharing of child care responsibilities between the mother and some other individuals; (3) since the mother role fits into a complex of relations and values within the larger society, it is necessary that a fit be achieved between the definition of the mother role and these larger forces; and (4) nursing organizations and nursing practitioners could serve the cause of primary prevention of role conflicts in working toward the reconstruction of the current ideas of motherhood and child care.

The second alternative for dealing with the conflict between the traditional and liberated notions of motherhood consists simply in encouraging women to take on more flexible styles of motherhood and child care. This alternative would stress the individuality of patterns of motherhood and child care within a family unit and deemphasize any dichotomous notion about the possibilities open to women. Although this second alternative sounds as though it could easily resolve the conflict problem, it does overlook the fact that carrying out patterns of motherhood occurs within a context of social and cultural influences that set constraints upon how individualized a given pattern might be without being considered deviant and, hence, subjected to various sanctions from the larger society.

Recognizing the importance and influence of the larger society's values and institutions on the definition of the mother and father roles, let us shift emphasis to the relationship between the mother and father. How the mother sees herself and her role and that of the father must be congruent or in harmony with how the father sees himself and his role and that of the mother. If the perceptions of each other and their respective roles are not in harmony, regardless of the larger society's role definitions, a conflictual relationship will be the result. For example, if a mother values the liberated concept of motherhood and her spouse does not, then their relationship will be in conflict. If the father values the traditional concept of motherhood, then he must see his wife primarily in the child caretaker role and not himself. When this conflict occurs, both mother and father will feel opposition or competition for the acceptance of their individual values. The relationship will be predominantly one of symmetry (that is, characterized by equality, competition, and a mirroring effect between individuals) especially in regard to child tending, and may well extend into other areas of the relationship. The symmetry is a product of the differing expectations of motherhood and fatherhood, and results in conflict between the individuals involved.[5]

The aim of a more individualized and flexible pattern of motherhood would be the development of a complementary relationship (that is, characterized by difference between individuals in which behavior of one individual complements that of the other) between mother and father in their function of child care. There are two distinct positions within a complementary relationship. At one time the father may be in the primary child-tending position, and at other times the mother may assume this position. One partner does not impose this type of relationship; rather each functions in a way that complements the other. In respect to child tending, the definition of their relationship is in harmony and results in a satisfying feeling for both. Whether or not the mother and father favor a liberalized concept of motherhood or the traditional is irrelevant, so long as they perceive their roles and child-caring functions in a way that complements the other; then their relationship will be harmonious and will allow each to develop their individual talents. A complementary relationship between the mother and the father would favor the development of an individual pattern of motherhood and child care within the family system. The father has been used here as an example of an alternate caretaker, based upon the assumption that in a highly mobile society frequently other alternate caretakers are not available.

Margaret Mead[6] has suggested three courses open to a society that has recognized the extent to which the male and female personality patterns are a social product.

1. A society can strive toward the standardization of sex-linked roles. Women would be taught certain functions and men different functions. The aim of all the society's institutions would be toward this end.

2. A society could strive toward a standardization such that men and women are completely equal and therefore can be shaped into one single form or pattern of human being. Children of both sexes would be taught the same attitudes, same emotional expressions and repressions, same functions, and same occupations. With these two courses above, the individuality of any person is lost to the standardization of the society, and a flexible family style would not be possible. A mother who found she could not fit into her standardized role would be classified as a social deviant. The lost talents of the individual members would be an even greater loss to the society as a whole.

3. Mead[6] suggests a final course toward

which a society can move that recognizes and highly values the potentialities and individual differences of its members. This course completely moves away from the standardization of sex-linked roles. The aim of the society would be toward greater development and expression of individual personalities, patterns, and functions, regardless of sex. In a highly complex and technological society, it seems imperative that movement is made away from standardization and toward maximizing differences. Both the individual and society would be the benefactor. Mead describes an approach open to such a society:

It [a society] might abandon its various attempts to make boys fight and to make girls passive, or to make all children fight and instead shape our educational institutions to develop to the full the boy who shows a capacity for maternal behaviours, the girl who shows an opposite capacity that is stimulated by fighting obstacles.*

When describing the benefits of a society adopting the course of maximizing individual differences, Mead says:

No child would be relentlessly shaped to one pattern of behavior, but instead there should be many patterns, in a world that had learned to allow each individual the pattern which was most congenial to his gifts.*

For the traditional conception of motherhood to change toward a more liberalized concept in this larger society, the idea of the nurturing role of fatherhood must also be brought about. The reconstruction of values and patterns of motherhood, including the fractionalization of the caretaking of children, is a slow process, but one in which the nursing profession must take a stand. Note that it is only within the past few years that the nursing profession has encouraged the respectability of the profession for the male. The nurturing male remains to be valued in the

---

*From Mead, M.: Sex and temperament, New York, 1935, The New American Library, p. 234.

overall society. Presently he too often is perceived as a social deviant.

Turning to the specific nursing implications that will contribute the development of a flexible pattern of motherhood, maternity and pediatric nurses have an ideal opportunity to study the existing relationship between the mother and father. If the mother and father roles are not in harmony, the nurse is able through counseling to help them identify and resolve the conflict. Whether or not the resolution is toward the liberalized or traditional concept or a combination thereof is the decision of the role members. The task is to help families develop a flexible and individualized pattern of motherhood and fatherhood and to alleviate conflict. Prenatal classes, doctors' offices, hospitals, and home visits all provide areas for the relationship to be studied and for the conflicts to be lessened.

Another very strong influence on the development of individualized patterns of motherhood are the role models within a given community or its institutions. Models are utilized in all cultures to promote the acquisition of socially sanctioned behavior patterns.[7] Imitative learning is related to the adoption of sex-linked vocational and occupational roles. Bandura and Walters[7] believe that not enough recognition is given to the influence of role models on behavior patterning:

The importance of social agents as a source of patterns of behavior continues to be largely ignored, despite evidence from informal observation and laboratory experimentation that the provision of models in actual or symbolic form is an exceedingly effective procedure for transmitting and controlling behavior.*

The successful mother who at the same time is successful in her chosen career serves as a figure for other mothers to imitate. The positive role model makes the dual role of motherhood and outside-of-home occupation more palatable and relieves a portion of the guilt for one caught in the double bind. The model also serves the function of gradually changing attitudes and values.

Unfortunately, the nursing profession on a national, state, or local level has few role models of this dual nature. Nursing must make explicit the high value it places on the combination of motherhood and professional nursing practice. The institutions within the nursing profession must give more than lip service to the dual nature of motherhood. One must ask the questions: Why are there so few role models in the nursing profession? Is it because few nurses have successfully combined a professional nursing career with motherhood? Has the profession itself encouraged or discouraged the dual role?

Finally, an individual maternity or pediatric nurse who is also a mother must comfortably accept the dual role before she is able to help other mothers caught in the double bind of motherhood. A nurse experiencing the double bind conflict herself will be so concerned with her own situation that she will have little energy to expend on lessening the conflict of other mothers.

The third alternative deals not with alteration of the patterns and values surrounding the traditional and liberated notions of motherhood, but rather takes a symptomatic approach toward the psychological conflicts to which the double bind gives rise, for example, self-depreciation, guilt, and depression. Since the treatment of these disorders is well documented, the intents here are (1) to make some observations about the way maternity nursing has dealt with psychological problems that arise from the two conflicting ideals of motherhood and (2) to point out some areas of practice where gaps have occurred.

---

*From Bandura, A., and Walters, R.: Social learning and personality development, New York, 1963, Holt, Rinehart & Winston, Inc., p. 51.

Perhaps most typical of the manner in which maternity nursing as a field has dealt with the value conflicts surrounding motherhood has been the philosophy of "have a good cry and the situation won't look so bad." While this approach is sometimes quite helpful at the moment, it tends to deal with the value conflicts that mothers experience in a superficial, symptomatic way; this approach tends to circumvent actively engaging in questioning and reappraising the values that may be causing the problems mothers experience. In assuming that the mother's problem is primarily psychological and not sociological in nature, one may safely avoid the kinds of value reappraisals this chapter is calling for.

The nursing profession has also been guilty of certain omissions in its practice. One major gap in nursing practice rightfully belongs with the symptomatic approach to the managing of psychological problems associated with motherhood. Consider the absence of formal or informal preparation of women for the separation from their children that occurs as women return to employment outside the home. Surely this period has its depressions and frustrations. It seems that women might legitimately expect to be prepared for coping with this event in parent education classes, along with the more traditional content that helps them deal with the various crises involved in parenthood.

Another gap in nursing practices occurs in the lack of preparation of fathers for assuming more of the nurturing role within the family. While men may of necessity have to take on such responsibilities when women seek employment outside the home, they may harbor unspoken feelings about their adequacy as providers and find the rearrangement of roles within their marriages threatening to their masculine identities. It seems that nursing might appropriately deal with this aspect of the changing roles within the family.

In conclusion the nursing profession in its practices within the field of maternity and pediatric nursing has tended to nurture the traditional values and expectations of motherhood, and hence to foster rather than alleviate the conflicts women experience in the mother role. The intent of this chapter has been to suggest how nursing as a profession might redirect some of its practices so as to serve as a positive social force in reducing the conflicts between the traditional and the liberated notions of motherhood. Three broad courses of action for achieving this goal have been proposed. These alternatives roughly parallel a primary, secondary, and tertiary preventive approach to the problem. A concurrent aim has been to suggest throughout this chapter what appear to be necessary issues for nursing to deal with if it is to have greater relevance to the contemporary family life.

References

1. Friedan, B.: The feminine mystique, New York, 1963, W. W. Norton & Co., Inc.
2. Radcliffe-Brown, A. R.: The mother's brother in South Africa. In the Bobbs-Merrill Reprint Series in the Social Sciences, reprinted from The South African Journal of Science, Vol. XXI, 1924.
3. Firth, R.: We, the Tikopia, Boston, 1957, Beacon Press.
4. Minturn, L., and Lambert, W. W.: Mothers of six cultures, New York, 1964, John Wiley & Sons, Inc.
5. Bateson, G.: Naven, Stanford, Calif., 1958, Stanford University Press.
6. Mead, M.: Sex and temperament, New York, 1935, New American Library.
7. Bandura, A., and Walters, R.: Social learning and personality development. New York, 1963, Holt, Rinehart & Winston, Inc.

Bibliography

Mead, M.: Towards mutual responsibility, J. Soc. Issues 4:45-65, 1950.
Nye, R. I., and Hoffman, L. W.: The employed mother in America, Chicago, 1963, Rand McNally & Co.
Walzlawick, P., Beavin, J., and Jackson, D.: Pragmatics of human communication, New York, 1967, W. W. Norton & Co., Inc.

Chapter 25

Adoptive parents need help

Shelley Horton

In 1967, 168,000 children were adopted in the United States. Seventy-four thousand of these children were adopted by persons related to them by blood or marriage, and 84,000 were adopted by non-relatives. Of these 84,000, 62,000 adoptions were arranged by social agencies. These will be referred to as agency adoptions. The remaining 22,000 were arranged independently; the adoptive parents secured the children from the natural parents or through intermediaries such as doctors, lawyers, or ministers. These will be referred to as independent adoptions.[1]

Review of the nursing literature, texts, and periodicals reveals little material regarding the role of the nurse in adoption. Does she in fact have any role? The literature of social work seems to indicate that the role of the professions, excluding law, is to refer the matter to a social agency. Do nurses prepared to work with mothers and children have more to offer these 22,000 children and their families at this critical time in their lives? While the percentage of children placed by agencies is increasing, the actual number of independent adoptions is also increasing and seems likely to continue to do so for some time. The position of the Child Welfare League of America is that children should be placed for adoption only by social agencies subject to the social and legal control of the state.[2] However, this may not be feasible for some time due to the limited number of social workers, the cost of agency placements, the length of time they require, and the current agency policy of attempting to achieve the best placement for each child rather than eliminating only those clearly undesirable homes. Legislation prohibiting independent adoptions might result either in agencies turning away mothers wishing to surrender their children and couples wishing to adopt or in boarding children in foster homes for long periods of time while agencies completed the necessary investigations. Does the failure rate of independent adoptions warrant this sort of action? In a study of 484 independent adoptions in Florida, Witmer and associates found a 70% success rate. They further note that reported agency failures range from 10% to 25% and conclude that an 85% success rate might be reasonably hoped for.[3] It would appear that here, in the area of increasing the success rate of adoption, the nurse would be in a position to use her professional skills. Since she is not charged with the evaluation and selection of adoptive homes, aspiring parents might find her more approachable and less threatening than a social worker.

Most couples desiring a child, but unable to conceive, eventually find their way to a doctor's office where they undergo a series of interviews and tests delving into an area that is usually considered as most private and personal. Should the tests reveal an untreatable problem that makes reproduction unlikely or impossible, the nurse realizes that this news will have a profound effect on the individual's self-concept and society's view of him or her. The couple will find themselves cast in a role for which they have not been prepared.[4] It is appropriate that the nurse encourage them to discuss their feelings and ask questions regarding their infertility just as she would in the case of the patient who has had surgery involving the reproductive system.

In working with these patients the nurse needs to be aware that attitudes toward childlessness are changing rapidly in our culture. Some young people seem to view a satisfying sexual relationship as an end in itself and not as a means to an end; others feel that there are already too many people on the planet and refrain from bearing children for that reason; still others do not wish to reproduce because of their genetic backgrounds. The nurse must therefore proceed with caution and not assume that failure to reproduce is deeply disturbing to all people, at least on a conscious level.

Once the couple has accepted their infertility, the nurse might explore with them the alternatives to bearing a child. For some couples, for instance, those who feel strongly about blood lines or illegitimacy, learning to accept their infertility and live with it may be the only alternative. Taking a foster child or becoming involved with the scouts, the Y, 4-H, or Sunday school groups may be an alternative measure for others. Volunteer work for children's hospital wards or sponsoring a child through an organization such as CARE, WAIF, or Save The Children Federation are other means of sublimating the desire for a child and may be the answer for persons too old to adopt or where one spouse does not really desire to adopt.

The most obvious alternative open to the infertile couple desiring a child is adoption. In coming to the decision to adopt, the couple needs to be helped to explore their feelings about raising, as their own, a child whom they have not borne. In addition to this, the woman needs to consider her feelings about missing what some people describe as one of the peaks of a woman's life experience, that is, pregnancy, labor, delivery, and breast feeding. In other words, is she more interested in the process than the product? If so, adoption will not satisfy her longing. If the couple does decide on adoption, many factors, including their age, race, religion, and geographical location will influence their chances of successfully adopting. However, the nurse can answer some of their questions and refer them to people more able to answer others.

Unfortunately, once the couple has made the decision to adopt, nurses may have little contact with them until they have obtained a child. This interval, sometimes five years or longer, between deciding to adopt and actually obtaining a child is a very stressful period for most people. If they go to an agency there is always the possibility that they will be rejected; if they try to arrange for an independent adoption, it may be some time before they can find an available baby. In either case there is seldom any clear-cut timetable by which they can pace their progress toward parenthood. The uncertainty of the child's arrival makes sharing of the news with family or friends difficult, thus depriving the adoptive parents of their support during this trying period. The lack of physical changes in the mother deprives her of the tolerance usually extended to the pregnant woman during what has been described as the "taking in" phase, a time during which she has to get ready to be able to give to a dependent and demanding infant. No one fusses over her, encourages her to rest, or caters good naturedly to bizarre food cravings.

By not having carried and delivered the child, the adoptive mother avoids the associated physical stress, but she is deprived of the two to four days of hospitalization and the attention of qualified staff available to answer questions as she is handling and feeding her new baby. The staff is equally deprived of the opportunity of observing the mother's interaction with her baby, identifying problem areas, and instituting corrective intervention. This situation could be corrected by a program, similar to those in premature nurseries, which encourages adoptive mothers to visit the hospital to learn to feed and handle their new babies prior to discharge. The nurse could use this opportunity to reassure her that mothering is a learned behavior and not a reflex reaction triggered by the birth of the baby and that even natural mothers experience a time lag between the birth of the baby and the development of warm maternal feelings.

Once the child is in his adoptive home the nurse is likely to have more regular contact with him and his family as they come to the clinic or doctor's office for well-child supervision. She will, of course, be concerned with his growth and development, but she also needs to be aware of some of the special problems of adopted children and their parents. Adoptive parents tend to be older than natural parents and adopted children are more likely to be only children.[3] As a result parents may tend to be overprotective, reluctant to set limits, or to use appropriate disciplinary measures. They need to be helped to see that freedom to develop within reasonable limits will result in making the child feel more secure and loved rather than in alienating him as they fear may result from being firm. Successful adoptive parents must tread a narrow path between maintaining a "normal" family life and at the same time accepting the fact that the adoptive family is different from the biological family. They must accept the child as their own, yet adopted. Kirk feels that adoptive parents who acknowledge the difference of their situation foster good communications with their children and, as a result, achieve order and stability in the adoptive family. On the other hand, rejection of the difference leads to poor communication between parent and child and to disruption of the adoptive relationship.[6] Accepting this difference begins with the couple's acceptance of their infertility and continues as they are able to discuss their plans to adopt with family and friends. The road becomes rougher as they tell and retell the child of his adoption and answer his questions about his natural parents.

In the past, adopted children were often told that the natural parents had died. This story had many advantages; it eliminated the problem of illegitimacy, the voluntary surrender of the child, and the existence of another set of parents. The obvious disadvantage to this story is that it usually is not true and as the child grows older he will certainly realize this. Another, less apparent, disadvantage is that the child may become very anxious whenever his parents become ill, fearing that they may die and he will be given up again. The approach most widely used at the present time is the story of the chosen child. Again, this is at best a misrepresentation of the truth. In addition, the child will soon realize that he was available to be chosen because someone had given him up. He may wonder if they did so because something was wrong with him and worry that his adoptive parents may give him up too if he is unable to live up to their expectations. Kirk proposes that in the long run the truth may be the best course of action. The child between 6 and 12 years of age is capable of understanding and accepting the idea that society makes it difficult for a single woman to provide a home for a child. This explanation need not be in direct reference to the child's natural mother but rather to the growing number of young people who, knowing the mores, nonetheless break them, which results in children for whom they prefer to find the homes that they themselves cannot provide.[4] Parents who have strong feelings about illegitimacy will find this approach difficult or impossible to use. There is no easy, proved way to tell the child of his adoption, but the nurse can support the parents as they strive to resist the temptation to deny the fact that they are not the child's natural parents. They need to be encouraged to become sensitive to the child's fears and doubts, realizing not only what it is to be an adoptive parent but also what it must be like to be an adopted child. They need to indicate to the child by their words and actions that he is wanted—acknowledging the adoption, but not making an issue of it.

Attitudes toward adoption have changed rapidly in the last twenty-five years. People used to and still do adopt to satisfy a need for a child they could not or did not have, to provide an heir, to carry on a name, or to provide a home for an orphaned relative. More recently people are adopting because they feel all children, even those who belong to minority groups or have handicaps, have a right to family life, because of a deep conviction that the world is becoming overpopulated and to produce more children is morally irresponsible, or because they do not want to perpetuate some genetic disorder. Although most people overtly express a favorable attitude toward adoption, Kirk

found that they also covertly feel it to be a second-best affair.[4] This may take the form of grandparents objecting to naming the child after a deceased relative or making a distinction between natural and adopted grandchildren or of friends remarking that the child looks so much like the parents that he could be their own or that the parents treat the child just like he was their real child. All these remarks indicate that the speaker is making a sharp distinction between adoptive and biological parenthood. While this behavior is likely to hurt or offend the adoptive parents, it can be minimized to some extent if they know that virtually all adoptive parents have similar experiences at one time or another and that the offense is usually unintentional. Here the sympathetic understanding of the nurse can be comforting.

In examining the status of adoption in the United States we have found it to be a widespread practice and predict that as a result of changing social factors the number of adoptions annually will probably continue to increase. It further appears that agency placement for all children will not be feasible for some time. Although the nurse is not prepared to assume the role of the social worker in the evaluation and selection of adoptive homes, she can, by maintaining an awareness of the unique problems of the adoptive family, foster healthy parent-child relationships, identify problems as they develop, institute intervention herself when appropriate, or refer the family to other professionals when necessary.

In addition she can help to find answers to some of the questions that remain unanswered. Are there developmental phases that adopters go through in becoming successful parents to their children? If there are, and if they can be identified, then we could assist parents through the process, guiding them toward optimal solutions much as Tanner has suggested we do when working with the pregnant woman.[5] Ways need to be found for helping the prospective parents to cope with the preadoptive stress as well as means for providing them with support as they assume the role of adoptive parents.

Yes, there is a role for the nurse in adoption. Eighty-four thousand children and their families need her help.

References

1. Statistical abstract of the United States, 1969, ed. 90, Washington, D. C., 1969, U. S. Bureau of the Census.
2. Child Welfare League of America standards for adoption service, rev., New York, 1968, Child Welfare League of America, Inc.
3. Witmer, H. L., Herzog, E., Weinstein, E. A., and Sullivan, M. E.: Independent adoptions, New York, 1963, Russell Sage Foundation.
4. Kirk, H. D.: Shared fate, London, 1964, The Free Press of Glencoe.
5. Tanner, L. M.: Developmental tasks of pregnancy. In Bergersen, B. S., Anderson, E. H., Duffey, M., Lohr, M., and Rose, M. H., editors: Current concepts in clinical nursing, vol. 2, St. Louis, 1969, The C. V. Mosby Co.

Medical-surgical nursing

With an introduction by
Betty S. Bergersen

The chapters within this section discuss selected concepts of major concern to medical-surgical nurses. Of prime importance is the concept of *adaptation*—to the aging process, to illness and disability, to cardiac surgery, to restrictive visiting privileges, and to medication therapy. These chapters direct attention to the importance of *anxiety* as a deterrent to or facilitator of optimal psychosocial and physiological functioning; of *touch* as a means of communicating information, acceptance, empathy, and caring; of *knowledge* and perceptivity as being vital for understanding and sound decision making; and of *individual differences* and experiences as being important to take into account when planning patient care. Each chapter has its own particular message to convey to medical-surgical nurses, and each imparts aspects essential to truly professional nursing.

This section of medical-surgical nursing is dedicated posthumously to Beulah Gingrich, R.N., B.S., author of the chapter "The Use of the Haptic System as an Information-Gathering System." Prior to her death from a brain tumor in the spring of 1970, Beulah Gingrich was a candidate for the master of science degree in nursing at the University of Illinois Medical Center, Chicago, Illinois; and an instructor in the School of Nursing at Cook County Hospital, Chicago, Illinois.

Qualities that Beulah Gingrich possessed—tenderness, empathy, warmth, sensitivity to the needs of others, sincere dedication to the nursing profession and to those in need of nursing care, belief in the dignity of all human beings—are those that provide kinship between nurses and their patients. These are endearing humanitarian qualities, and thus this section is dedicated to Beulah Gingrich.

Chapter 26

The use of the haptic system as an information-gathering system

Beulah Gingrich

Medical technology has advanced to the point where an increased life expectancy is an accepted fact. However, there is a social lag between the quantity and the quality of these bonus years. Indulgent tolerance or outright irritation with the idiosyncrasies of the elderly frequently permeates the attitudes of personnel administering care as well as the attitudes of relatives and friends. Little effort is expended to try to understand how these behaviors and activities may be related to incomplete or inadequate messages obtained from the environment and to an attempt to use a substitute means of obtaining information to function securely. "The difference between successful and unsuccessful aging lies in the ability of the individual to make . . . necessary adjustments to both the external social environment and the organic changes within himself."[1]

Nurses receive messages and gather information from a rich supply of varied sources. These messages are not all on a consciously perceived level, but nursing decisions are effective only when based on sound knowledge and increased perceptive awareness of the information present in the nuances surrounding the aging individual. This chapter is based on the belief that the personal integrity of an individual is a priority in interpersonal relationships and in the administering of a service. This integrity can be strengthened and guarded more effectively if the demonstrated activities and behaviors are understood as an adaptation of the individual to the organic changes within himself and the social changes in the external environment. Moreover, an awareness of these factors would assist in providing a therapeutic environment, one of the responsibilities of nursing care.

How do individuals obtain information about their environment that enables them to adapt to it, be secure, move around, and survive within it? The continuous array of information they derive from the environment is essential for adaptive living. "The perceptual systems, including the nerve centers at various levels of the brain, are ways of seeking and extracting information about the environment from the flowing array of ambient energy."[2] When the senses are considered as perceptual systems, their function is "to detect something" or to "make us perceive."[2] There is a dynamic exchange taking place in which the individual can take account of the environment to cope with objective facts. The information coming to us from the environment is incessant and of many different kinds—sight, sound, touch, odor, temperature, and position in relation to gravity. These perceptions occur at the same time. We sort out of these multiple sensory stimuli the specific details that enable us to determine their source, meaning, and threat or nonthreat to our well-being. Our responses are usually based on these assessments.

An individual is stimulated by the kinds and density of physical energy in the environment as well as by the energy activity of his own body. Not only do his internal organs provide stimulation, but so does his position and his movement in space. "There is always some discoverable variable in stimulation . . . which determines the character of the perceptual process aroused by it."[6] Internal and external stimuli are the means by which an individual perceives his environment and maintains contact with it. He is an active participant in this process and not a passive recipient regardless of whether the response is one of performance or merely contemplative perception. Stimuli can be selected or enhanced by adjusting the sense organs. When a sound is detected, the head is turned in the direction of the source to balance the sound waves in both ears. A bright light causes one to turn either toward or away from it. A sharp object elicits a moving away action, whereas a soft pressure may stimulate a movement toward the object. "The passive detection of an impinging stimulus soon gives way to active perception."[2] Vision, hearing, and touch function in essentially the same way. They provide in-

formation that permits a person to either respond to or simply be aware of an object.

Our environment is, in a very real sense, a language containing messages that constantly convey information to us. These messages are decoded by intact senses. The older person has a serious problem because his sensory channels are no longer functioning at full capacity and not all of the information registers. He may be receiving only partial messages or, in some cases, distorted ones. Depending on the seriousness of the situation, this can lead to disorientation or hallucinations.[4] If environmental information is to be meaningful, it must travel the complete circuit: the energy input of sensory stimulation, the feedback route of interpretation, collation, and organization, and the energy output represented by behavioral manifestations.[5]

Percept is established by input. What is done with it is determined by experience and culture. Interference anywhere in the circuit means an alteration in the quality of the information as it is perceived by the individual. The source of alteration in the kinds of information received may be located in one or more of a number of sites. There may be a break in the afferent part of the circuit through interference of neuronal pathways by tumors or hemorrhage, or through interference of metabolic pathways by development of heart block or the use of drugs. The effector part of the circuit may be interfered with by disease processes such as arthritic joints or bone changes. Whatever the cause or wherever the site, there is a decrease in available information for the aging individual and he must substitute for this deficit through other sources.

How well he copes with these alterations determines his level of adaptation—the change whereby he retains his integrity within the realities of his environment. Change is stimulating.[2] In fact, a controlled amount of change is essential for individual well-being.[7] Studies of isolation have demonstrated that if exploration of the world around the isolate does not contain change, the individual provides his own stimulation by hallucinatory experiences to maintain his identity as an individual.[8, 9]

The perceptual systems

Gibson states that we must view the external senses ". . . in a new way, as active rather than passive, as systems rather than channels, and as interrelated rather than mutually exclusive."[2] He proposes five perceptual systems. The *basic orienting system*, with receptors in the cochlear and vestibular portions of the inner ear, responds to the forces of gravity and acceleration and stabilizes the individual in relation to gravity and body position. The *auditory system* functions by detection of sound as well as orientation to the direction of the source. The *haptic system* responds to touch and information received by skin surfaces, body orifices, as well as the joints and their associated muscles and tendons. It enables the individual to explore his environment, including his stability on the surface he walks on and the shape of objects around him. The *taste-smell system* provides information essential for adequate nourishment by recognition of acceptable foods. The *visual system* permits him to look, to scrutinize, and to be vigilant. These systems are interdependent in obtaining environmental information. "The two-eyes-with-head-and-body system, in cooperation with postural equilibrium and locomotion, can get around in the world and look at everything."[2]

The world has meaning only as we experience it, and these experiences are mediated through the tissues of our bodies as we interact with our environment. Whitehead wrote, ". . . our only exact data as to the physical world are our sensible perceptions . . . . The physical world is, in some general sense of the term, a deduced concept. Our problem is, in fact, to fit the world to our perceptions and not our perceptions to the world."[3]

The haptic system and its component parts

The haptic system permits an individual to obtain information about his environment and his body. "He feels an object relative to his body and the body relative to an object."[2] Unlike the other perceptual systems, the haptic system includes the whole body, most of its parts, and all of its surface. The two main parts are the skin and the mobile body. The cutaneous appendages are receptive units that protrude into the environment and are capable of feeling things at a distance. A man using a cane as an extension of his arm can detect mechanical variations in his environment. This is felt at the end of the cane but the hand, acting as a perceptual organ, obtains the information, including the length and direction of the extension of the appendage.

Body members are built around a bony skeleton in an organized pattern of joints and articulations so that the movement of any bone is relative to the next bone inward. In this way a person sitting may feel the shape of the wheelchair as well as the shape of his body in the wheelchair. Likewise, the upright posture is maintained by an organized arrangement of head to trunk, trunk to thigh, etc., all cofunctioning with the inner ear orientation to gravity. In this way the body members are oriented to the frame of the body as well as oriented to space.[2] The individual who has suffered a cerebrovascular accident loses this capacity of basic orientation on the side affected and must periodically look to that side to determine the presence and location of the affected member.[10] In many respects the haptic system parallels vision. "Animals with little vision depend on a sort of primitive haptic system for their orientation to the adjacent environment, the muscles and skin cooperating with gravity detection to yield whatever they have in the way of space perception."[2]

The eye scans the environment by looking at parts of an array in succession. In like manner tactile scanning is accomplished by successive exploratory movements of the hands. Information from the environment is obtained by these samples of external stimulation and is useful for purposes of detecting the layout, detecting changes, and detecting and controlling locomotion. The feeling of an object by the hand involves the feeling of position of the fingers, hand, arm, body, and even the head in relation to gravity . . . "all being integrated in some hierarchy of positional information."[12] When vision and touch are considered as channels for information, they seem to register the same kind of information. The simultaneous input of many stimuli permits the substitution of information when that which is being received via one system is inadequate for secure functioning and a sense of well-being. Most individuals have experienced this upon entering a dark room. If the area is familiar, a mere scanning touch of articles, furniture, or wall immediately orients the person so that he is able to navigate safely due to previous experience and knowledge. If the area is an unfamiliar one or if the furniture has been rearranged, ambulation is accomplished with difficulty, more slowly and cautiously, and with increased stress.

The skin, as part of the haptic system, is an information-gathering device that is highly sensitive to radiated heat. Hall cites the blind as a good source of data on this sensitivity, although they are not aware of it in a technical sense until alerted to it. He emphasizes the importance of windows to the blind for purposes of nonvisual navigation. Windows provide currents of air and variations in temperature, thereby transmitting information that orients the blind to their location in a

room as well as helping them to maintain contact with the out-of-doors. An incident is cited in which the blind passing along the streets reaffirmed their location by means of a high brick wall located on the north side of the street at a specific corner. The brick wall had absorbed the rays of the sun and consequently radiated heat over the total sidewalk. This subtle change in temperature aided navigation.[13]

Eric Hodgins had suffered a cerebrovascular accident and although he had recovered the motor use of his left side, the proprioceptive sense was absent. He suggests that the skin has a definite assistive function which extends beyond the body. As he walked along the street with a lady companion he sensed her presence on his right side, but if she switched to his left side this sense of her presence was absent. It may be that a slight touching of clothing or a radiation of body heat below the level of conscious perception keeps the senses reassured.[10] The lack of perception of this environmental information on the affected side requires visual documentation. Likewise, decrease in visual acuity requires increased use of this thermal perception of space.

"Man's sense of space is closely related to his sense of self, which is an intimate transaction with his environment."[13] The criteria for distance are established by the type and reception of stimuli, but what will be done once they are received is determined by cultural and past experiences. These behaviors are subject to much variation, but are fairly well established in the older person. His daily life is established around the patterning within his space, which supports his integrity within the familiar framework. Aging is accompanied by a loss of tissue and functioning reserve. Fewer stimuli are perceived and frequently partial stimuli transmit inadequate messages leading to misinterpretation.

The apparent stubbornness of resistance to change in the older individual may be caused by a confrontation of a new environment that demands a change in lifestyle and by his inability to assess the situation as thoroughly and as readily as he once might have done. "Any paucity of input, any failure of integration which alters the effective feedback, and any limitation which threatens the behavioral output results in a crisis of identity which may be accompanied by profound physiological and emotional components."[5] Only after sufficient information has been gathered does he feel safe and secure.

A decrease in the information that comes through the precise sources of sight or sound requires the individual to depend on less precise sources for information. The haptic system is the most diffuse and the most primitive. Infants depend almost entirely for information on this source. The aging person utilizes it increasingly as a gradual reduction in other sources occurs. Eric Hodgins, after his cerebrovascular accident, elaborated on the assistive function of the skin in normal daily activities. "Not by hands alone does a man remove his clothing: his skin, if it feels, assists."[10] Removal of his right sock with his affected left hand posed no problem, but removal with his unaffected right hand required tugging of his left sock, which seemed to cling to his foot as if it were glued there.[10]

Adaptation becomes more difficult and longer to accomplish. Familiar space with familiar objects and familiar arrangements of these objects support the maintenance of adaptability and promote optimal functioning for the individual. Institutions for the aged often have strict rules regarding the number and placement of personal possessions that the person may bring with him. These rules increase the problem of adaptation, depriving the individual of sentimental ties with the past as well as the familiar landmarks of a familiar environment that serve the purpose of substitution for the familiarity of his previous space.

Some biological, social, and environmental aspects related to aging

Progressive loss of functional capacity in the aging interferes in his interaction with the environment. Balance and gait are affected by pathological conditions in nerve tissue such as vascular defects or senile parkinsonism. The world is circumscribed by impairment of the special senses. Macular degeneration, cataracts, and other ocular diseases of primary origin or secondary to systemic conditions decrease visual acuity so that other sources must be substituted for obtaining information in the environment. Bone changes and cartilage aging affect the posture, ambulation, and alignment of the entire skeletal structure. Loss of joint integrity due to osteoarthritis as well as impairments in posture decrease amount, ease, and sureness of mobility and increase discomfort of the aging individual. In addition, vascular degeneration causing arteriosclerosis or hypertension results in syndromes affecting brain, kidney, heart, and peripheral tissues.[1]

"Changes are greater in complex performances than in simple isolated systems."[1] Simple reaction times are increased in the old when compared to the young, but the effects are greatest in complex reaction times involving the higher centers of the nervous system.[1] Aging is accompanied by a slowing of perceptual and response processes. It takes longer for each item to be registered and it takes longer for the response to occur. As a result, there is less information to be processed and a decrease in the amount of output. Constant interaction with the environment requires attention to many aspects of the environment simultaneously, and adaptation occurs as they relate to past experience or anticipated future events. The intensiveness of an individual's behavior in time and space is an important determinant in the aging process. The habit pattern and information that he possesses may be antiquated and less effective and result in a slowing of the handling of both incoming data and the response.[1] Caution and studied deliberateness of action are evidence of this impairment and represent an effort to obtain sufficient information to function safely within the situation.

Aging also affects sleep patterns. Sleep is generally considered to be basically a physiological regenerative process, but in a real sense we sleep because we like to sleep. An individual living in a hypodynamic environment could conceivably find sleep less rewarding and might alter his sleeping pattern to the lowest level necessary for regenerative purposes. In a hypodynamic environment in association with reduced physiological activity, normal sleep becomes unnecessary.[13] It is not uncommon for elderly persons to vehemently defend the declaration that they did not sleep all night, despite the fact that snores issued from their room. Likewise, observations from the corridor in midmorning demonstrate motionless, apparently dozing persons who can be readily aroused from their light withdrawal from contact. "Findings indicate that . . . sleep and wakefulness . . . [are] regulated largely by environmental factors. Variations in sensory input appear to be the main factor governing normal rhythmic processes. . . ."[13]

Although the amount of personal touching is determined in part by cultural factors, there is, in the elderly, an increased use of this mode of communication and receiving of information. Just as children use touch as a dominant means of communication, so the elderly resort to touch to substitute for incomplete messages received through failing sensory channels. Diminished sensory capacities also alter the distances at which the elderly must interact to maintain an adequate level of incoming messages. Thus social distance, as described by Hall,[13] may need to be within the limits of personal distance or intimate distance for the aging person. Separation from normal environmental stimuli of family and friends and a lack of knowledge

of activities of significant others also increases the feeling of isolation and further deprives the aged of rewarding stimuli.

Environments

New residents of institutions for the aging experience a threat to their integrity similar to that experienced by scientists involved in studies of isolation and confinement. "Byrd, Bombard, Slocum and others found that the greatest threat to their survival was not the hazard of their particular environs, but their aloneness and the monotony of their surroundings."[14] Removal of individuals from their accustomed environment results in a form of isolation that can be viewed as representing some degree of sensory deprivation or sensory paucity. They may be subjected to any of a number of conditions. Burns and associates[14] specify four such categories of sensory deprivation: (1) single modality in which one sensory channel is blocked as a result of increasing age, (2) multimodality deprivation by means of decrease in visual, auditory, touch, or physical contact, (3) absence or decrease of input patterning that is of great importance to adaptive behavior, and (4) separation from normal environmental stimuli. Categories 1 and 2 have been discussed earlier, but 3 and 4 require further elaboration.

Normally the environment provides stimulus variability and density. These form a baseline for adaptation either by nonspecific arousing properties via the brainstem or by evoking and guiding certain behavior. In the absence of variation of stimuli, long lapses of attention have been demonstrated. Under monotonous conditions, radar observers failed to respond when changes occurred on the radar screen. Isolation studies conducted at McGill University demonstrated that subjects were unable to concentrate on any topic for a long while and consequently resorted to daydreaming and letting their minds wander, abandoning all attempts at organized thinking.[14]

There is an increasing tendency to decrease the number and variability of stimuli in the environment of the elderly thereby further depriving the aged person of picking up environmental information. Carpeted floors, acoustic ceilings, air conditioners, and noiseless carts eliminate background information necessary for assessment of threat or safety. Subdued lighting, long empty corridors, and impersonal arrangement of furniture increase the monotony of the environment and deprive the individual of adequate cues as well as nonspecific input on which the cortex depends for normal functioning. Limiting the stimuli in the environment, therefore, reduces the number of primary responses as well as associative responses that are indirectly initiated by the stimulus. Over the passage of time "the organism now attends to certain less well-defined aspects of the particular stimulus (such as shadows . . .) and reads into the environment other stimuli that physically do not exist."[14]

Use of the haptic system

In the process of aging there is a normal attrition in the number of cells. The special senses and aptitudes become impaired and no longer function in an optimal way. Even in the well-aged person, failing vision represents increasing difficulty in receiving information, but these changes occur slowly so that the individual adapts to them gradually and reaches adequate function in his familiar environment. As long as he remains alert and involved with life, the individual must constantly seek the information that orients him so that a failure in one perceptual system creates increased activity in another system, as substitute, to obtain vital information. DeLong[4] suggests that the older person relies on quite different sensory information in dealing with his environment. Our culture is a highly visual one, and as visual acuity decreases, the older person gathers a considerable amount of information through the modality of touch.

DeLong[4] has emphasized the fact that the aging individual is greatly dependent on touch for obtaining information. With decreasing visual acuity along with further haptic loss through osteoarthritic changes in the joints, the older person "feels" his way through his environment to obtain sufficient information for assurance of safety and well-being. DeLong ascribes the older person's tendency to prefer crowded rooms and cluttering artifacts to the need to use the haptic system to substitute for a failing visual system in order to read the language of the environment. The relationship of the objects one to another, their arrangement, is of great importance. DeLong also suggests the need for increasing the amount of information available by cluttering the environment with irregularly placed objects. If the room looks about right to you, add more furniture. In this way the older person will be near something he can lay his hands on at all times to use as landmarks for points of reference.

The gaining of information from the environment by using the haptic system is the first, most diffuse and least differentiated method, and is characteristic of the way an infant explores his environment. As the infant becomes older he becomes more visually oriented. Our society is visually oriented and as people grow older and begin to lose the acuity of information coming to them via these systems, they begin to substitute via the haptic system.

There is a substitution of haptic information to maintain equilibrium when basic information is deficient. The following behaviors evidence this fact:

1. Skimming of articles of furniture or corridor walls by elderly people to orient themselves in an upright position. Tactile information from articles allow them to remain upright because it gives another dimension of information.

2. The use of a cane is an extension of haptic information.

3. The walker is similar in principle

to the cane; it provides a more diffuse source of information through the four legs and crossbar.

4. The shuffling gait of the individual represents an effort to increase environmental information through increased length of contact with the floor surface when sufficient detail is lost to him due to an inadequately functioning visual system.

5. A light touch on the arm of a companion increases information and aids in ambulation through barren spaces.

Substitution of haptic information when the acuity of the visual system is decreased may be effected by the following modes:

1. Organizing the furniture in the room and maintaining this plan enables them to move through the room without bumping into furniture.

2. A cluttered room provides information readily available and is both direction and reality orienting.

3. Organizing the artifacts of the environment so that they are within reach or easily found increases environmental information.

There is need for increased human contact as a means of communication and gathering of information.

1. Holding hands or sitting within touching distance of those for whom they care aids in transfer of information.

2. Kissing is basically a haptic sensation and conveys a need for physical sensation of acceptance. It is a means of establishing contact.

Observations on the use of the haptic system

To obtain data on the use of the haptic system, the author visited several homes providing care for a high population of nonsenile, well-aged persons. The author assumed the role of a detached observer in the corridors, sitting room, dining area, and personal rooms of ambulatory and mobile elderly residents. The author's purpose was to observe for evidence of the use of the haptic system as a substitute information-gathering system when other systems did not provide adequate environmental information.

Those behaviors that occurred repeatedly are discussed in this chapter. Additional isolated behaviors that could be attributed to haptic use as a substitute were noted, but because of their infrequent occurrence during observation periods they are not recorded.

Musculoskeletal adaptation to maintain equilibrium was frequently noted. Some stiffening of the knees and ankle joints along with limitation in cervical range of motion results in a characteristic posture of body and head bent slightly forward. An accompanying shuffling gait prolongs contact with the walking surface and represents the need to increase information via the haptic system. The variations in texture between tile, wood, and carpeting convey information in a familiar environment relative to space use—sitting, dining, or public hallway areas. A lack of sureness in ambulating is compensated for by the shuffling gait in relation to both maintenance of balance and also in mobilization. The surface underfoot varies in level and angle. A gentle slope or ramp, the edge of a step or doorsill, and a solid, soft, smooth, or lumpy surface all convey information via the feet as part of the haptic system to assist in making judgments that promote safe ambulation through the environment.

Various extensions of the haptic system in the form of canes, walkers, and wheelchairs were commonly used. As previously discussed the probing end of a cane detects information that is received and transmitted through the hand and eventuates in a behavior based on judgment. The angle of the surface, the distance, and the texture and consistency all are detected by the cane and are added to other information to assist in the behavior desired. The four-legged walker is often carried and touched down briefly and lightly to either reinforce or add to insufficient information coming from other sources. Some lean heavily on the apparatus for support when an obvious impairment is present. Progress is, therefore, slower, and longer contact aids perception of informational messages. Wheelchairs were used in a variety of ways. One gentleman wheeled his wife up and down the corridors, pausing at the glass door each time for an appreciative observation of the lawns and woods outside. His posture and gait were typical of that previously described when he walked alone in the hallway, but when he pushed the wheelchair he had an added dimension of information that increased his sureness and speed. Besides information relative to the surface over which they traveled, there was an added message of movement. This sensation would be quite different to him than it was to his wife who was riding. The smoothness of a modern wheelchair eliminates many of the sensations in the environment and adds to stress and anxiety until the experience becomes a familiar one and it is possible to anticipate or predict the course of events. Some residents wheeled themselves. Information that is received by the feet in walking is absent, and there is a resultant greater dependency on vision. A normal attrition of the older person's vision makes self-propelled movement more hazardous and until the environment becomes familiar, he will move slowly and cautiously.

Grab rails in halls, toilet areas, and bathrooms are considered a means of support to prevent falling. In observing their use, I consider them also a motivation to mobilization. The user often merely skims his hand along the rail as he goes for a walk. Sometimes the walk is for the purpose of exercise, and sometimes it is for the purpose of socialization. A light touch orients him in relation to gravity, the sensation of the wall indicates a protective barrier from unexpected dangers, and he is guided toward his destination of living

room or dining room or whatever the case may be, away from the mainstream of personnel traffic in the center of the corridor. Grab rails aid in independence and a sense of self-determination.

A variety of wall textures also provided additional information through haptic use. Painted walls in personal areas, wooden doors and window frames, and embossed covering in hallways all gave information as to the location or the direction in which the resident was going. He had no problems in zeroing in on a light switch or doorknob because the information was obtained within a familiar setting, and he could anticipate the locations due to past experiences.

Institutions for the aging seriously restrict the number of personal belongings that an individual is permitted to bring with him. These objects not only represent sentimental ties to the past but are familiar landmarks of a familiar environment. The few that are permitted are arranged in a specific way and if a visitor picks them up, they must be replaced in exactly the same place and manner in order that they can be located with a minimum amount of vision or movement. The clock, magazines, drinking water, books, and chairs— all artifacts in the environment—have a specific arrangement that conveys information of safety and security.

In one of the homes visited the lounge area was adjacent to the dining area. They were separated by arrangement of the furniture and texture of floor covering. There were two approaches to the lounge area— one was located directly off the main corridor and the other was through the dining area. In coming to the lounge the majority of residents came through the dining area where the clutter of tables and chairs provided information immediately at hand as they skimmed the surfaces lightly in the course of their walk. An additional factor to be considered here is one of distance. The cluttered environment with chairs readily available decreases the sense of distance in comparison to a long empty corridor. A similar sensation is experienced if one stands with arms extended in front of him, having one arm facing a long corridor and one facing a wall. The arm extended toward the corridor is perceived as longer than the other.

The type of chair that was preferred by the majority of residents is also significant. Chairs having a high back, arms, a seat low enough to permit feet to be firmly planted on the floor yet high enough to prevent sitting on the sacrum, and minimal firm padding were observed to be preferred. The shape of these chairs is felt relative to the body and the moulding of the body is felt relative to the chair and both are perceived in relation to gravity. A soft, overstuffed chair decreases the number of environmental messages available and adds to the deficit of information perceived by the aging individual. A low, tilted chair holds the occupant captive and increases dependency and insecurity. Many also chose a straight type of chair located at a table, which permits them to lean lightly on the table. The table provided an added dimension of information and orientation relative to position.

The need for increased human contact was obvious. Residents strolled down the corridors holding hands. Visitors had their hands grasped and clung to, communicating unspoken messages of appreciation, affection, and intense need. Conversation with family and friends often lagged, but a companionable silence prevailed as they held hands or sat closely together. Nonverbal communication was obvious to the detached observer. Spacing of individuals in the groups was arranged so that they could easily reach out and touch each other as they conversed. Although children were sometimes reticent about kissing the one being visited, they submitted on the urging of their parents and to the obvious delight of the older person. Af-

fection and acceptance are conveyed via the haptic system, and the information that people care is a message all humans need regardless of their age.

If aging inhibits adaptation due to a loss of tissue and functional reserve, those concerned with the overall well-being of the elderly should combat the influences that interfere with adaptation and support those that tend to maintain it as closely as possible to the optimal level. This study concluded that the aging individual uses the haptic system as a substitute for information-gathering when other systems do not provide sufficient information for safe and secure function. The environment of the older person needs to be an environment of touch, in which the messages available convey a meaningful language in the interaction taking place.

Promoting adaptation through use of the haptic system

A thorough orientation to a new environment decreases the time needed for adaptation. Changes in textures of the floor and walls speak definitely to the shuffling gait and the scanning hand. These should be identified and tested personally under the guidance of the one doing the orienting. Furniture should be spaced irregularly and closely so that a searching hand may have the reassurance necessary at all times.

There should be space enough for the individual to move among his personal belongings. We should arrange them as he desires and not impose our own idea of orderliness. Artifacts should be put back the same way so that he has ready access to them without having to go through a process of searching. Past experience will lead to anticipation and predictability and will promote a sense of security and well-being.

Socialization and mobilization should be encouraged; each can influence the other. Grab rails, canes, and walkers should be considered as motivation to socialization. These are the means whereby the older person seeks out variety from his environment, increases the amount of information perceived, and interacts in a social way. Personal and social integrity are maintained through interaction and a measure of independence. Long corridors frighten those who ambulate with difficulty. There has to be a good reason for walking the endless course before it is attempted. Breaking the distance with chairs and little tables or benches spaced at intervals reduces the sense of distance and encourages more frequent efforts at walking. The individuals who are dependent on wheelchairs for mobilization should be placed within the mainstream of activity. They should not be placed facing an empty, dead-end corridor, but in the corridor where they can watch their world interacting and participate in this interaction themselves. People passing by can smile, touch, or converse, all adding a dimension to the information obtained by the one confined to the chair.

Wheelchairs and stretchers should be used thoughtfully. Because the rider is not receiving information usually obtained through the feet, a sense of rapid movement is added. The ability to handle multiple stimuli simultaneously is greatly reduced in the older person. The rapid passage of walls and ceiling, apparent near collisions, and sense of movement are frightening. Wheeling the elderly backward is absolutely terrifying!

The amount of assistance that is required by the hesitant aging person should be carefully evaluated. More assistance than necessary increases dependency and results in some social deprivation. An observation noted was that a light touch on the arm or shoulder by the one being assisted may be adequate for safe, secure ambulation. One individual perferred to merely hold onto the uniform button of the nurse. This extra dimension of information was all that was necessary to orient her in an upright, mobile position.

The diminished sensory capacities of the older person alter the distance at which he must interact to obtain the messages from his environment. Nurses should become aware of this so that they will increase the amount of touching while administering care. Many of the activities in which the nurse engages with her patient require her to interact within a close range. This frequently makes her feel uncomfortable and results in behavior that may be interpreted by the patient as rejection. Normal social distance to her is perceived as public distance by the aging individual and connotes lack of involvement. The nurse must move into the personal zone for social interaction to maintain the intensity of the messages and prevent distortion or inadequately transmitted messages.

There are many additional ways of increasing the amount of information the older person receives from his environment—color, lighting, odor, and sound—all enrich his world and provide stimuli that add quality to his extended years. Nurses must become aware of the necessity for providing these stimuli as they care for the aging individual who has a decreasing acuity of the information-gathering system.

As I visited elderly persons in nursing homes and as I observed the long-term elderly person in hospital wards, I had been developing the uneasy feeling that we, as nurses, were neglecting some vital aspect in caring for the aging individual. In this neglect, we were contributing to the early senility so prevalent in our society today. Institutionalization and subsequent disorientation or withdrawal from reality appeared to be an accepted sequence of events and were shrugged off as seemingly natural by a large majority of people.

During my course of reading for this

study, I became sharply aware of specific ways in which the nurse can increase the intensity and completeness of the messages in the older person's environment. The potential for giving meaning and enjoyment is exciting and challenging, and the effort invested would be rewarding. We, as nurses, need to sharpen our awareness of the decreasing abilities for information gathering in those for whom we care so that we may support all those influences which tend to maintain adaptability as closely as possible to the optimum. This concept is also applicable to the younger patient who has interference due to a disease process or surgical procedure. The nurse must sharpen her awareness so that her plan of care will be based on meaningful observations.

In conclusion it can be stated that the use of the haptic system enables the elderly to orient themselves to reality, and being reality-oriented decreases the likelihood of confusion and disorientation. Nurses need to be knowledgeable about the haptic system and foster its use in elderly persons. Thus nurses can promote successful adaptation to the aging process and unfamiliar environments.

References

1. Shock, Nathan W., editor: Aging: some social and biological aspects, Washington, D. C., 1960, The American Association for the Advancement of Science.
2. Gibson, James J.: The senses considered as perceptual systems, Boston, 1966, Houghton Mifflin Co.
3. Whitehead, Alfred North: The aims of education and other essays, New York, 1959, The Macmillan Co.
4. DeLong, Alton J.: An outline of environmental language of the older person, unpublished paper presented at the Sixth Annual Meeting and Conference of the American Association of Homes for the Aging, Oct., 1967.
5. Levine, Myra E.: Proxemics and patient cure, unpublished paper presented at the Annual Meeting of the National Conference of Jewish Communal Service, Detroit, Mich., June 9, 1968.
6. Koch, Sigmund, editor: Psychology: a study of science, vol. 1, New York, 1959, McGraw-Hill Book Co., Inc.
7. Gibson, J. J.: The useful dimensions of sensitivity, Amer. Psychol. 18:1-15, 1963.
8. Solomon, Philip, et al., editors: Sensory deprivation, Cambridge, Mass., 1961, Harvard University Press.
9. Linton, Patrick H.: Sensory deprivation in hospitalized patients, Alabama J. Med. Sci. 2:256-258, 1965.
10. Hodgins, Eric: Episode, New York, 1964, Atheneum Publishers.
11. Harris, Charles S.: Adaptation to displaced vision: visual, motor or proprioceptive change? Science 40:812-813, 1963.
12. Gibson, J. J.: Observations on active touch, Psychol. Rev., 69:477-491, 1962.
13. Hall, Edward T.: The hidden dimension, Garden City, N. Y., 1966, Doubleday & Co., Inc.
14. Burns, Neal M., Chambers, Randall M., and Hendler, Edwin, editors: Unusual environments and human behavior, New York, 1963, The Free Press of Glencoe, Inc.

Chapter 27

The nurse—the patient—and touch

Shirley Farrah

Touch is an all-pervasive phenomenon in nursing. Early educational experiences of nursing students involve patient situations requiring touch. Nurses employed in medical and surgical-clinical areas repeatedly use the touch gesture as they administer direct physical care to the hospitalized patient. For example, the nurse comes into direct physical contact with a patient while giving a backrub, inserting various catheters, and administering parenteral medications. In each of these nursing interventions touch is dominant. When administering this type of patient care, touch becomes a routine part of the nursing procedures.

On the other hand, medical-surgical nurses have been observed by the author to use touch less frequently in situations involving other than direct physical care; for example, supportive touch to convey concern and understanding to a frightened or lonely patient. In addition to physical contact, this form includes another dimension—nonverbal communication. At times there seems to be almost complete interdiction of this form of touch between nurse and patient.

For this chapter communication includes all modes of behavior an individual employes to affect another—not only verbal behavior, as written or spoken words, but also nonverbal communication as facial expressions, posture, body movements, and gestures such as touch.[1] Verbal communication is difficult, if not impossible, in the absence of nonverbal behavior; the latter adds meaning to what is said. Thus a verbal response might become more meaningful if accompanied by a touch gesture. However, if verbal and nonverbal communication are incongruent, communication moves into a position of conflict.[2] For example, gently touching the patient on the shoulder while speaking in a harsh angry voice might make him question the nurse's true feelings.

Communication is a highly personal process taking place each time the nurse interacts with the patient; it occurs in nurse-patient verbalizations as well as in periods of silence. Communication occurs between the nurse and patient whether or not they are aware it is happening. Thus social interaction and social influence between nurse and patient depend on communication. It is the medium through which the nurse builds her relationship with the patient.

Touch is operationally defined for this

chapter as a gesture involving physical contact of the nurse's hand with the head, shoulder, arm, or hand of the patient. It is a form of nonverbal communication used in nursing interventions to convey caring and concern from the nurse to patient. Critchley[3] mentions a group of gestures, including touch, that have universal meaning; he states they form a "silent lingua franca," meaningful to all regardless of age, race, religion, mentality, or socio-cultural background. Touch must convey a message from one person to another if it is to be considered a form of communication. Touch is a primitive mode of communication among humans and frequently has meaning for an individual when no other form of communication does.[4] Both tactile and emotional elements are recognized in the symbolic expressions "I am touched" or "I feel."[5]

Literature review

Since the nurse performs a major portion of her functions through touch and since nursing has long been considered a service involving the "laying on of hands,"[2] it is surprising that a review of nursing literature disclosed a paucity of information concerning the use of touch as a particular form of nonverbal communication. No research directly related to the use of touch was reported in medical-surgical nursing literature from 1952 to 1970. Only three investigations pertaining to touch were found in nursing literature—two in journals of psychiatric nursing and the third in a psychiatric nursing textbook.

In psychiatric nursing literature Cashar and Dixson[6] say, "It seems that much emphasis is placed on verbal communication, but the nonverbal is seldom considered. This is unfortunate, since nonverbal communication is generally more accurate in reflecting emotions. . . ." They further report that nurses are most often not aware of their own feelings relevant to touching patients and being touched unless it is brought to their attention.[6]

In an extensive study concerning medical-surgical nurses' response to a need for the relief of pain, it was found that nurses used touch infrequently as a specific action to relieve pain. Although touch was not the major focus of the study, it was reported that the nurse was more likely to use a verbal or silent response than touch in patient situations involving pain.[7]

In a before-after exploratory study of ten adult female medical patients, it was found that deliberative nursing interventions involving touch can be effectively used to significantly alleviate and, at times, completely eliminate the pain experience.[8] This occurred regardless of the personal characteristics of the patient or the location, duration, nature, or intensity of pain. Supportive touch seems to be a specific need for a patient experiencing pain; and he often initiates the gesture. It is effective for conveying concern and alleviating anxiety as well as for relaxing tense muscles. There appears to be a relationship between increased relaxation, decreased anxiety, and decreased pain.

Analysis of general nursing and psychiatric textbooks reveals touch is mentioned merely as a means of nonverbal communication. Most often the authors state only whether touch should or should not be used in patient care. Statements relative to touch tend to reflect personal opinions and subjective experiences of the authors. Use of physical contact has also received little attention in general psychiatric literature. The most sophisticated research has been conducted on subhuman species and reports on man are mostly incidental findings not derived from systematic studies.

Before proceeding with analysis of nursing literature relevant to touch, a brief discussion of one's need for human contact is presented in an effort to emphasize the importance of touch to nursing.

Need for human contact

The young infant has a need for tactile experiences that constitute the "very beginning of purely human or interpersonal needs."[9] The need for physical contact is "innate and consistent from the time the human leaves the womb and is physically separated from his mother."[10]

The need for human contact, although normally not as active in the adult as the infant, can become more intense in stressful situations.[11] It thus seems the hospitalized patient might have an even greater need for tactual communication. The need to touch is greater than the need to verbalize, particularly for geriatric or regressed schizophrenic patients who have been hospitalized for long periods.[12] These patients want physical contact to reassure themselves of their continuity and existence.

Data concerning the need or wish to be held or cuddled from fifty-four female adults—twenty-seven paid volunteers and twenty-seven psychiatric patients—revealed no significant difference in responses of the two groups. The majority of subjects indicated a marked or moderate desire to be touched.[13] Perhaps, then, the seemingly well-adjusted, mature patient might need tactual experiences as does the anxious, depressed, and schizophrenic patient.

Tactile experiences in personality development and contact deprivation

Tactual sensitivity appears even before birth as probably the first sensory process to become functional. During gestation the fetus receives continuous tactile stimulation from the maternal heart beat as it is transmitted and amplified through the surrounding amniotic fluid. Thus even the infant becomes accustomed to tactile experiences in a rhythmically pulsating environment.[5]

During birth the fetus is subjected to intense tactual stimulation as he emerges from the birth canal into an environment with a different pressure, temperature, and surrounding medium. Shortly after birth the newborn infant is again subjected to touch as he is handled, fed, and bathed.

The infant's need for physical contact may be largely derived from these antepartal experiences that exercise his tactuality.[5]

For the newborn infant, incoming sensory stimuli are mediated almost exclusively by the skin.[14] The child feels mother's touch before he sees her. He experiences touch as a behavior communicating comfort, warmth, security, and love.[2] He begins to know mother through her touch by the way she suckles and caresses him. Through these experiences the infant communicates with mother in a reciprocal way, each evoking responses from the other. The infant elicits from mother the close bodily contact he needs and responds by sucking. Mother, in turn, responds to this lip to breast contact with lactation.[5] Although nourishment comes from the breast, the contact manipulations the child has with the breast are as psychologically important as the nourishment itself.[12] These bodily contacts establish the infant's early patterns of love, trust, and confidence, which forms the basis for his first interpersonal relationships.[5]

Studies concerning development of marasmus indicate direct skin contact after birth is absolutely essential for survival. Spitz's classic study[15] concerns a contrast between a group of children raised in a foundling home and a second group raised in a prison by their own mothers. The latter group did well despite the unfavorable environment. The orphanage babies, although well cared for, were seldom touched. They became anxious, cried easily, slept and ate poorly, lost weight, did not manifest normal exploratory behavior, and were quite susceptible to infections; withdrawal and regression to earlier patterns of behavior occurred.

Prolonged maternal deprivation where there is an extreme diminution of rewarding tactual stimulation may have lasting serious impact on the infant's character. For example, a study of the call girl revealed the girls discovered at an early age they could satisfy feelings of loneliness and needs for affection through sexual gratification. Physical contact was one way of obtaining the closeness denied them by their parents. Perhaps many of today's personality disorders are due to deprivation of essential tactual experiences.[5]

Touch is regarded by some as the earliest means of reality contact for the infant.[16] The infant first learns about and relates to objects in the outside world as he explores with his hands and lips. He orients himself to the spatial dimensions of the world as he tests size, shape, texture, and density of whatever he touches.[5] Touch is the "only sense of immediate outer perception, hence also the most important and the one that informs with greatest certitude."[17] This is exemplified when an adult touches an object to make sure it is really there.

Thus the infant's perception of the world is determined by his initial tactile experiences, and these experiences have a significant influence on personality development as the child forms his first object relations.[5] If denied the opportunity to learn and test his environment through touch, the child must presumably wait until vision and audition develop sufficiently for him to enter into communication with others. He will have limited tactile experiences on which to develop more mature symbolic communication. Moreover, he must arbitrarily accept prescribed meanings of visual and auditory symbols rather than validating them independently through touch. The child's future learning, speech, cognition, and symbolic recognition are hindered if he is deprived of tactual experiences.[5]

Touch in patient care

Nursing literature is in accord with literature of related disciplines that there are three schools of thought concerning the use of touch in patient care.[18] Proponents of one school of thought strongly advocate the use of touch. Supporters of the second school strongly oppose the use of touch, whereas those of the third school state touch may be valuable when the nurse is aware of the patient's dynamics and his interpretations of touch, that is, cognizant use of touch.

Strongly advocate use of touch

One group of authors in nursing and related disciplines strongly advocate the use of touch as a communication tool. One writer cites an example from her nursing experience when she used touch in tying a patient's shoelaces and states there was a subsequent strengthening of the relationship.[19] The schizophrenic girl analyzed by Sechehaye felt secure when she was with her therapist, especially when the therapist put her arm around the patient's shoulders.[37]

Greenhill[21] says physical contact seems to act as a powerful catalyst in communication. He maintains nursing procedures involving touch can strengthen the nurse-patient relationship. Hayes and Gazaway[22] state an important part of nursing care involves touch to provide firm support for the patient needing courage in some effort he must make. McCaffery and Moss[23] say a firm touch may be used to communicate to the patient that dependency is allowed during stressful periods. Lockerby[24] states in *Communication for Nurses:*

> Touch is instinctive. The clasped hand, tightening fingers relieve tension . . . the physical communicates understanding, a desire to help. This language is universal, more meaningful than words.*

In direct opposition to those who strongly sanction touch are those who strongly oppose touch.

Strongly oppose use of touch

Whereas the proponents of touch emphasize the caring, support, and understanding which touch can convey, the op-

---

*From Lockerby, F.: Communication for nurses, ed. 2, St. Louis, 1963, The C. V. Mosby Co.

ponents cite examples involving purely intimate or sexual connotations of physical contact. Authors of one psychiatric nursing textbook show a picture of a female nurse half-embracing a female patient and state, "Intimate relationships with patients are not conducive to a therapeutic atmosphere."[25] Although further explanation of this statement is not presented, the authors seem to equate close physical contact with "intimate relationships." In discussing the management of an aggressive patient, authors of another psychiatric nursing textbook caution, "Women nurses, especially young students, should not touch a male patient, merely walk beside him with a male aid or nurse."[26]

Another source believes the therapist must not respond to the physical contact of a patient but encourage him to verbalize his feelings. He comments, "It goes without saying that physical contact with the patient is absolutely taboo."[27]

However, the majority of literature in nursing and related fields condones cognizant use of touch.

Cognizant use of touch

Psychiatric nursing research. Authors of each of the three nursing research studies concerning the use of touch with psychiatric patients recommend the cognizant use of touch as a means of establishing and maintaining effective communication. One study revealed the use of simple, appropriate touch gestures resulted in increased verbal interaction and rapport between the nurse and patient, as well as positive changes in attitudes of patients toward nurses.[18]

A second investigation indicated the touch gesture carries with it an array of diverse meanings, some of which may be misconstrued by the recipient. It was further found that in any single instance there is an equal chance for touch to be interpreted correctly or incorrectly.[17] However, the largest group of touch gestures were interpreted by both psychiatric personnel and patients as "tender feelings." Hand touches most often indicated tender feelings. In addition, cultural influences, maturation levels, and recent personal experiences affected one's use and interpretation of touch. Those who frequently used touch viewed it as a pleasurable and satisfying experience. It seems, then, that one's perception of being touched may relate to one's comfort in touching others. The touch gesture is, therefore, a powerful technique of nonverbal communication when it is appropriately timed in the appropriate context with the appropriate individual.

The third study reported frequent touch gestures among nurses and adult patients in a psychiatric hospital.[6] Touch often appeared to be used without planning or apparent therapeutic value and staff nurses could not identify their reasons for touching patients.

Patient characteristics and cognizant use of touch. Other authors of psychiatric nursing literature also recommend the use of physical contact only if the initiator is aware of its potentialities and limitations. One source says the nurse can impart reassurance through touch. However, they continue, some touch gestures may be threatening to the psychiatric patient, particularly a patient having homosexual tendencies who avoids any close relationship with members of the same sex.[28]

Authors of another psychiatric nursing textbook likewise contend the nurse must be aware of possible meanings touch has for a patient.[29] Similarly, another psychiatric nursing publication states, "The nurse must determine when closeness is acceptable and when it is not; she must determine how the patient might interpret and respond to it."[30]

Some authors of psychiatric and psychoanalytic publications also condone the cognizant use of touch and state that adhering to the severe tradition of not touching the patient may be due more to the therapist's fears than to those of the patient. Another psychotherapist maintains touch may convey better than words to some patients the therapist's knowledge and appreciation of their emotional conflicts, whereas even the slightest physical contact may be very frightening for other patients.[31]

Fromm-Reichmann,[10] who is known for her genuinely warm relationships with patients, also sees touch as an important communication technique that should be carefully considered before using it with psychiatric patients. Data from Hollender's[13] recent investigation, referred to previously, revealed patients most commonly interpreted touch to mean *security, protection, comfort, contentment, love,* and *affection,* and felt that touch helped overcome feelings of being lonely. Common reactions to frustrated bodily contact wishes included feelings of *tension, "let down," rejection, hurt pride,* and *loneliness.*[13] Hollender further reports there is possibly a correlation between a woman's desire to be touched and her femininity as well as her attitude toward sex. It seems likely the more secure one is in her feminine role, the more comfortable she might be with physical contact. One study revealed that women more accepting of sexuality are more likely to express a desire for touch.[13]

Research concerning medical-surgical nurses' reported cognizant use of touch. Just as one allows for individual differences in the patient's perception of touch, one must also allow for individual differences in the nurse. She too varies in degree of comfort she feels as the initiator and recipient of touch.[2] The nurse may feel that touching the patient indicates she is becoming too involved with him or vulnerable to his demands.[4]

The only study known to the author concerning medical-surgical nurses and touch was an investigation by the writer of forty-nine female registered medical-surgical nurses in which vignettes were used to determine the nurses' reported use of touch in patient situations not involving direct physical care.[32] Touch was reportedly used to a much greater extent than was predicted. The touch gesture was ranked as the third most preferred behavior out of five possible nursing interventions, and when touch was accompanied by a verbal response, it was reported as the most preferred nursing intervention. The three remaining nurse interventions that the subjects could rank order from "most likely to use to least likely" included verbal responses alone (ranked second), silent responses (ranked fourth), and suggested activities not involving touch (ranked fifth).

Subjective responses to a touch questionnaire were likewise favorable toward touch and revealed several themes that added depth and clarification to the study findings. Touch was generally seen as a therapeutic gesture that:

1. Communicates a feeling of "I care"
2. Establishes and maintains openness of communication and development of rapport
3. Transcends oral communication in some patient care situations
4. Promotes contact with reality
5. Should be used more in nurse-patient relationships

Touch was seen by all but one of the forty-nine nurses as a gesture capable of conveying to the patient *security, understanding, sincerity, respect, support, warmth, feeling, concern, caring, reassurance, interest, sympathy, empathy, comfort, kindness, closeness, encouragement, acceptance, willingness to help,* and *willingness to become involved.* In other words, touch communicates to the patient a feeling of "I care."

Although nurses generally described touch favorably, they reported the following limitations in its use with their patients and these limitations may explain why "touch in conjunction with verbal responses," and "verbal responses alone" were rank ordered as more preferable nurse interactions than was "touch alone":

1. Touch may easily be misconstrued
2. Social mores and taboos
3. Individual nurse's comfort as the initiator of touch
4. Individual patient's comfort as the recipient of touch

Nearly one third of the total sample reported the possibility of misinterpretation limited their use of touch or they would use touch only in conjunction with verbal communication. Apparently the chance of misinterpretation was seen by these nurses as being greater with touch than with spoken words. This finding is in contrast to a previous statement by Cashar and Dixson that nonverbal communication generally expresses one's true feelings more accurately than do words.[6]

Over one third of the nurses felt the individual character of the nurse was important and stated the nurse should not use touch unless she feels *natural, comfortable,* or *genuine* in doing so. Some nurses specifically stated their use of touch depended on the individual patient, length and stage of the nurse-patient relationship, and the patient's feelings concerning touch and being touched.

Subjective responses to the touch questionnaire further revealed how age, sex, and medical circumstances influenced the nurse's reported use of touch. Nurses were reportedly more likely to touch older than younger patients, regardless of sex, and more likely to touch female than male patients. Physical contact was reportedly used more frequently with the elderly because "touch helps bridge the communication gap" and "the elderly seem to appreciate this form of nonverbal support and respond to touch—they actually initiate the use of touch by reaching out for the nurse's hand." Some nurses saw touch with the male patient as being too personal or in some way detracting from the male patient's masculinity.

Cultural patterning and cognizant use of touch

The patient variables of age and sex may further be explained by cultural influences on the nurse's reported use of touch. This is based on the assumption that one's behavior is determined by the rules of the particular culture with which he is dealing.

Each culture has specific rules of how, where, and when persons may touch one another. These cultural expectations differ widely from one culture to another. In a study of childrearing practices in American and Finnish cultures, a striking difference was found in the use of touch by parents to demonstrate affection toward their children.[33] The Finnish infant received far less fondling and kissing, but affection was displayed through voice fluctuations and eye glances. In some cultures men are not permitted to touch other men except in greeting, handshakes, or athletic competition. In that same culture, however, women touching one another as an expression of support or joy might be sanctioned.[2] Chinese students commonly hold hands with students of the same sex.[34] One investigator watched pairs of people in coffee shops in San Juan, Paris, and London. The scores, indicating the number of times one person touched the other at one table, were 180, 100, and zero, respectively.[34]

The appropriateness of the touch gesture can be evaluated only in terms of a given situation. Certain kinds of touch are used by the mother figure to communicate restraint. Such behavior might be appropriate with her children but not with her peers. Certain kinds of touch used between husband and wife might not be appropriate between brother and sister.[2] Thus, to use touch cognizantly, the nurse must be familiar with the mores of the particular culture with which she is dealing.

Western culture is governed by many obsessional taboos with regard to people touching one another. Burton and Heller[12] illustrate this taboo when they say, "An infant can be fondled with social approval, but once the infant is grown the taboo asserts itself." Small children are no longer allowed to touch and explore their mother's body and, very often, not the genital areas of their own. The child is repeatedly told, "Don't touch." To touch is not only admonished but loaded with overtones of disgust and fear.[34]

As cultures progress, tactual communications are usually exchanged for more conceptual ones such as language. Burton and Heller[12] contend, "There is, of course, nothing wrong with conceptualizing, but we sometimes forget that a concept, in order to be truly communicative must . . . have an emotional meaning."

Touching the body is often looked on as deviant without necessarily exploring its meaning or purpose.[12] This is particularly true in nursing if the initiator is of the opposite sex and in the same age group as the recipient.[17] Therefore one might expect, as was found in the subjective responses to the touch questionnaire, the young female medical-surgical nurses in this investigation to reportedly use the touch gesture more frequently with an older female patient than with a young male patient. Young female nurses seemingly have an anticipatory fear of their touch being misinterpreted by the patient, particularly the young male patient. It may be that in the author's investigation the crucial factor in avoiding misinterpretation of the touch gesture by the young male patient is not simply whether or not the young female nurse touches him but rather how, where, and when she touches him.

In relation to medical circumstances, nurses were reportedly more likely to touch in situations involving pain, anxiety, rejection, loneliness, fear, and the dying patient. Medical-surgical nurses commonly encounter all these situations. It has previously been stated that supportive touch can be effectively employed to alleviate the pain experience of selected patients and, further, that anxiety is a frequent concomitant of pain.[8] Perhaps nurses see touch with an anxious patient, whether or not he is experiencing physical pain, as conveying, "I am concerned for you and want to help." For a patient experiencing feelings of rejection, such as frequently occurs with patients placed on isolation precautions or with *problem patients*, touch possibly means, "I do care for you," or "I'm not afraid of you and I don't think you're dirty." For the lonely or fearful patient touch may mean, "I am here and want to be with you." For the unconscious and dying patient touch may be used as a means of reality orientation to remind the patient he is still in contact with reality and someone is willing to share the experience with him.

Further evaluation of the subjective portion of the touch questionnaire indicated baccalaureate degree graduates described touch more favorably than did diploma program graduates, and nurses with three or more years of experience described touch more favorably than did the new practitioners. The first of these findings is possibly due to increased emphasis in baccalaureate nursing programs on psychosocial needs of the patient.[35] Second, the person who has been practicing nursing for a number of years often generates an understanding type of warmth and is frequently seen as a mother figure; thus the more experienced graduate nurse might reportedly view touch more positively. The nurse's marital status and number of children did not significantly influence the nurse's subjectively reported use of touch.

The objective portion of the touch questionnaire has been found to be a reliable instrument. Unlike the subjective portion, it indicates that patient variables of age, sex, and medical circumstance as well as nurse characteristics of educational background and length of professional experience do not significantly influence the nurse's reported use of touch. Like the subjective portion, the objective portion reveals personality traits, marital status, and number of children do not significantly affect the nurse's report. Exactly how the interpersonal behavior of the nurse affects her reported use of touch could not be ascertained from this investigation. Perhaps the crucial elements in the nurse's reported use of touch are not the specific variables dealt with in this investigation but, for example, how satisfied the individual is with her job in general and with herself as a nurse. The individual who is comfortable and competent in her role as a woman and as a nurse and who has successfully worked through her own feelings toward touch, might be more likely to employ touch and risk the possibility of misinterpretation, knowing it is potentially an effective means of nonverbal communication. On the other hand, the individual who is more anxious in her role as a nurse may be more fearful of the possible risk of the patient misconstruing her gesture. Her primary goal might be avoidance of difficulty instead of patient comfort. It would seem either the nurse sees touch as an important and effective means of nonverbal communication and feels comfortable using it, and therefore reports its use, or she does not feel it important and thus does not use it.

Summary of literature concerning use of touch

Review of literature pertinent to touch in patient care indicates three viewpoints in relation to touch: (1) those who advocate the use of touch; (2) those who strongly oppose the use of touch; and (3) those who advocate the cognizant use of touch. The latter view stresses touch as a means of establishing and maintaining therapeutic communication if it is used with foresight and knowledge about the patient and with an understanding of the possible interpretations of touch.

Touch is the most important and immediate contact experience with environment. It forms the foundation of language, learning, mental growth, and personality development. Touch is a form of nonverbal communication and a tool for social interaction that makes meaningful and rewarding interpersonal relationships possible.

The need for physical contact is a basic interpersonal need. The infant uses touch almost exclusively as a vehicle for communicating with other persons. Through physical contact with a mother figure, the infant establishes his first interpersonal relationship. Touch is a vital part of man's interaction with others, and satisfying tactile experiences during infancy and childhood have implications for physical survival as well as emotional well-being and self-esteem.

Touch is an integral part of nursing care. It is an interpersonal and therapeutic behavior that has the potential of conveying concern and understanding from nurse to patient. The touch gesture is interpreted in a highly personal manner and has a unique meaning for each individual. How one interprets the touch of another depends on each person's cultural background and personal characteristics and on the nature of the relationship. It is therefore important the nurse realize that when, where, and how she touches a patient will most likely affect their relationship. Whether or not the relationship will be strengthened depends on both the patient's and nurse's interpretation of the situation in which the touch gesture occurred.

Criteria concerning touch as a valid nursing intervention

If touch is not shunned as taboo, it might be helpful to consider when touch may be used therapeutically in medical-surgical patient situations and when it is likely to be ineffective. The following situations are presented for individual questioning and evaluation rather than dogmatic rules.

Inappropriate situations

Situations in which touch might not be appropriate are as follows:
1. Using touch in any sexually suggestive way
2. Using touch without conveying a genuine message—most patients can recognize insincerity instinctively
3. Using touch with a patient having extreme fear of dependency and who is unable to request assistance from anyone
4. Using touch with a patient who sees physical contact as a form of nonverbal communication reserved only for children or the handicapped
5. Using touch with a patient having an aversion to sex
6. Using touch with an angry or suspicious patient
7. Using touch with a patient who obviously does not desire to touch or be touched
8. Using touch when the initiator obviously feels embarrassed or unnatural in doing so

Appropriate situations

1. Depression. A common factor among depressed patients is an increased need or wish for touch.
2. Anxiety. When a patient fails to respond to oral communication, he may be reached on a physical level.
3. Courage. Touch imparts support to a patient needing courage in some effort he must make, such as a paraplegic patient who is frustrated in his attempts to walk again.
4. Fear. Touch can help calm fears; for example, a frightened patient during grand rounds of the medical staff; a patient who has received unfavorable laboratory results—one who has just been told by the physician that the colon biopsy suggests malignancy and a colostomy is indicated; and new procedures such as a young girl's first pelvic examination.
5. Joy. Touch can express joy in situations, such as with an aphasic patient who has just spoken his first words.
6. Difficult to verbalize. Touch can display empathy in any situation where it is difficult to express one's thoughts and feelings orally. In any extremely stressful situation touch can often express the nurse's appreciation of the patient's needs and feelings more than verbal attempts, such as with a terminally ill and dying patient and his family, a patient experiencing meaningless suffering, or an extremely distraught and crying patient and family.
7. Meet mothering needs. Touch may be viewed as symbolic mothering[36]; when mothering needs are met, there is increased meaning in verbal communication for the patient.
8. Patient reaches out. Some patients reveal their need for touch by reaching out for the nurse; touch communicates to a patient that dependency is allowed during stressful periods.
9. Demonstration of affection and acceptability. The patient who is uncertain of her or his desirability can be reassured; for example, the patient who has just had a mastectomy or facial plastic surgery.
10. Disoriented, unconscious, terminally ill, and dying patient. Touch is a means of reality contact and assures the patient "you are really there," a means of integrating the hospital environment as a part of the patient's real world; a physical reminder of the patient's existence and continued life.
11. Pain. Touch helps to alleviate the patient's pain experience and indicates the nurse is willing to share the patient's experience.
12. Rejection and loneliness. Touch assures the patient the nurse is not afraid of

his disease; even a gloved hand is a hand. For example, a patient placed on isolation precautions often feels "unclean" and feelings of rejection and loneliness are exaggerated.

13. Sensory deprivation. To the geriatric, blind, deaf, or immobilized patient, touch provides an additional source of orientation to reality as well as meaningful stimulation.

Implications for nursing education and nursing service

The following implications for nursing education and nursing service can be derived from this chapter:

There should be greater emphasis in present in-service programs on the judicious use of the touch gesture as a therapeutic nursing intervention. Such programs should be geared toward increasing the nurse's awareness of the many different meanings and feelings that touch can convey to the patient. By becoming more cognizant of the touch gesture as a powerful tool of nonverbal communication, the nurse can effectively use it for many different purposes in many different patient care situations. This might be accomplished by showing films involving touch as a means of nonverbal communication. It would be beneficial to stop the films at specified intervals and have the nurse viewing the film write her interpretation of the interaction between the filmed nurse and patient to determine if she even recognized the use of touch. A discussion focused on the nurse's observation from the film could then follow. The films could foster the nurse's understanding of what touch means to different people and what effect it has on specific patients in specific situations. The nurse should be encouraged to explore and express her feelings toward the use of touch (1) as demonstrated in the film, (2) when she is touching others, and (3) when she is being touched. The discussion group could work together to set down some guidelines to use when the nurse finds herself in a situation where she deems touch appropriate. The nurse needs to understand herself and her motives, as well as the patient's, to be truly cognizant of the therapeutic use of touch.

To be truly effective in her nursing care and to avoid misinterpretation of the touch gesture, the nurse needs to know how, when, and where the patient desires to be touched. Does she stroke him gently on the forehead or touch him firmly on the shoulder or arm? Similarly, is there a difference in the patient's interpretation of physical contact during a backrub where the nurse brushes lightly over the patient's back and one where she uses continuous firm strokes? Touching the patient roughly when awakening or positioning would certainly not convey the same message as a firm touch on the arm during certain stressful periods.

Deliberative touch interventions should be a tool of all persons rendering nursing care, not just the registered nurse but the practical nurse, technician, and aide. One does not need formal advanced preparation to administer an effective touch intervention.

The importance of the many different uses of touch with the depressed, anxious, frightened, joyful, uncommunicative, dependent, insecure, disoriented, unconscious, terminally ill, dying, suffering, rejected, lonely, and sensory deprived patient should be increasingly emphasized in both nursing practice and nursing education.

The importance of meaningful, rewarding physical contact for the very young in terms of emotional, intellectual, and personality development cannot be overemphasized. Present practices in newborn nurseries in many hospitals need to be reevaluated. Infants are frequently isolated from mother, fed at specified intervals for certain lengths of time, and given minimal bodily contact.

The concept of touch as a nursing intervention should rightfully be stressed early in undergraduate education programs and can be discussed with the concept of nonverbal communication. It is necessary for the student to distinguish between her own feelings concerning a particular form of touch and its application to the nurse's role. For example, the student should have an opportunity to express her feelings toward touch before she is assigned to perform specific patient care procedures such as giving a patient a bath or catheterizing a patient.

Seminars would be helpful for focusing upon the critical use of touch as an asset to the nurse's communication tools. Practice and thought are used to increase the nurse's effectiveness with verbal communication. The same should be true with nonverbal techniques as touch.

It is particularly important for the student to differentiate between her own perception of how she has touched a patient and the patient's perception of how he has been touched. Role playing might be a meaningful experience to assist the student to appreciate the importance of how and where she touches the patient as well as when touch is permitted and when it should be avoided.

Students should be encouraged to explore with the patient his feelings toward touching and being touched. Nursing is one of the unique professions where the "laying on of hands" is permitted. Students should be assisted in seeing themselves as professionals who have been given this special privilege and therefore be able to effectively use touch for the benefit of the patient.

Although this chapter focused on medical-surgical nurses, the concept of touch and its use with psychiatric patients should be dealt with in greater depth in undergraduate nursing programs, particularly since the use of touch with psychiatric patients is such a controversial issue among psychiatric nurses.

Conclusion

There is no intention on the part of the author to suggest that touch be used indiscriminately as a way of relating to patients. It is the author's belief, however, that the judicious use of touch can be a valuable asset in nursing care. The avoidance of touch should not be taken for granted as taboo by the nurse, rather, it should be recognized, discussed, clarified, and evaluated within the general framework of the nurse-patient relationship. The use of touch should be determined according to each patient's individual needs and wishes and not by the nurse's predetermined bias. It is hoped that each reader, regardless of area of practice, will become increasingly aware of the significance of touch and his or her feelings about touching and being touched. It is also hoped that more scientific explorations into the therapeutic use of touch will be forthcoming.

References

1. Davis, A. J.: The skills of communication, Amer. J. Nurs. 63:66-70, 1963.
2. Johnson, B. S.: The meaning of touch in nursing, Nurs. Outlook 13:59-60, 1965.
3. Critchley, M.: The language of gestures, London, 1939, Edward Arnold (Publishers) Ltd.
4. Mercer, L. S.: Touch: comfort or threat, Perspect. Psychiat. Care 4:20-25, 1966.
5. Frank, L.: Tactile communication, Genet. Psychol. Monogr. 56:209-255, 1957.
6. Cashar, L., and Dixson, B. K.: The therapeutic use of the touch, J. Psychiat. Nurs. 5:422-451, 1967.
7. Newton, M., and McDowell, W. E.: A study of nurse action in relief of pain, second printing, Columbus, 1966, Ohio State University Research Foundation: Division of Nursing, United States Public Health Service.
8. Farrah, S. J.: Effect of deliberative nursing intervention upon the alleviation of pain in selected female patients, unpublished paper, Chicago, 1968, University of Illinois Medical Center.
9. Sullivan, H. S.: The interpersonal theory of psychiatry, New York, 1953, W. W. Norton Co., Inc.

10. Fromm-Reichmann, F.: Principles of intensive psychotherapy, Chicago, 1950, University of Chicago Press.
11. Bowbly, J.: The nature of the child's tie to his mother, Int. J. Psychoanal. 38:350-373, 1958.
12. Burton, A., and Heller, L. G.: The touching of the body, Psychoanal. Rev. 51:122-134, 1964.
13. Hollender, M. H.: The need or wish to be held, Arch. Gen. Psychiat. 22:445-453, 1970.
14. Cohen, S.: Contact deprivation in infants, Psychosomatics 7:85-88, 1966.
15. Spitz, R.: Childhood development phenomena: The influence of mother-child relationships and its disturbances. In Soddy, K., editor: Mental health and infant development, New York, 1956, Basic Books, Inc., Publishers.
16. Brody, S.: Patterns of mothering, New York, 1956, International Universities Press.
17. DeAugustinis, J., Isani, R. S., and Kumler, F. R.: Word study: the meaning of touch in interpersonal communication. In Burd, Shirley, and Marshall, Margaret A., editors: Some clinical approaches to psychiatric nursing, New York, 1963, The Macmillan Co.
18. Aguilera, D. C.: The use of physical contact (touch) as a technique of nonverbal communication with psychiatric patients, exploring progress in psychiatric nursing practice. From a Series of Papers presented at the 1965 Regional Clinical Conferences Sponsored by the American Nurses' Association, New York, 1966, American Nurses' Association.
19. Robinson, A. M.: Communication with schizophrenic patients, Amer. J. Nurs. 60:1120-1123, 1960.
20. Aguilera, D. C.: Relationship between physical contact and verbal interaction between nurses and patients, J. Psychiat. Nurs. 5:5-21, 1967.
21. Greenhill, M. H.: Interviewing with a purpose, Amer. J. Nurs. 56:1258-1260, 1956.
22. Hayes, W. J., and Gazaway, R.: Human relations in nursing, ed. 3, Philadelphia, 1964, W. B. Saunders Co.
23. McCaffery, M., and Moss, F.: Nursing intervention for bodily pain, Amer. J. Nurs. 67:1224-1227, 1967.
24. Lockerby, F.: Communication for nurses, ed. 2, St. Louis, 1963, The C. V. Mosby Co.
25. Matheney, R. V., and Topalis, M.: Psychiatric nursing, ed. 3, St. Louis, 1961, The C. V. Mosby Co.
26. Render, H. W., and Weiss, O. M.: Nurse-patient relationships in psychiatry, ed. 2, New York, 1959, McGraw-Hill Book Co., Inc.
27. Wolberg, L. R.: The technique of psychotherapy, New York, 1954, Grune & Stratton, Inc.
28. Steele, K. M., and Manfreda, M. L.: Psychiatric nursing, Philadelphia, 1959, F. A. Davis Co.
29. Hofling, C. K., and Leininger, M. M.: Basic psychiatric concepts in nursing, ed. 2, Philadelphia, 1967, J. B. Lippincott Co.
30. Schwartz, M. S., and Shockley, E. L.: The nurse and the mental patient, New York, 1956, The Russell Sage Foundation.
31. Varley, B. K.: Reaching out, therapy with schizophrenic patients, Amer. J. Orthopsychiat. 29:407-416, 1959.
32. Farrah, S. J.: The nurse's reported use of touch, unpublished master's thesis of surgical nursing, University of Illinois at the Medical Center, Chicago, Ill., 1969.
33. Elonen, A. S.: The effect of child rearing on behavior in different cultures, Amer. J. Orthopsychiat. 31:505-512, 1961.
34. Bosanquet, Camilla: Getting in touch, J. Anal. Psychol. 15:42-58, 1970.
35. French, J. G.: A delicate balance, Nurs. Outlook 16:52-53, 1968.
36. Mintz, E. E.: Touch and the psychoanalytic tradition, Psychoanal. Rev. 56:365-376, 1969.
37. Sechehaye, M.: Autobiography of a schizophrenic girl, New York, 1951, Grune & Stratton, Inc.

Chapter 28

Nursing assessment of the aging

Lily Larson

The integrity of the aging American has long been threatened by the values society regards as important. Two of these values are efficiency and achievement in the world of work. By declaring "statutory senility" on persons over 65 years of age, society has negated basic rights of the individual—the right to live independently and with dignity. Supporters of disengagement theory have compounded the problems of the aging population by assuming that older people anticipate death by being freed from participating in the mainstream of life.[1] Removing oneself from the mainstream of society is not necessarily a choice of the elderly; it may actually be a method of coping with the loss of former ties, jobs, friends, decreased energy, and death of significant others.

Most elderly persons want to be a part of the living, dynamic society. If an individual is preoccupied with separation from this world, there is little point in planning for future gratification, since the future has already been expended and incorporated into the past and present. Activity theory states that maintenance of activities is important to individuals as a basis for obtaining and maintaining satis-faction, self-esteem, and health.[2] Maddox's findings in a longitudinal study of elderly subjects support activity theory as the basis for preservation of vigor and satisfaction.[3]

These two contrasting theories, disengagement and activity, have far-reaching practical implications for the aging population. Present-day society is manifesting its concern for the aged by building retirement and nursing homes and developing protected environments. It appears that such endeavors support disengagement theory by further separating the aged population from society. On the other hand, some things are being done that support activity theory, such as providing opportunities for involvement of the aged in further education, hobbies, and community projects. In addition, the trend is to extend the retirement age.

A generation ago aging persons were not as visible as they are now. An important reason for their increased visibility is that of increased numbers. Thus the aged have suddenly become a major economic and social problem. Since 1900 the percentage of the United States' population for ages over 65 has more than doubled, from 4.1% in 1900 to 9.4% in 1968. The actual number of aged persons has increased from approximately 3 million in 1900 to nearly 19 million in 1968. For the same year, the female aging population was approximately 10,600,000 as compared to approximately 8,070,000 males.[4]

Longevity is influenced by a complex of interacting factors that are environmental, nutritional, psychological, economic, and genetic. The sharp increase in life expectancy since 1900 has been due largely to advancements in medical technology, which have resulted in a decrease in deaths attributable to infectious disease, early detection, and inhibition of pathological phenomena.

Although it appears that the projected number of persons in the aging group will continue to increase in the United States during this century, the life-span probably will not increase markedly, since advances in scientific knowledge are not easily disseminated or put into practice. Therefore progress in controlling the killers of the aged, the degenerative diseases, probably will not be realized in the near future.[5]

Since the elderly constitute a sizeable portion of the population, it is surprising that the elderly are subtly referred to as a minority group. If one accepts the view that elderly Americans comprise a deprived minority, then it is important to understand how they acquired that status. They differ from other minority groups in that they were not born into it nor did they decide to achieve this status—rather it is due to the accumulation of years of living and to the value society places on younger individuals. The "minority group" status of older people may also be related to the early separation of children from their grandparents, which affords little opportunity for the young and the elderly to share experiences. This is one reason why young people have not learned to appreciate or understand the elderly. It appears that adjusting to the

new status of aging is more difficult for the white aged than for the black aged. One reason is that the white aged generally take a reduction in income, whereas many elderly blacks acquire a more stable income than they had formerly.[6]

The health professions have reflected to a large extent the values and attitudes of the larger society. Many individuals within these professions have had little opportunity for enriching experiences with an aging person. Therefore many persons have difficulty relating to the elderly person, perhaps because they are reminded of their own physical and mental decline and their own vulnerability to death. In addition, health professionals are committed primarily to curing illness and overcoming or alleviating disability; thus progressive degeneration and death often denote failure. Therefore the consequence is avoidance of the problems of aging persons. Comfort has coined the term "gerontophobia" to describe the resistance on the part of some health professionals to become involved in the problems of the aged.[7] It would follow that those who work with the elderly should be mature persons who not only understand their intimate and interdependent relationship with the universe in which they live and with their fellowmen, but who also have resolved, to a fair extent, their feelings about their own life and death.

For various reasons, which include increased visibility of the aging American and the fact that he has become a socioeconomic problem, a White House Conference on Aging was held in 1961. Out of this conference evolved the Senior Citizen's Charter that enumerates the rights and obligations of senior citizens, which includes the following: the rights for employment, usefulness, and freedom from want; a right to a fair share of the community's recreational, educational, and medical resources; the right to live the way one wants to live; and the right to live and die with dignity.* The individual's obligations include the following: to remain self-supporting as long as health and circumstances permit; to learn and apply sound principles of physical and mental health; to make available the benefits of one's experience and knowledge; to adapt one's self realistically to the aging process; and to attempt to maintain relationships with family, neighbors, and friends.

After the White House Conference on Aging and with increased federal monies for research in the field of gerontology, members of the disciplines of sociology, psychology, physiology, and related fields became more actively involved in investigations into various aspects of aging. Recent research findings have important implications for health professions for improving the care of the aged.

In the past thirty years the knowledge explosion in medical science has brought about specialization and subspecialization in medical practice. However, geriatrics has only recently been accorded a prominent place in medicine. Although the first medical book on geriatrics in the United States was published in 1914, it was only during the past two decades that the American Medical Association formed its Committee on Geriatrics, an example of changing attitudes toward aging. This committee later changed its name to the Committee on Aging, and more recently it became known as the Committee on Living. After seven years of study, the Committee on Living made this statement: "Compulsory retirement is a waste of human resources that the nation can ill afford—it contributes measurably to ill health resulting from lack of work, exercise and responsibility."[8]

The nursing profession has been slow to focus on the aging population to any

great extent. The first nursing textbook on geriatric nursing was published in 1950. However, it was another ten to fifteen years before a number of baccalaureate programs in nursing began to include in their curricula courses focused on geriatric nursing. In 1966 a Division of Geriatric Nursing Practice was formed within the American Nurses' Association that gave impetus to increased concern for the practice of geriatric nursing. Project grants under the Nurse Training Act of 1964 were initiated to spark interest in nurses for the health care of older people and to disseminate new knowledge in geriatric nursing to the profession at large. The increased need for nursing care of the elderly, plus the public's demand for this service, makes it imperative that nurse educators include teaching the care of the aging in the nursing education program. Birren warns that the sin of our present generation is to ignore existing knowledge, whereas the sin of former generations was not to seek knowledge.[9] Some new knowledge of the aging is contradictory to many of the stereotyped beliefs of the aged. Emerging concepts from the field of gerontology are applicable to nursing and are useful for assessment and intervention on the secondary and tertiary levels of prevention and cure. However, at this point in time we do not have the knowledge for primary prevention of degenerative diseases that plague the aging population.

Attitudes toward the aging and nursing education

Attitudes of nursing students as well as nurse practitioners toward the elderly patient can be summarized as follows: "Old age is synonymous with senility. Caring for older people is dull, routine, and depressing."[10, 11] Assuming that overt behavior is consistent with attitudes, the author's observations, conducted over a two-month period, tend to validate that nursing students' and nurse practitioners' attitudes

---

*From the 1961 White House Conference on Aging.

toward the aging person are less positive than are their attitudes toward the younger person.[12]

On a thirty-five-bed adult hospital unit where 40% of the patients were in the above 65 age group and 60% in the age group ranging from 30 to 65, both baccalaureate nursing students and graduate nurses (that is, registered nurses) chose to have more continuity of care with the younger age group. Students had experience on this unit 4 out of 7 days a week and were permitted to choose their own patients. Students had experience with all age groups. Average number of days of continued care for the same patient over 65 was 3 days, although average length of hospitalization for this age group was 11.5 days. For patients under 65, average number of days of continued contact with the same patient was 5 days with average length of hospitalization being 7.5 days. Students choosing more aged patients and longer continued experiences with the aged patient had previous experience with aged grandparents, relatives, or friends. Their attitudes toward the aged, as revealed by their communication in diaries, indicated less stereotyping than that of their peers who had chosen less experience with the elderly and who revealed that they had little previous interaction with grandparents or other elderly persons. These latter students' verbal and written communications about the elderly were more stereotyped than was their communications about younger patients. Nurse practitioners on the same unit had an even less impressive record; the average number of days of continued contact with the elderly patient for six nurses on the day shift was 1.5 as compared with 3.5 days with the patient under age 65.

One of the important functions of a teacher in nursing is to create an environment in which desirable attitudes can develop. The behavior of the teacher toward the aging patient influences the behavior of the student. The young activity-oriented nursing student finds it difficult to adjust to the slower pace of the aged individual. Lack of previous involvement with aging individuals by nursing students creates anxiety and frustration with which the instructor must cope.

An effective approach to teaching nursing of the aged person is to use developmental theory. Erikson describes the healthy aging person, at the last maturational level, as having reached ego integrity and fulfillment.[13] The aged person having attained this fulfillment is described as one who has accepted responsibility for what life is and was and its place in the flow of history. At the other end of the spectrum, as opposed to integrity, is despair and dysphoria.

Continued contact with older healthy people in the community and experiences in communication with the elderly in order to learn about their life-style and their adjustment to aging may foster in the student an appreciation for the need to increase her understanding of the aged person. Having students read biographies and autobiographies of aged persons provides vicarious experiences and serves to illustrate the wide range of individual differences in aging. Mark Van Doren, now past 75 years of age, describes the healthy aging person as one who likes himself and one who does not think about himself.[14] "He thinks about the world and other people." Van Doren compares his own feelings of old age with the feelings of younger people:

> It's nice to be old
> Old people feel things
> So much more deeply
> And passionately.

He further adds that old people can afford to be simple; young people are complicated. The despair and dysphoric state of aging are illustrated by Shakespeare.[15]

> . . . a world too wide
> For this shrunk shank; . . .
>
> .   .   .   .
>
> Is second childishness and mere oblivion,
> Sans teeth, sans eyes, sans taste, sans everything.*

Persons with over a half-century of experience to form their personalities, to adopt a life-style, and to develop ways of coping with everyday life as well as crises have greater opportunity for individual

---

*From Shakespeare, William: As you like it, II, vii, 160, 161, 165, 166.

differences than may occur in other age groups. Nurses working with aged persons need to consider these differences.

The following was written in a diary by one of the author's nursing students who had been avoiding the aged patient, but who tried to meet the objectives of the course requirements:

Mrs. J is a 72-year-old woman who has been hospitalized for ten days. During her hospitalization she had a permanent colostomy as a result of cancer of the rectum. Her husband died six months ago. She has social security and a 'substantial life savings.' She owns the house in which she resides. It is situated in a middle class neighborhood consisting predominantly of middle-aged and younger families. Mrs. J's only daughter and her family live in a small town, about a two-hour drive from Mrs. J.

I'm very ambivalent about taking care of Mrs. J. I know I need this experience with an older person and I know I'll have some help from you. On the other hand, I am so discouraged about what I found in the nursing notes. The only comments I've found about her are 'disoriented, confused, got out of bed and fell, shows signs of senility.' The only positive notes are 'eats well, cooperative, no complaints.' The nurses have given her colostomy irrigations, sitz baths, and a bed bath every day. Mrs. J is ambulating, but only when the staff persuades her to do so.

With this information, I went to visit Mrs. J to tell her I would be working with her nearly every day if it would be okay with her. She looked at me and nodded. I remembered that by really being concerned and communicating this to the patient is one way of establishing a trusting relationship so I proceeded to talk with her about things that I thought might concern her. . . . My assessment thus far is that this lady is hard of hearing. I had to speak in a lower tone of voice and get close enough for her to see my face. I also learned that she feels abandoned by her daughter even though her daughter visits her daily. She made one angry, tearful statement that everyone is too busy to bother about old people like her. I'm sure that it is true and I am guilty of it—and here I am expecting to be a nurse! I have to work on this.

After working with this student and the patient for a period of over a week, the author noted the following entry in the student's diary:

I feel so good about Mrs. J. My last visit with her at home was yesterday. What a contrast to my first meeting with her! She is still living alone and wants it that way. Her daughter comes to see her and plans to buy groceries for her until she can do so herself. Mrs. J's neighbors and church circle friends see that she has a hot meal a day. Mrs. J did say she could take care of this herself but likes the attention. Yesterday she called the bakery where she had worked on Fridays and Saturdays previous to her illness. She was so delighted to find they could use her as a sales clerk Friday and Saturday afternoons. She is also going to get a hearing aid. She is very proud that she is able to regulate her colostomy. She still refers to it as 'that thing.'

My own feelings now about older people are entirely different. I'm glad you persuaded me to have more continued contact with them. I know all older people aren't as interesting as Mrs. J, but I've learned they want to be accepted and appreciated like everyone else. I can't help but think I made a difference to Mrs. J but it was only after she had learned to trust me.

The above account of a process of change in attitude is typical of other students' entries in their diaries. It is apparent that conferences focused on behaviors and feelings of the aged as well as the students' own feelings about aging are necessary to bring about a change in behavior.

Another student wrote in her diary:

Caring for older patients more than anything else has taught me to have an open mind and patience. Older persons have taught me to enjoy the beauty around me, to appreciate their wisdom, and to value all people. I am less superficial in my dealings with all people and like myself better for it. I think we should be required to care for older people and learn more about them earlier in our nursing courses. Most students avoid older people so our instructors should see that we have experiences with them.

Development of a nurse's ability to care for the geriatric patient is probably the same as for other age groups, with emphasis on understanding, empathy, and patience. The nurse needs flexibility, since some older people have developed fixed habits of daily living. She may need to be more persuasive to help the patient manage and sustain himself; and there is need to be particularly observant of both physical and psychological aspects of behavior. The nurse also needs to be especially perceptive of and sensitive to the aging person's desires and needs for privacy, independence, and dependence and to assist him in his attempt to maintain or increase his integrity.

The ability to empathize with individuals is an essential characteristic of a nurse. It entails the ability to put one's self in another's place—an I-thou relationship.[16, 17] It is difficult for a young person to enter into an I-thou relationship with an older person whose living experiences and feelings are vastly more varied and moored in time periods unexperienced by the young. It is necessary then for the nurse to comprehend how the elderly person feels, thinks, and perceives the situation in which he finds himself. The nurse needs to intellectually examine the situation with the person, deal with it honestly, and at the same time communicate that she appreciates his feelings and experiences. This kind of communication is an important element in a trust relationship. Furthermore the actions of the nurse must be consistent with her verbal communication. Continuation of a trust relationship is fostered by continued interaction with a significant person. On the other hand, when an everchanging stream of nurses give care and interact on a superficial level, the older person's anxiety and dissatisfaction increase. One elderly person said, "The other nurses mean well but they don't allow me to do the things by myself the way my real nurse does." Her "real nurse" was the nurse who had cared for her daily over an extended period of time. This patient slept poorly at night and became confused and uncooperative on the days that her "real nurse" was absent.

Nursing assessment

The nurse, to be empathic, must also have knowledge of the dynamics of psychological aging as well as the physiological processes of aging. Both processes take place within the person and are therefore interrelated and cannot be separated when making assessments and decisions about nursing intervention. Assessment is a continuous process, not a onetime incident that might occur during a hurried admission interview. An organized method of assessment and an assessment guide are useful. These should be an essential part of the patient's record, with continuous reassessment and reevaluation.

Since nursing is involved with the patient's activities of daily living, a patient history is a useful tool. If the patient is hospitalized for a physical illness and is seeking relief, this may be his first concern and this is where the nurse should focus—on his concerns. Hospitalization for most older people creates increased anxiety, and the initial concern of the nurse may be to decrease the patient's anxiety. It is important to remember that information given by the highly anxious person may be distorted or even inaccurate. Interviews may focus on the patient's usual eating, sleeping, resting, elimination, and activity patterns. It is essential to know how he copes with what he considers discomforts arising from circulatory, respiratory, or neurological decline or impairment. Some patients may view themselves more ill than they really are, and some may view their illness merely as an annoyance. The interviewer, or nurse, needs to communicate to the patient that information is needed to help the nurse be of assistance to him during hospitalization. The nurse's understanding that most elderly people want to maintain as much control as possible over their environment will be communicated by her words and actions. A skilled nurse can evaluate the patient's ways of coping and the defense mechanisms that need to be supported. The level of maturity a person has achieved can be assessed only in part. Observation of hearing and visual function are evaluated grossly to determine the best means for the patient to receive input and need for environmental modifications.

If the elderly person is slow in responding or misinterprets a question, the nurse needs to determine if it is due to a diminution of hearing, a slowing of thought processes, or both.

An essential part of the interviews is focused on the patient's family or significant others. The person may desire to have some member of the family with him or nearby during periods of hospitalization. It is important that members of the family know the nurse is concerned about the welfare of both the patient and his family, and they should be encouraged to participate in the patient's care insofar as it is mutually beneficial to both.

Loss of significant others occurs frequently in the elderly person's life and creates additional stress for the aging person. The nurse must determine the kind of supportive environment needed to assist the elderly patient through the grieving process, thereby promoting the patient's "psychological equilibrium."

Maintaining physiological equilibrium in the elderly is a problem. Studies indicate the aged (1) on exposure to cold lose body heat more rapidly and have a greater increase in oxygen consumption than in the young; (2) on exposure to heat or with elevated body temperatures are unable to quickly dissipate body heat; and (3) following glucose tolerance tests have a greater rise in blood sugar levels with a return to normal taking longer than that occurring in younger persons. These findings along with others indicate that the compensatory responses of the aged are at times slower and less effective than those in young individuals. Special attention should be focused on room temperature for persons with circulatory problems, since extremes of temperature may be hazardous. A hot bath for a young person can be invigorating, but it may cause confusion in the elderly due to excessive peripheral vasodilation and delayed vasoconstrictor response that causes a slowing of blood flow to the brain and a resultant cerebral anoxia. Sudden changes of position from horizontal to vertical can also result in cerebral anoxia due to delayed pressor receptor response and vasoconstriction in the lower extremities. Decreased cardiac output, together with decreased vital capacity and a less efficient vascular system, contributes to the elderly patient's confusion. The nurse must be aware of these factors in assessing physical abilities and disabilities. An appropriate protective environment is needed for the elderly with muscle weakness, osteoporosis, poor coordination, or failing eyesight. The nurse also needs to be aware of the gradual diminution of pain sensations. Since an elderly patient often has vague feelings of discomfort and may not experience pain when injured or ill, he should be observed for clinical signs that indicate a loss of or threat to tissue integrity. These include a slight rise in baseline temperature, changes in skin temperature or color, slight increase in pulse rate and respiration, or changes in blood pressure.

With the possible decrease in effectiveness of the autonomic nervous system, stress resulting from too much or too little sensory input must be avoided. Decreased auditory and visual receptions shut out sensory input and thus increase the importance of touch. However, too much sensory input, such as overactive, overtalkative visitors or the entourage of medical personnel, may cause the elderly person to act in such a way that he becomes classified as being uncooperative, confused, or even senile. It is important for the nurse to know that either sensory deprivation or overstimulation can cause an altered state of consciousness. It is the prerogative of the nurse, who should be the patient's advocate, to protect the patient from environmental stress that threatens his integrity.

If the nurse's orientation has been to

focus on disabilities of people, she may underestimate the abilities of the aging person. To rely on limited knowledge and intuition and to omit deliberative assessment of the aging person's abilities and strengths result in either a lack of intervention or in nursing intervention that is less than beneficial for the patient and highly dissatisfying for the nurse. Continuously emerging concepts that are proving to be significant for health care of the aged make it no longer acceptable for the nurse to deprive the older person of high-quality care. Information used in providing care for the aging should be based on documented data. The nurse, in her assessment, must be aware of what is myth and what is fact.

New findings in the area of learning do not give credence to the myth "you can't teach an old dog new tricks." It is true that whereas some elderly persons have a narrowing of intellectual skills, others show little or no decline. In a longitudinal study of aging, memory recall for simple material showed relatively little decline, but an increasingly greater lapse in recall for the more complex.[18] The aging person's fear of failure when attempting something new often results in poor performance. These findings are important for the nurse to remember when teaching the elderly person. Pacing of inputs, prevention of overloading, and realistic expectations will do much to enhance the elderly person's self-confidence and decrease his anxieties, thus freeing him for new learning.

Selected physiological aspects of aging

Although the brain gradually decreases in weight, evidence shows that intellectual loss does not correspond with the loss in weight.[18] It may be that the brain has a compensatory mechanism for this gradual loss of nerve tissue. Some cells in the human body, that is, the fully differentiated cells, lack the power to divide and even-

tually cease to exist or function. Many of the body cells exist for relatively short periods and are continually replaced from reservoirs of unspecialized cells that persist and continue to function. Neuron, cardiac, and skeletal muscle cells, which are examples of fully differentiated cells, are not replaced during the lifetime of the individual. The reservoirs for "short lived" cells also diminish with age and finally lose their capacity to divide so that life processes cease.[19]

The rate of decline in ability to do physical work depends on the following variables: muscle strength, coordination involving the nervous system, and adequacy of the heart and vascular system. Shock[20] reports the following estimates of tissue dimensions and functions remaining in "average" 75-year-old persons when compared with "average" 30-year-old persons: 70% of his former work ability, 90% of brain weight, 63% of nerve trunk fibers, 90% of nerve conduction velocity, and 56% of his former vital capacity.

One could speculate that Americans have not been prone to physical exertion and that the decrease in functional capacities may be due in part to too much physical inactivity. More rapid aging may involve faster deterioration of neuronic control and loss of neurons if neurons are not activated and reactivated.[21] Activity for the elderly depends in part on their conviction of usefulness to others and their state of health. The nurse needs to take into serious consideration the theory of atrophy of disuse and activity theory when planning for the aged patient.

Although almost every kind of heart disease encountered in earlier decades of life can still be found in old age, atherosclerotic and hypertensive cardiovascular diseases are far more numerous. Heart rate has a tendency to decrease between the ages of 60 to 85 years.[22] Thereafter a slight increase occurs. Although hearts vary in size, all hearts tend to decrease in weight after the sixth decade. Heart muscles at autopsy vary in tone; some muscles are firm and well-developed, and others are thin or flabby. Fibrous and fatty tissue as well as calcification may be present in "normal" hearts at autopsy. The increase of cardiac fibrous tissue along with decreased vascular elasticity diminishes cardiovascular functioning. Circulation is also dependent on the muscle tone of the trunk and extremities. An efficient diaphragm assists, as does exercise, the return of blood to the heart.

Lung tissue decreases in weight and effective functioning with age.[22] Average right lung weight for young adults is 570 grams, whereas for the aged it is 440 grams; average left lung weight is 430 grams for young adults and 350 grams for the aged. It is well documented that tidal volume is decreased, elasticity and recoil ability are reduced, and oxygen consumption is diminished in the elderly. These alterations may be due to primary body cellular loss, increased pulmonary fibrosis, and decreased pulmonary elasticity. It is difficult to determine changes in the lung that are due to normal aging as opposed to those caused by pathology.

The functional decline of the kidneys in old age, because of the reduction of neurons and nephrons, is made more serious by the corresponding decline in effectiveness of the cardiovascular and respiratory systems.[23] All these systems are interdependent—the decline of one system affects the efficiency of the others.

With diminution of nerve fibers, significant changes affecting sensory input are present. Proprioceptors, pain, and temperature sensations are decreased in varying degrees. These receptors are important in considering the older person's safety, and the nurse needs to consider the status of the receptor system when caring for the aged.

Research on hearing indicates much variability, but the hearing loss incidence is nine times greater in the 60-year-old group than the 30-year-old group.[24] Factor analysis of data derived from physical examinations, neurological investigations, and laboratory studies indicated that hearing loss was the most important variable related to overall deterioration.[25] Those persons over 60 with hearing loss in the range of twenty decibels or more showed marked deterioration both in cognitive functioning and personality. Age-related hearing loss is characterized by a progressive loss of high tones; such loss usually becomes stabilized after the seventh decade. If the high tones lost are within speech range, those communicating with that person need to speak in a lower pitch. A hearing aid may also be needed. Hearing loss from other causes can be avoided by (1) preventing acoustic trauma from loud noises, (2) preventing ear infections, (3) keeping ear canals open by removing wax plugs, and (4) avoiding use of ototoxic drugs such as streptomycin.

Visual function declines with aging: the pupils react to light more slowly; the lens becomes less transparent resulting in lessened illumination of the retina; the lens loses its capacity to focus objects clearly on the retina; tolerance to glare is diminished; and speed of adaptation to a dark environment is decreased.[26] For these reasons nonglare illumination and night lights should be provided for the elderly. It is important to remember that the aged have difficulty in perceiving outlines of objects, especially if color contrast is absent.

Deep sleep, or stage four sleep, is reduced considerably in the elderly.[27] Awake periods are also more frequent in elderly persons. Both of these factors may account for some older persons' statements that they sleep poorly—even though the total sleep time per night is reduced insignificantly.

Nutritional status of the elderly is influenced more by social and economic factors than by physiological changes. However, physiological changes do occur, as evidenced by decreased numbers of lingual papillae and taste buds and by a decrease in saliva output. Sensitivity to taste qualities of sweet, sour, salty, and bitter is noticeably decreased with age. Thus elderly persons have less zest for food and often complain of "tasteless" food. As a result they tend to add a greater amount of salt, sugar, and other condiments to their food than they did in their earlier years. Since salt is a pressor substance, caution should be exercised in the amount used by those with hypertension. In addition, advancing age is associated with decreased production of hydrochloric acid and slowed gastric motility. Foods served to the elderly should be moderate in amount, of proper consistency, and easily digested.

Good bone texture of proper strength is the result of appropriate nutrition. Vitamin C is indispensable for effective function of connective tissue, and minerals are vital for proper bone density. Nutritionists recommend an upward revision of dietary protein, particularly those foods rich in lysine and methionine. Subclinical osteoporosis is demonstrated in about 20% of aged women and 10% of aged men.[28] Patients with osteoporosis have had inadequate intake of calcium their entire adult life. Increase of sedentary life may also contribute to loss of calcium from the bones. Thus the implication for the aging person is that exercise is imperative for preventing the complications that result from loss of calcium and that adequate intake of vitamins and minerals is vital for tissue strength and function.

Studies in psychophysiology indicate that the autonomic nervous system of the aged person is considerably different from that of the 30-year-old.[29] Psychological stress initiated by the same stimuli produced higher levels of blood fatty acids and remained higher for a longer period of time in the aging person than in the young, which may indicate a more labile homeostatic mechanism. Eisdorfer predicts that "if this proves to be the case, adre-

nergic blocking drugs may be used to modify autonomic responsivity with resultant sustained activity and interest levels."[29] Since the aged person's autonomic and central nervous system responses can be erratic, his emotional and physiological responses may be unpredictable and at times uncontrollable. Thus, the aging person may avoid emotional involvement and situations requiring rapid expenditure of physical energy.

Several recent longitudinal studies on "healthy" aging persons demonstrated that those persons curtailing their activities suffer a reduction of satisfaction, mental deterioration, and loss of vigor.[30-33] On the other hand, those persons who continued the same type of activity in which they formerly participated or who substituted new activities displayed mental flexibility, vigor, and high satisfaction. One could speculate that nervous system responses may be less effective in those persons who decrease their activities. However, ongoing research in psychobiology may give us more definitive answers about autonomic and central nervous system responses in aging persons.

Conclusion

Concepts useful for nursing of the aged are emerging from interdisciplinary gerontological studies. Some of these concepts have been incorporated in this chapter to illustrate their relevance to nursing assessment of aging persons. However, much more needs to be learned about the multidimensional aspects of the aging person that have an impact on his welfare. This knowledge of the whole person needs to be added to nursing's changing body of knowledge. Nurse educators need to reevaluate the nursing education program to include care of *all* age groups. Nurses who are already practitioners should have the opportunity to renew, revise, and further their knowledge, understanding, and skills in geriatric nursing. The nurse's positive attitude and the extent to which she uses knowledge and skill in working with aging persons may not only add years to the individual's life, but, more importantly, add quality of life to those years.

References

1. Kastenbaum, R.: The foreshortened life perspective, Geriatrics 24:121, 1969.
2. Palmore, E.: The effects of aging on activity and attitudes, Gerontologist 8:259-263, 1968.
3. Maddox, G. L.: Activity and morale: a longitudinal study of selected elderly subjects, Social Forces 42:195, 1963.
4. Brotman, H. B.: Who are the aged: a demographic study, useful facts. Washington, D. C., 1968, United States Administration on Aging.
5. Palmore, E.: Sociological aspects of aging. In Busse, E. W., and Pfeiffer, E., editors: Behavior and adaptation in late life, Boston, 1969, Litle, Brown and Co.
6. Jackson, J. J.: Social gerontology and the Negro: a review, Gerontologist 7:168-178, 1967.
7. Comfort, A.: On gerontophobia, Med. Opinion Rev. 9:30-37, 1967.
8. United States Department of Health, Education, and Welfare: Social and rehabilitation service administration in aging, Quarterly Report, Region 9 10:18, 1967.
9. Birren, J. E.: Research on aging: a frontier of science and social gain, Gerontologist 8:10, 1968.
10. Brown, M. I.: Attitude of nursing personnel toward aged patients, Gerontologist 6:19, 1966.
11. Coe, R.: Professional stereotypes hamper treatment of aged, Geriatric Focus 5:1, 1966. (Reported from speech presented at Seventh International Conference on Gerontology in Vienna.)
12. Larson, L.: Unpublished study, 1968.
13. Erikson, E.: Childhood and society, New York, 1963, W. W. Norton & Co., Inc.
14. Van Doren, M.: Interview by Israel Shenker, Kansas Chity Star, June 22, 1969.
15. Shakespeare, W.: As you like it. In Clarke, W., and Wright, W., editors: Great books of the western world, Chicago, 1952, Encyclopaedia Britannica, Inc.
16. Katz, R. L.: Empathy; its nature and uses, New York, 1963, The Macmillan Co.
17. Giffin, K.: Recent research on interpersonal trust, paper presented at annual convention of the Speech Association of America, Los Angeles, 1967.
18. Eisdorfer, C., and Wilkie, F.: Intellectual changes with advancing age: a 10-year follow-up, paper presented at symposium on longitudinal changes with advancing age, at the annual meeting of the American Psychological Association, San Francisco, 1968.
19. Loofbourrow, G. N.: Physiological aspects of aging, paper presented at conference on sociobiology of aging, at University of Kansas Medical Center, Kansas City, Kan., 1968.
20. Shock, N. W.: The physiology of aging, Sci. Amer. 266:100-110, 1962.
21. Mead, S.: A century of the abuse of rest, J.A.M.A. 182:344-345, 1962.
22. Howell, T.: A guide to geriatrics, Springfield, Ill., 1963, Charles C Thomas, Publisher.
23. Loofbourrow, G. N.: Physiological aspects of aging, paper presented at conference on sociobiology of aging, at University of Kansas Medical Center, Kansas City, Kan., 1968.
24. Bell, B.: Maintenance therapy in vision and hearing for geriatric patients. In Busse, E. W., and Pfeiffer, E., editors: Behavior and adaptation in late life, Boston, 1969, Little, Brown and Co.
25. Eisdorfer, C.: The implications of research for medical practice, Gerontologist 10:65-66, 1970.
26. Stone, V.: Nursing of older people. In Busse, E. W., and Pfeiffer, E., editors: Behavior and adaptation in late life, Boston, 1969, Little, Brown and Co.
27. Katz, A., Kales, A., Wilson, T., Kales, J. D., Jacobson, A., Paulson, M. J., Koller, E., and Walter, R. D.: Measurement of all night sleep in normal elderly persons—effect on aging, J. Amer. Geriat. Soc. 15:405-412, 1967.
28. Todhunter, E. N.: The evaluation of concepts, perspectives and new horizons, J. Amer. Diet. Ass. 46:125, 1965.
29. Eisdorfer, C.: The implications for research in medical practice, Gerontologist 10:65-66, 1970.
30. Butler, R. N.: Aspects of survival and adaptation in human aging, Amer. J. Psychiat. 123:233-243, 1967.
31. Maddox, G. L.: Activity and morale: A longitudinal study of selected elderly subjects, Social Forces 42:195, 1963.
32. Palmore, E.: The effects of aging on activities and attitudes, Gerontologist 8:259-263, 1968.
33. Smith, K. U., and Smith, F. G.: Cybernetics principles of learning and educational design, New York, 1969, Holt, Rinehart, & Winston, Inc.

Chapter *29*

Stages of adaptation to illness and disability: a psychosocial view

Jurate A. Sakalys

Man's physical, emotional, and social survival is largely dependent on the nature of his interaction with the environment in which he lives. In constant transaction with his environment, the individual is constantly apprehending stimuli, interpreting these stimuli on the basis of a number of characteristics unique to him, and deciding on action in relation to the stimuli. Change, in both external and internal environments, is a constant, inevitable, and universal aspect of life, and man's well-being is dependent on his ability to reorganize his behavior in relation to change.

Illness is an example of an universal experience of change to which some adaptation must be achieved. Until recently, there has been limited exploration of an individual's reaction to the experience of illness. At present, however, accumulating evidence indicates that perceptions of illness and ways of adjusting to illness influence the effectiveness of the curative regimen and of future health-oriented experiences. Given that adaptation is interactional in nature and that the environment of the

ill individual is partly composed of health professionals, it seems evident that the nature of adaptation to illness is influenced by an individual's interaction with the health professionals. Of interest to health professionals, therefore, is that very process of adaptation; that is, how does one adjust to the perception of being ill? How does one adjust to the interpersonal and intrapersonal stresses illness entails? The ways in which one adapts must be studied and must be understood for adaptation to be facilitated. In the context of illness as a psychosocial phenomenon this means that health professionals must be able to identify and to modify factors that affect how a person adopts the sick role, how he functions having assumed it, and how he emerges from it.

This chapter will explore psychosocial stresses (change forces) in illness that necessitate some adaptation for a valued goal (wellness or resolution) to be achieved. Several stages of transition, or adaptation, have been identified as part of the illness experience. It may be safe to assume that every individual who becomes ill experiences these stages, but that these stages will differ according to the type of illness. This chapter will focus on differences in stages of adaptation to illness and sick role behavior in relation to three major types of illness—temporary, progressive, and permanent. The frame of reference directing this exploration is of a psychosocial nature, and it must be stated that the following thoughts are generalized, abstract, and out of context of specific diseases. Highly variable factors, such as diagnosis, intrapersonal stress-coping mechanisms, demographic factors, and cultural factors, which also influence adaptation to illness and sick role behavior, are not explored in favor of a more heuristic view.

Illness as a socially defined phenomenon

Illness can be viewed from many perspectives that focus on a failure to maintain a dynamic equilibrium with the environment. Broadly, an illness can be defined as an event or accumulation of circumstances that temporarily, progressively, or permanently interrupts and alters an individual's physical, psychological, and social equilibrium. Illness, therefore, represents an unsuccessful adaptation to biological or behavioral norms (or both) and produces some dysfuncion in any or all spheres of life.

The social components of a definition of illness derive from the fact that physical and behavioral norms are, to some extent, socially determined. Each society defines distinct physiological and psychosocial norms of health; emerging concepts of illness represent some functional deviation from those norms. Parsons' sociological examination of health and illness in America alludes to the flexibility of these norms. If mental health is defined as the capacity to engage in social interaction, then, he states, mental illness can be defined as an incapacity to meet expectations of social roles. Somatic illness, in contrast, is defined as an incapacity for task performance, a task being a set of external or internal physical operations that are the actions of the individual interacting with his physical world.[1] Although the operations of interacting with the physical world may be more consistent cross-culturally, the operations of social interaction vary greatly from one social group to another. It is apparent, then, that definitions of deviance from health norms are, at least in part, socially determined. William Faulkner[2] describes this aspect of the concept of deviance vividly:

Sometime I ain't so sho who's got ere right to say when a man is crazy and when he ain't. Sometime I think it ain't none of us pure crazy and ain't none of us pure sane until the balance of us talks him that-a-way. It's like it ain't so much what a fellow does, but it's the way the majority of folks is looking at him when he does it.*

Society views as deviant those behaviors (or forms of being) that are dysfunctional or harmful to the normal processes and survival of the group. The deviant individual is then usually excluded from the group until his deviance is rectified. It is important to note that deviance in this context is defined as a digression from behavioral or biological norms. As such, it refers only to a "health-illness" perspective and not to a "goodness-badness" perspective, which relates to social problems of crime, delinquency, etc.[3] An ill or disabled individual is defined as deviant by his social group, but his deviance can be rendered socially acceptable or legitimized by fulfillment of a number of expectations society places on his behavior. These expectations in our society are defined as the sick role, which Parsons[1] describes as follows:

1. The individual is not held responsible for his incapacities (he did not choose to violate the norm).

---

*From Faulkner, William: As I lay dying, New York, 1930, Random House, Inc.

2. The individual is released, to varying degrees, from normal role obligations.

3. The individual must recognize that illness is undesirable and have an expressed desire to "get well."

4. The individual must seek competent help, cooperate with treatment, and relinquish the right to make decisions to the doctor or to other health professionals.

Parsons' concept of the sick role identifies normative expectations pertaining to sick role behavior. Normative expectations in relation to any role, however, will always vary in their fulfillment because of the unique characteristics of each person and his environment. Therefore, although Parsons' model is a valuable conceptual tool, it does not take into account a number of factors that may influence the fulfillment of the sick role, such as the individual's well roles, his cultural background, his demographic characteristics, and the effect of interpersonal influence, among others. In addition to these variables, adaption to illness will be largely influenced by the nature, severity, and progression of the illness, factors that have been selected as the focus of this chapter.

Types of illness

Illnesses have long been broadly typed as either acute or chronic, and these categorizations have some suggestive significance apart from their explicit meanings. Because this classification is subject to a number of imprecise and differing interpretations, the typology of temporary, progressive, and permanent illness or disability has been selected.[4] This framework is viewed as more discriminating in that it holds implicit acknowledgement that different stressors affect adaptation to an illness type by incorporating the illness dimensions of differential time and progression. It also allows for the superimposition of the illness dimension of severity, or acuteness, on any of the time dimensions; that is, either a temporary, progressive, or

permanent illness or disability can have acute periods, such as an episode of acidosis in the progressive disability of diabetes mellitus.

Definitions of temporary, progressive, and permanent illnesses

Temporary illness can be viewed as an impermanent deviance from a norm of health that renders the individual disabled for role or task performance. There is a definite time limit to this illness; the duration usually is relatively short, with rapid improvement and ultimate removal of etiological factors. Adaptation to usually unimposing changes engendered by illness is transient, and recovery of premorbid levels of function is the goal. Temporary illness may vary in intensity and may be sudden or insidious and short-term or long-term. It may be sudden and severe, constituting an emergency situation, such as a ruptured appendix; it may be insidious and mildly incapacitating, such as an upper respiratory infection; or it may be long-term, such as the length of incapacitation with a fracture. Hospitalization may or may not be required, but when it is necessary, it is most often of short duration. Since a temporarily ill individual recovers and returns to his normally productive social role and manifests no residual behavioral or physical aberration, temporary illness is a deviant role that usually bears no stigma* and that can be legitimized with relative ease.

In permanent illness or disability a permanent pathophysiological or a psycho-

---

*Goffman defines stigma as "an attribute that is deeply discrediting . . . an attribute that makes him different from others . . . and of a less desirable kind." Central to the concept of stigma is the feature of acceptance: not only does the stigmatized individual find himself disqualified from full social acceptance because of the discrediting attribute, but the stigma also tends to "spread" to "uncontaminated" aspects of his identity.[5]

pathological alteration occurs, and the individual never regains premorbid levels of function (even though he may regain some of his former abilities). Profound and extensive adaptation is necessary in relation to a permanent change, and goals are not "cure," or recovery of premorbid function, but relate to maximizing remaining function. Function and appearance may be grossly different from the premorbid state. The duration of this disability is lifelong, and progress toward a higher level of wellness, if any, is slow. Lifelong medical treatment can be an inevitable circumstance, and repeated hospitalizations for long periods of time may be necessary. The deviance of permanent disability is less acceptable to society and therefore stigmatized for a number of reasons: (1) the individual may not be able to return to a fully productive social role; (2) existing vestiges of social feelings link physical and emotional disability to evil; (3) there is a high degree of social emphasis on the appearance and integrity of the body; and (4) social interaction is governed by strict social norms, and the individual may not be able to interact "normally."

Progressive illness or disability is characterized by a deviance advancing in stages that subjects the individual to a state of constant transition in all spheres of life. Remissions and exacerbations leave the patient vulnerable to periods of extreme stress, and the time perspective of the illness is infinite. Adaptation must be in relation to ongoing, often dramatic, and unexpected changes. Bodily or functional changes occur, necessitating intermittent or constant medical supervision. The disability is likely to be insidious, slow, and, when overt or revealed, subject to stigma. Like permanent disability, progressive disability is generally irreversible and frequently leads to permanence or death.

Both progressive and permanent disabilities can be congenital, acquired, insidious, or sudden. Some can be controlled to a high degree, permitting almost normal role and task performance, albeit with dependence on some therapeutic measures, as is the case with epilepsy. Whether the disability is overt or covert, stigma is rarely escaped.

Unlike temporary illness, progressive and permanent disabilities frequently cause gross changes in appearance or function, requiring adaptations in self-concept, in social interaction, and in life-style. In the genesis of self, one of the first perceptions of being an entity separate from the environment is an awareness of one's body through sensorimotor experiences. The bodily self remains a keen configuration of the sense of self throughout life, although by no means all of the self. Other aspects of self-concept are partly determined by an individual's perception of others' responses to him, by his perceptions of his own abilities, status, roles, and by his aspirations. All these aspects are threatened and even assaulted in progressive or permanent psychosocial or physical disability. In bodily or functional alterations that part of the self-image relating to the alteration may be foreign, and that foreignness is often further enhanced by deprivation resulting from sensory deficits and decreased motor activity. Progressive and permanent disabilities deprive the individual of the means for normal role and task performance and cause another aspect of one's self, self-esteem, to be threatened by dependence and feelings of unworthiness. Exclusion from former social groups leads to the process of disengagement—the mutual withdrawal of the individual and significant others in his social system—that deprives the individual of the social interaction necessary for maintenance of the integrity of self. In view of these events, premorbid conceptions of one's self are no longer tenable. Since self-concept is a vital determinant of behavior, the individual is then faced with the stress of

Table 7. Medical diagnostic examples of illness

Temporary	*Progressive*	*Permanent*
Simple fracture	Atherosclerosis ⟵————⟶	Atherosclerosis
Acute anxiety state	Rheumatoid arthritis	Hemophilia
Neoplasms ⟵————⟶	Neoplasms	Paralysis
Some infectious processes	Emphysema	Epilepsy
	Multiple sclerosis	Amputation
	Schizophrenia ⟵————⟶	Schizophrenia
	Renal failure	Some sensory defects

reassessing and reorganizing (or adapting) his self-concept and his conception of others in such a way as to incorporate the fact of disability.

Progressive and permanent alterations may no longer be defined as illnesses, since illness, as it is usually defined, implies a temporary state of dysfunction. Once an illness becomes progressive or permanent, it tends to disable the individual's interaction with his environment—physiologically, psychologically, or socioculturally—and therefore becomes a disability subject to varying interpretations.

These categorizations are not consistently clear-cut differentiations, since they may blend or merge (Table 7). Some illnesses, if treated early and properly, are temporary; if untreated or if treatment is delayed or inappropriate, they become progressive. Other conditions progress constantly, never stabilizing into what can be defined as a permanent disability and never reaching a finality. Some cardiovascular and renal dysfunctions may fall into any category, depending on whether treatment is administered and on the patient's response to treatment. It is just such modification of this schema that gives it added meaning and serves to avoid stereotyping of illness as acute or chronic.

Stages of adaptation to illness or disability

Regardless of the nature of the illness, all individuals who become ill experience a similar sequence of psychosocial adaptation. This sequence includes both illness behavior and sick role behavior and occurs in stages. Illness behavior has been defined as "the way in which symptoms are perceived, evaluated and acted upon by a person who recognizes some pain, discomfort or other signs of organic (add emotional) malfunction."[6] As such, illness behavior determines whether diagnosis and treatment will begin at all. Sick role behavior may be defined as the activity an individual who considers himself ill performs for the purpose of getting well.[7]

Lederer[8] defines three time periods in one's experience of illness: (1) the transition from health to illness, (2) the stage of accepted illness, and (3) the stage of convalescence. More currently, Suchman[9] identifies these stages similarly, but clarifies points that Lederer subsumes: (1) symptom experience, (2) assumption of the sick role, (3) medical care contact, (4) the dependent patient role, and (5) recovery or rehabilitation.

These stages are generally experienced by all ill individuals whether their illness is temporary, progressive, or permanent, although they may not be manifested in the same way. Some major differences in the experience of the stages of illness are (1) the duration of each stage, (2) the degree of emotional or physical energy invested in each stage, (3) the relative necessity of reidentifying self, and (4) the relative necessity of reorganizing interaction with one's environment. These latter factors are largely dependent on and vary with the temporary, progressive, or permanent nature of the illness. Experience of these stages also varies with the demographic factors and cultural background. In some cultures, for example, the medical care contact stage may be totally bypassed and the entire illness experience may take place within the family. Socioeconomic status factors have been found to influence how readily an individual identifies his feelings as illness as well as how readily he seeks and accepts medical assistance. This chapter will not explore demographic or cultural factors, but will be concerned with generalizations regarding stages of illness in middle-class North America.*

Lederer's first stage, the transition from health to illness, is similar to Suchman's stages of symptom experience and assumption of the sick role. Notable characteristics of adaptation in this stage, if illness is insidious, are a perception of unusual, unpleasant, or even painful bodily or emotional changes with accompanying anxiety. Coping with this anxiety and unaccustomed feelings is partly dependent on individual patterns of dealing with similar previous problems and may result in a variety of behaviors. Mechanic[3] identifies the following among factors instrumental in affecting illness behavior at this stage:

1. Visibility and recognizability of deviant signs and symptoms
2. Extent to which the symptoms are perceived as serious and deviant
3. Extent to which symptoms disrupt family, work, and social activities
4. Frequency and persistence of signs and symptoms
5. Tolerance threshold of those who are exposed to and evaluate signs and symptoms
6. Available information, knowledge, and cultural assumptions and understandings of the evaluator
7. Availability and physical proximity of treatment resources and psychological and monetary costs of seeking treatment

Lederer and Suchman agree that denial may be prominent during this stage and may be demonstrated by a "plunge into health," but effectiveness of denial is minimal if symptoms are alarming. During this stage the individual may also attempt self-treatment, but as symptoms progress, neither self-treatment nor denial can be maintained as effective measures for adapting to the situation. Continuing discomfort and increasing symptomatology usually force the individual to seek assistance. It is at this point that the socially instituted aspects of illness become more apparent. As the individual seeks assistance, he generally first consults his reference group about his symptoms. The reference group concept refers to a group with which an individual identifies and the values and norms of which he shares. Reference group relationships are significant in forming judgment about one's self, a perspective of the world around one, and in regulating behavior. This group reflects status, roles, and norms and in so doing helps the individual to arrive at a decision about his signs and symptoms. Several sociologists stress the significance of reference group behavior at this stage of illness. Freidson[10] describes a "lay referral system" composed of those lay persons closest to the individual who play a major role in decision-making processes. The influence of significant social relationships in the individual's assumption of the sick role is paramount and can reinforce or challenge that assumption. Attempts to verify one's perceptions of being ill through the reference group is a process

---

*For elaboration of responses to illness differentiated by demographic factors, see Koos, E.: The health of regionville: what the people thought and did about it, New York, 1954, Columbia University Press, and Saunders, Lyle: Cultural differences and medical care, New York, 1954, Russell Sage Foundation.

that can result in any of four possible outcomes:

1. The individual attempts to enact the sick role, and his behavior is validated by his reference group.

2. The individual attempts to enact the sick role, and his behavior is not validated by his reference group.

3. The individual does not attempt to enact the sick role, but his reference group behaves toward him as though he were ill.

4. The individual neither attempts to enact the sick role, nor does his reference group identify it as an appropriate role for him.[11]

In elaboration of these possible outcomes, Hadley[11] states, ". . . whatever characterization of the sick role is derived . . . [is] dependent upon one or more relevant other roles toward which it would be oriented." That is, the sick role identifies some social regulation of behavior of the ill, but the development of characteristics of the sick role is dependent on the interaction between the individual and his reference group.

However, there are some exceptions to the general patterns of behavior during this stage as, for example, the individual who bypasses the "lay referral system," contacts professional helping persons, and tells his spouse that he is ill only after consulting a physician. Patients in emergency situations may experience this stage of illness in a condensed and critical way, which also bypasses the "lay referral system."

Whatever route is taken, the individual eventually arrives at the stage of accepted illness (Lederer) or the medical care contact stage (Suchman). That is, he abandons any pretext of being well and relinquishes the lay care system, actions that reflect a conscious choice on the part of the individual to define himself as ill (or deviant). It is probable that help-seeking behavior or the arrival at this stage is more comfortable in physical illness than in emotional illness. Not only are physical symptoms often perceived as more urgent, but they are also less likely to provoke rejection.

If agreement is reached between the individual and the physician that the former is ill, legitimation of the sick role occurs. Again, however, the aforementioned possibilities of verification (or non-verification) of illness are present. In mental illness the process of this stage is especially testy. Although many people have developed superficially understanding and tolerant attitudes toward the mentally ill, traces of the social feeling that these individuals are "not really sick" or "really cured" remain not only among lay people but also among some health professionals. Erikson states that a mentally ill person ". . . acquires recognition as a 'sick' person only at considerable pride, if at all; later he is able to withdraw from this recognition only with extreme difficulty."[12]

If consensual validation regarding illness does not take place between the individual and the physician, the deviation of illness is not legitimized and two outcomes may result: (1) the individual does not define himself as ill although the physician does or (2) the individual judges himself ill, but the physician does not. The latter situation leads to the stigmatized role to which the label of malingerer, hypochondriac, or crock is applied. Either outcome may indicate maladaptation and necessitates intervention.

Ideally, the period of accepted illness gradually ends after optimal regression and when medical treatment has reversed or controlled the pathogenic process. In reality, this stage often ends with pathogenic control or reversal only; the patient is then whisked into the stage of convalescence, with all of its expectations, without having been optimally allowed or assisted to resolve either the dependency state or regression characteristic of the stage of accepted illness.

The stage of convalescence (or recovery and rehabilitation) is a transition from illness to a state of optimal wellness and reflects another adaptive change in role. Again, there are four possible options in this stage. The individual can do one of the following:

1. Continue to enact the sick role and have his behavior validated by his reference group
2. Continue to enact the sick role and not have his behavior validated by his reference group
3. Attempt to relinquish the sick role and have his performance validated by others
4. Attempt to relinquish the sick role and not have his performance validated by others[11]

In her study of children who had corrective surgical procedures for congenital heart defect, Hadley identifies the role change in convalescence as being partly dependent on (1) the length of enactment of the sick role and (2) the reinforcement of that role by one's reference group; that is, the longer the sick role has been enacted and the more reinforced it is through interaction with significant others, the more difficult it will be for the patient to abandon this role.

If both the individual and his reference group are ready to allow transition out of the sick role, convalescence is marked by a return to optimal functions, an emotional reintegration, and the beginning of any necessary changes in life-style. It may be a turbulent stage for the individual, who must gently experiment with renewed strengths and adapt to remaining incapacities while working through his feelings about his illness. As Norris states, "the major work of convalescence is a reassessment of life's goals, modifying one's purposes and goals; looking and working toward new meaning and redirecting one's energy toward the development of one's potential for living."[13]

In concluding the discussion of stages of adaptation to illness, it must be said these stages are seldom as orderly as depicted. An enormous range of variations exists and these are only abstractions regarding some common elements of the illness experience. The stages identified are likely to occur in the presented order, but some may be condensed and others may be manifested differently.

Effects of hospitalization

Although in some cultures it is possible for an individual to experience all stages of illness without hospitalization, in America hospitalization often accompanies the sick role, necessitating additional adaptations. Differences between illness in the home and illness in the hospital are largely due to the social system of the hospital, which is reminiscent of Goffman's concept of "total institutions." In total institutions the three spheres of life (sleep, play, and work), which are generally separated by the places where they occur, the people with whom they occur, and the types of rational plans by which they are directed, are blended; that is, there is a breakdown of the barriers that normally separate these spheres of life. Consequently, Goffman defines a total institution as a place of residence in which large number of people live their lives together characterized by segregation from wider society and by a formal administration.[14] Moreover, individuals in total institutions are subject to a "mortification process"; the individual entering such an institution is divested of roles, possessions, privacy, and autonomy. He is placed in a position so that he can be "worked upon" by representatives of the institution; objects of self-image (body, thoughts, and possessions) are violated; and a defensiveness is often created in the individual. In brief, all symbols of self are assaulted, depriving the individual of security and trust in his self-concept.

Upon entering a new social situation

an individual usually begins to adapt by trying to define the situation; that is, he must be able to define his position in the situation, the positions of other participating individuals, and the symbols (language and gestures) used in the situation. All behavior that follows is a function of such definitions. Moreover, for adaptation to take place, there must be congruence of such definitions, that is, symbols and expectations must be similarly defined by the individual and participating others. In addition, the individual must develop the ability to take on the roles of others in the group. He must develop the ability to anticipate the responses of others in the situation and to include these roles in his repertoire of behavior. If there is incongruence in definitions and expectations, personal disorganization or maladaptation may result. These basic elements of social interaction in any setting also hold true in the hospital environment. The hospital social system may be totally foreign; roles are unclear, as are language and gestures. Easy entry into the social system of the hospital is not only complicated by its total institution-like, regimented characteristics, but also complicated by widely held conceptions of the hospital as a place for the very ill, a place where people go to die, to be mutilated, or to suffer, and a place where trust in those who care for one is often tenuous at best. Thus some degree of anxiety, fear, or even personal disorganization is probably not uncommon among individuals who are hospitalized for the first time. Coe[15] identifies four major ways by which an individual may adjust to the experience of hospitalization: (1) psychological withdrawal; (2) aggression in the form of resistance to rules and regulations or to therapeutic efforts; (3) integration into the institutional setting; and (4) acquiescence, or compliance with procedures, rules, and regulations. Integration into the institutional setting is, perhaps, the only mode of adjustment that is founded

on a socialization process; the other modes of adjustment are characterized by a probable absence of effective interaction and communication. Moreover, there seems to be limited assistance to the individual in socialization to this new social system. What adaptation does take place is most often facilitated or accomplished through patient relationships, not usually by patient-health professional relationships. Types of adjustment may overlap and vary with a number of factors such as the individual's personality, his perception of hospitals and health professionals, and the nature of his illness.

Stages of adaptation in temporary illness

A person with a temporary illness may move rapidly through all illness stages with relatively minimal stress and with effective, independent adaptation. Although the experience of symptoms may cause anxiety, adaptation is generally facilitated by the following factors: (1) the symptoms are common and familiar to laymen; (2) others in the "lay referral system" either know of effective home remedies or can comfortably recommend medical care on the basis of past experience, personal or vicarious; and (3) the deviance from a standard of health is socially acceptable and carries little stigma. However, social perception of temporary illness may vary with the nature of the illness and the organs or functions involved. Because certain areas of the body and certain functions assume good and bad connotations in early childhood, illnesses afflicting these areas are likely to evoke emotionally laden responses or provoke stigmatization.

In temporary illness, there is usually little need for prolonged denial, consensual validation regarding entry into the sick role is easily achieved, and medical care is sought and accepted readily. Acceptance of the sick role is facilitated for a number of reasons: (1) diagnosis is readily made; (2)

the course of illness is relatively predictable; (3) the diagnosis carries the connotation of recovery and cure; and (4) deviance is temporary and reversible. There is some threat to self-image by virtue of dysfunction, but the temporary nature of the dysfunction is reassuring and conducive to facile adaptation.

The patient may or may not need to be hospitalized; if he is hospitalized, it is usually for relatively short periods of time, so that the impact of the total institution-like system is neither severe nor sustained. Adjustment to hospitalization may be by acquiescence, since this route is the most expedient and undemanding. The effects of hospitalization are further ameliorated by the fact that the individual need not define a vast number of positions in the hospital social system, since a variety of health professionals are usually not involved in therapy and the primary physician's role is often constant. Dependency during the stage of accepted illness generally lasts for short periods of time because the patient's progress constantly decreases the need for it.

Convalescence is also likely to be rapid and is recovery in literal meaning: a regaining of the premorbid state of health and function. The adaptive role change of convalescence, like the role change in transition from health to illness, is usually marked by consensual validation as the patient, his reference group, and his physician agree regarding relinquishment of the sick role. So the deviance is socially acceptable and temporary; the sick role is totally abandoned; and the individual regains ability to fulfill normal expectations.

This is not to minimize the potential stress of temporary illness. For some individuals, temporary illness may constitute a crisis situation, and adaptation to illness may not be as fluid as described. Circumstances surrounding the illness may be of crisis proportions, especially if the illness is sudden, is unexpected, and affects crucial family interaction. Other factors, such as a predilection for aspects of the sick role, may contribute to a difficult adaptation to temporary illness.

Nursing implications in temporary illness

In preface to all discussion of nursing implications, it needs be said that it is not within the scope of this chapter to identify specific problems and related nursing interventions. Nursing functions will differ not only according to types of illness and stages of illness, but also according to specific diagnoses, illness contexts, and nurse-patient interactions. Given examples of intervention are general, abstract, and not intended to be comprehensive or indicative of priorities. A basic premise underlying exploration of nursing implications is that, through interaction, a nurse has the potential to create, to modify, or to control a therapeutic environment that will guide or support a patient's adaptation to the disequilibrium he is experiencing. Nursing function may be necessary in all stages of illness and may be performed either outside or within the hospital. In all stages, in all types of illness, the nurse must help the patient to define himself and his environment in order for adaptation to occur. Whenever and wherever the nurse functions, her goals must relate not only to the exigencies of adaptation to a particular stage of a particular type of illness, but also to facilitating the patient's progress to ultimate adaptation in optimal wellness.

In temporary illness nursing function is most commonly observed in the stage of accepted illness and in the hospital environment. Generally, a nurse's function in this type of illness is subordinate to that of a physician, who makes the decision regarding the presence and type of illness. In addition to being supportive of the medical regimen, nursing interventions with hospitalized, temporarily ill patients tend to be relatively standardized, technical, and largely oriented to the goal of cure. If the illness is severe and the health team disease oriented, the primary concern is that of saving life or preventing suffering. The health team often becomes concerned with other aspects of the patient's disequilibrium and adaptive deficits only when these reach crisis proportions. Intervention then is often directed to the goal of overcoming the crisis with secondary concern for the patient's long-term resolution. In other words the nurse often focuses on maintaining the patient's effective adaptive abilities and strengthening those that are inadequate for the present situation, but rarely focuses on helping the patient to develop adaptive mechanisms to deal effectively with future stressors.

A community nurse, for example, may be instrumental in a patient's stage of symptom experience by reflecting a highly discriminating norm of health and so guiding transition from health to illness. As a practitioner in the community she may also be called on to guide and to support a patient's recovery or convalescence. In any stage, in any setting, the nurse may derive her function from the "situational aspects" of illness, that is, those aspects deriving primarily from the patient's reaction to being ill.

From the health professional's perspective, temporary illness is usually relatively nonthreatening. It is common and predictable, progress is apparent, and recovery is ensured, making rewards to health professionals high and speedy. Recoveries generally outnumber deaths (except in emergency rooms and other specialized units), and because hospital stays are often short, deaths are most frequently responded to on the basis of social loss and not as loss of someone in whom there is a high degree of personal investment.

Stages of adaptation in progressive disability

Since many progressive disabilities have an insidious onset, the transition from health to illness may be prolonged and traumatic. Signs and symptoms are often vague, inconsistent, and difficult to classify, making denial a highly functional adaptive mechanism. Because of the limbolike nature of progressive illness, stress is severe and sustained; the individual does not know what to expect, when to expect it, or what it is. The patient's adaptation to the relentless diminution of ability depends in part on the timing of the progressions of the disability and the final expectation of the illness; that is, expectation of permanent disability or death. It is sometimes difficult to decide which is worse: to be in a state of exacerbation or not to know when symptoms will begin again and to live in constant, tense expectation. Because of often obscure symptoms, consensual validation regarding entry into the sick role is achieved with difficulty, and it is possible that arrival at the medical care contact stage is predominantly a product of the sophistication of the individual and the lay referral system in evaluating signs and symptoms. Morover, it is likely that medical care contact is postponed longer in progressive disability than in other types of illness, since symptoms, although persistent, do not quickly become alarming or grossly limit role and task performance. Even at the medical care contact stage, lack of clarity of signs and symptoms in early stages of illness make it difficult for physicians to intervene therapeutically or, sometimes, even to diagnose the disorder. Thus legitimated assumption of the sick role may be a lengthy and ambiguous process.

The sick role may be assumed with relief by the individual who has been struggling to achieve some equilibrium of self. Yet the sick role identified may be qualitatively unstable. Remissions and exacerbations cause fluctuation in states of relative illness and wellness, in capacities for role and task performance, and in dispensation from normal role obligations. Because the individual is often defined neither as "well" nor "ill," role conflicts may occur. There arises the necessity and extreme stress of selecting between adapting to these two organized perspectives for defining the situation, each perspective presenting contradictory expectations of behavior. The individual is, therefore, viewed as being in a "marginal role."

Inevitable functional or bodily changes compound the stress of maintaining integrity of self-concept. Because predictability of interaction with the physical environment is limited for persons with progressive disability, stable reformulation of body image is difficult. Role and task performances may become difficult, leading to at least a partial divesting of roles and generating feelings of unworthiness. Interaction may become increasingly stressful due to the patient's stigmatized function or appearance, which becomes gradually evident. The state of being "marginal" in itself may add to the stigma, and stigmatization may lead to participation in fewer social roles as well as a change in the nature, amount, and quality of interaction. The patient's reference group participates in this psychosocial disequilibrium and is often unable to help the patient.

Since progressive illness is often long term, medical treatment is prolonged and sometimes life long. Hospitalization is almost certain, repeated, and, at least initially, a highly stressful experience. A patient with progressive disability is more vulnerable to the effects of total institutions and mortification processes because his self-concept already may have been severely assaulted before hospitalization. By virtue of longer stays in the hospital, the effect of its total institution-like system is more apparent. There are more positions to define and more persons with whom to interact. The primary physician may need consultants; occupational and physical therapies may be required; financial assistance and vocational counseling may be necessary, all requiring the patient to identify a number of roles and counterroles. Moreover, the persons occupying these positions vary from one hospitalization to the next. The stripping process continues, although during severe exacerbations the patient may be too ill to notice. With repeated hospitalizations, a unique lay familiarity with the social system of the hospital may emerge as the patient becomes more adept at defining situations and roles. If the latter experience is a positive one, it may compensate for some of the more negative effects of hospitalization. Initially, however, with the patient's selfhood ill-defined, reference groups changing, an ever-lasting variety of other positions emerging, adaptation is difficult, and hospitalization may result in temporary retardation of the adaptive process.

Although the patient with temporary illness may adjust to hospitalization most expediently by acquiescence, the patient with progressive disability may respond differently. In fact, any continued acquiescence may be pathological and indicative of "overdependency." Due to acute anxiety, adjustment by psychological withdrawal may be common initially; this ultimately may be resolved through integration (socialization) into the hospital culture.

There is no one stage of convalescence or rehabilitation in progressive disability. Much time and energy are spent moving in and out of the stage of accepted illness, with any number of temporary remissions or "convalescent" periods. Some emotional, physical, and social equilibria may be reached during these periods, but these are tenuous at best, since every identified progression of the disability creates crisis and necessitates recycling of the adaptive process.

Some of the aforementioned elements of the illness experience are common to patients with progressive or permanent disabilities. Of particular note are the commonalities of need for adaptation to an irreversibly changed or changing state of being: need for lifelong medical care; stigma; lengthy hospitalization; and mourning for loss of function or appearance. The most salient difference may result from the continuous or recycling process of adaptation to a constantly changing state that is characteristic of progressive disability. Patients with progressive disabilities experience repeated and profound crisis situations that result in continued diminution of various capabilities; thus, there is the need to recycle the entire process of adaptation to integrate each new loss. In patients with permanent disability, the sudden and overwhelming loss of functions and role change occur only once, albeit extensively and profoundly. (Recycling of adaptation to illness in permanent disability may occur on another level, that of adaptation to secondary complications of the primary disability, such as urinary tract infections, decubiti, etc.)

Crate[16] writes of her experiences with patients with multiple sclerosis, stating that adaptation to the illness seems to follow a pattern of grieving, which she applies to all chronic illness. Using George Engel's model of the grieving process, she describes patients working through disbelief, developing awareness, reorganizing relationships with others, and resolving the loss and identity change. To this perspective, one may add points from the recent work of Elisabeth Kübler-Ross[17] on death and dying. Persons who are dying (or who are progressively or permanently ill) may initially respond with denial, "no, not me." As it is unconsciously impossible for us to conceive of our own deaths, so too it is distressing to conceive of one's own disability. Although few people go through life without experiencing temporary illness, progressive and permanent disabilities are less common and are generally thought of as events that befall "the other fellow."

Kübler-Ross also states that denial is used intermittently by dying patients throughout their illness, and she identifies this denial as a healthy way of dealing with a prolonged, intensely uncomfortable situation. With developing awareness of reality and decreased ability to maintain denial, anger (extroverted or introverted) may be a subsequent emotional response. Essentially the patient asks, "why me?" "What have I done to deserve this?" The patient may direct his anger at everyone around him—at health professionals for not restoring him and at God for letting it all happen. Before reorganization of relationships and resolution of loss, Kübler-Ross includes two other stages of adaptation— those of bargaining and depression. As he bargains, the patient says, "yes me, but . . ." and proposes an agreement in which he will receive a postponement of the inevitable in exchange for "good behavior." Depression is of two types—reactive and preparatory. Reactive depression is characterized by an active bemoaning of one's fate. The patient is aware of his inabilities to function and overtly mourns his loss(es) by complaining and crying. Preparatory depression is quiet and marked by overt sorrow as the loss is assimilated.

Persons with progressive or permanent disabilities grieve their losses. The person with a progressive disability, however, may find resolution illusive as the loss progresses.

Nursing implications in progressive disability

Except in acute phases of illness, most common nursing functions in progressive disability derive from care and coordination goals, as opposed to the cure goals that direct actions with temporarily ill patients.

Although the nurse may be functional during the patient's role transition from health to illness, she may be faced with the same vagaries of signs and symptoms as is the patient. In this stage major needs for intervention may derive from the patient's emotional reactions. While the patient seeks to assume the sick role, his reference group and, indeed, health professionals may dispute this adaptive behavior. The patient's trust in his perception of reality is thereby threatened; trust in others may falter; overt anxiety may be prominent; and emotional disorganization may occur. After illness is verified, remissions may lead to another situation in which nursing intervention may be necessary. In such instances, denial may be resorted to and should be accepted, although not supported.

In the stage of accepted illness, intervention partly derives from specific diagnoses and should include early rehabilitative measures. Included among such early rehabilitative measures is the nurse's assessment of the patient's and family's adaptation to the progressing disability. In addition to supporting presently adequate coping mechanisms, the nurse possesses a unique opportunity and responsibility to help the patient and his family develop coping mechanisms to adapt to often unpredictable future progressions.

As stated previously, there is no one stage of convalescence or rehabilitation in progressive disability. Indeed, the patient is in constant transition in and out of the sick role. More precisely, perhaps, the sick role, with its vicissitudes, becomes a marginal role; that is, the patient continues to enact that role intermittently and incompletely, and his behavior is intermittently validated. After acute episodes the nurse may need to function in a sustained, if frequently interrupted, stage of rehabilitation directed at maintenance of present function and prevention of further dysfunction. Moreover, because progressive disability is likely to affect all spheres of the patient's life, intervention by other helping professionals is often necessary. Family relationships, for example, are usually more severely disturbed in progressive disability than in temporary illness. As questions of continued abilities for role and task performance, of shifting family roles, and of vocations arise, such changes in life-style may necessitate referral to and coordination with other services.

Once the progressive nature of the disability is known to the patient, aspects of the grieving process and beginning resolutions of identity appear throughout all stages of adaptation. The skilled and knowledgeable nurse has the potential to help the patient in his struggle to reorganize his self-concept. As previously stated, the self develops only in relation to others, and thus a revised concept of one's self can emanate only from interaction. The significance of interaction with health professionals cannot be underestimated. It is in these interactions that the first meanings of disability are gleaned, and it is these interactions that set the stage for life as a person with a disability. It is important that the nurse facilitate communication and, in so doing, reflect reality to the patient. This is not to say that she imposes reality; rather, she represents a reference group whose perception of the patient is altered and whose definition and expectations the patient must define and incorporate. In socialization processes an individual first internalizes the attitudes of those closest and most important to him (significant others). Therefore the nurse may need to work with those significant to the patient, or she herself may eventually become a significant other to the patient. The nurse's function in this area includes many aspects, all of which must be decided on with the patient and some goals which may not be reached in that particular nurse-patient encounter. The nurse can help the patient to assess the following: (1) his feelings toward himself, (2) his perceptions of others' responses to him, (3) his identification with a new social group and his need to adopt the attitudes and the norms of revised and new reference groups, and (4) development of new roles to replace non-functional ones. She may also help him to identify an attainable ideal of being, supporting and guiding him as he strives toward it.

Continuity of care in progressive disability is a highly desirable goal and the nurse who enters into the patient's adaptation process when the illness is not new must first explore previous attempts at adaptation before beginning interventions. In progressive disability, however, these adaptive processes may not be sustained long enough for effective resolution, especially if remissions of the disability occur. Thus the nurse must help the patient not only to arrive at some equilibrium between progressions of illness, but also to be better prepared to cope and adapt to future events.

Caring for progressively ill individuals produces vastly different satisfactions and vulnerabilities than does caring for temporarily ill persons. Nursing of patients with progressive and permanent disabilities is necessarily marked from the start by a high degree of concern and empathy for the patient. Just as families often experience stages of illness conjointly with patients, nurses are also highly susceptible to the same experience. Since it is stressful for the nurse to be compassionate, to participate in the patient's world without losing awareness of her helping role, and to participate in his emotion, these patient care situations can be identified as nursing in "high emotional risk areas."[18] To readjust her perspective or to find sustenance the nurse may need to retreat periodically to be sensitively and comfortably therapeutic. For this, she will need the help of her colleagues.

Stages of adaptation in permanent disability

Two classifications of permanent disabilities can be identified: (1) those disabilities that become permanent after a prolonged progressive stage and (2) those that occur suddenly. (Congenital permanent disabilities have distinct characteristics and merit more exploration than lies within the scope of this chapter.) If the disability is the result of a long progressive process, it is possible that the progressiveness may have strengthened coping, but this is an issue meriting more investigation. The stages of adaptation to sudden disability more closely parallel the grieving stages described previously, each stage having major importance: (1) transition, including crisis, shock, and disbelief; (2) accepted illness, including mourning (including denial, anger, grieving, and depression) and self-devaluation as the loss feature of the new state of being predominates; and (3) resolution or adaptation. In sudden permanent disabilities (such as cerebrovascular accidents, paralysis resulting from accidents, or traumatic amputation) transition from health to illness is unexpected, unmistakable, and readily verified. The individual may bypass the elaborate decision-making process of the stage of symptom experience and may experience this stage as an overwhelming crisis. Denial is often a predominant feature of this stage and may continue for indefinite periods of time. It may begin with total denial of symptoms, followed by conditional acceptance—"yes, I'm disabled but not permanently." Further stages of adaptation may blend and be undifferentiated. Adaptation, although always a dynamic process, is not as constantly changing as in progressive disability and eventually attains more stability. The patient may revert from one stage to another, but eventually he arrives at some more or less stable resolution of, or adaptation to, the disability.

An individual with a permanent disability never leaves the sick role which, to varying degrees and in varying characterizations, becomes a major role in his life. Although the patient may resume some normal role obligations, he is also forever defined as deviant from health. Society nevertheless expects him to display a desire to "get well" and to cooperate with treatment, as is evidenced by elaborate rehabilitation planning. The deviance of permanent disability is ameliorated by rehabilitation—"doing something about the disability." Dependence, to varying degrees and in various ways, is also a permanent state, and some patients always remain grossly dependent on others for vital functions. Lifelong medical supervision and care tend to become absolute necessities, with complications requiring frequent, prolonged hospitalizations. Hospitals for the permanently disabled patient frequently bear a closer resemblance to total institutions than do general hospitals in some situations and may become the patient's permanent living environment. Adjustment to hospitalization is likely to be turbulent and may be aggravated by the occasional need to transfer from a long-term institution to a short-term institution (as for example, when surgery is required for a contracture). All types of adjustment may be experienced, ideally resolving in integration into the patient culture.

Permanent disability is socially perceived as a major deviance, is often severely stigmatized, and frequently becomes the focus for interaction. As stated previously, individuals entering a new interactional situation respond to it initially by defining the situation. Participants look for signs and symbols conveying social information about each other. It is, at least initially, on the basis of this perceived information and interpretation of this information that interaction proceeds. This process, which structures expectations of others, is the first and foremost basis of social interaction. This phenomenon becomes particularly poignant in the situation of the individual who is permanently disabled. Information regarding him is evident and often interpreted as stigma; it then becomes the focus for interaction. Goffman[12] stated that the stigmatized individual is, at least initially, perceived and interacted with

on the basis of his changed appearance and/or functioning alone. At best the disability leads to strained interaction in which the individual and others try to cope with the deviant aspect of being by trying to ignore it, thereby inadvertently and severely hampering interaction. If disability is sudden, the often drastic but inevitable change in roles, task performance, and self-conception may be overwhelming. Changes in self-image and modes of interaction are an eventual necessity: new roles and new modes of interaction must be formed. The sudden onset of a disability that was not anticipated may make the process of adapting body image and ego identity more difficult than when disability advances in stages. Intense and painful examination of the meaning of the disability is sustained and, when supplemented by other long-term psychological factors such as guilt, depression, and feelings of "nonbeing," may necessitate psychiatric intervention.

The stage of accepted illness "ends" when the patient indicates motivation toward resolution, an event that may precede or succeed any degree of physical progress. The final stage of adaptation to progressive or permanent disability is ideally one of physical or psychosocial rehabilitation or resolution. The stage of convalescence for persons with progressive or permanent disabilities is more correctly identified as a stage of rehabilitation from a medical frame of reference. Convalescence, recovery, and rehabilitation have distinct, functional differences, but are often used interchangeably. Convalescence, derived from a Latin word meaning, "to become strong" shares the static, indistinct quality of the word "chronic." Recovery, strictly defined, means a regaining of a former state of health and should be used only in relation to temporary illness. Rehabilitation, on the other hand, ideally begins with the patient's first medical care contact and is the process of guiding an individual to maximal capacity and independence in all spheres of life. Wright identifies factors in overcoming the process of mourning and moving toward resolution as the enlargement of one's scope of values, that is, the emotional realization of the existence of values other than those destroyed by the disability.[19] This enlargement of value scope needs to include a change of values in relationships. Old reference groups are no longer appropriate reflectors of self and status, and slowly yield in importance to others that more accurately reflect new meanings, values, and expectations.

To these resolutory factors, one may add the words of Frankl[20]:

Again and again we have seen that an appeal to continue life, to survive the most unfavorable conditions, can be made only when such survival appears to have meaning. That meaning must be specific and personal, a meaning which can be realized by this one person alone. . . . Man should not ask what he may expect from life, but rather understand that life expects something from him.*

This is perhaps the most basic and most difficult aspect of rehabilitation for the patient, his reference group, and health personnel. Until all accept that the patient's life has meaning, the process of adaptation to disability cannot be facilitated.

It can be said, then, that the individual with a sudden permanent disability may expend the greatest amounts of time and energy in the stage of rehabilitation. More so than for the individual with a progressive disability, the sick role becomes adaptive and a primary basis for interaction that is both consistently accepted by the patient and reinforced in his reference group relationships. Variations in this adaptation process are significantly due to individual differences, the degree of preparation for disability, the degree of the

disability, the age at which disability occurs, and the meaning the disability holds for the patient.

Nursing implications in permanent disability

Nursing functions in permanent disability are generally concentrated after medical care contact has been made and are usually oriented to care and coordination. Because complications of the primary disability may produce recycling transitions from health to illness within the disability (for example, the patient with paraplegia who develops a urinary tract infection), the nurse may also be functional in this stage. The permanence of the disability suggests a lifelong process arriving at some equilibrium of adaption and suggests potential nursing functions in all stages of illness. In all stages the nurse's major role is oriented to facilitating the patient's adaptation to permanently and profoundly changed external and internal environmental circumstances. The patient's disability naturally affects his perception of the environment, and his perception, in turn, affects his decision making. Old cues and symbols previously used to structure physical and social environments and to give them meaning are no longer valid or reliable. The nurse can help the patient to reassess them and to reorganize new meanings with the goal of developing trust in the changed environment. This process requires the nurse to be able to perceive the environment as the patient does, an endeavor that cannot be accomplished without expending a great deal of empathy and energy.

Providing nursing care for those permanently disabled can be a difficult and depleting endeavor. In addition to the requisite ability of perceiving the environment as the patient does, emotional states of intense dependence, regression, denial, anger, and grieving are difficult to deal with over long periods of time in a close

---

*From Frankl, Viktor E.: The doctor and the soul, New York, 1965, Alfred A. Knopf, Inc.

relationship. The nurse's skill and sensitivity may help her to recognize the function of these feeling states and to accept them, but her skill and sensitivity may be exhausted, necessitating temporary withdrawal. To provide effective and supporting care of patients regardless of their illness, the nurse must know herself; this is particularly true in "high emotional risk areas." Prerequisite to the nurse's "therapeutic use of self," a major facet of nursing in progressive and permanent disability, is identification of herself—who she is, her motivations, her aspirations, the meaning of life to her as well as the meaning of loss; all these beliefs and attitudes merit exploration and identification to permit her to recognize her feelings as being distinct from those of the patient and at the same time demonstrate respect for both. It is only through frequent and even uncomfortable self-examination that the nurse becomes an other-directed individual, able to interact with the patient, to enter into his world, and to allow the nursing process to evolve from this interaction. And it is only through such interactions that the nurse can assess the patient's perceptions and capacities, promote a mutual definition of goals, and enhance the patient's involvement in his own therapeutic process. The patient's involvement in the therapeutic regimen cannot be underestimated as a necessity. The individual is an active agent in maintaining a stable environment, a fact that health professionals do not consistently note. The inadvertent imposition of goals on the patient often results in disappointment for both and, if repeated, may lead to a gradual diminishing of trust and interaction. Mutual cooperation, on the other hand, can have the highly valued results of the patient's pride in his strengths and coping abilities and of positive expectations of the future. Ultimately, as Crate has stated, "it is the patient's illness and his adaptation."[16]

Other emotional hazards are basic to the "high emotional risk" phenomenon. First, despite socialization into a helping profession, health professionals do not always internalize the knowledge gained and may react to a disabled individual solely on the basis of his deviant appearance or function. The stigma attached to disability is partially the result of some answers to the question, "why did it happen to him," and partially the result of the threat "it could have happened to me," which affects health professionals no less than it affects lay persons. Second, as mentioned, health professionals are also susceptible to experiencing a patient's adaptation to illness as well as the patient, but the consequences of such empathy can be the immobilization of professional skills. Finally, responses to patients who are permanently disabled may reflect a nurse's motivations for entering a health profession. Nurses are dedicated to "help sick people get well" and often equate recovery with success in meeting this goal. When the goal of cure cannot be achieved, feelings of failure are often experienced, forgetting that part of that stated goal is to nurture. Bettelheim states, ". . . I believe that the true virtue, the true calling of the nurse . . . [consists] in the two aspects contained in the very name of the profession: to nurse and to nurture." He further states that nursing is one of the few professions with which every human being has direct, meaningful contact, but that nursing comes first because it stands at the very beginning of our lives.[21] So it is with nursing in progressive and permanent disability. The nurse is present at the beginning of a restructured life and is in a position to affect the very course of the life by giving of herself.

Summary

Since psychosocial adaptation to illness may affect the physical course of that illness, it is significant for health professionals to understand how individuals are de-

Table 8. Stages of adaptation to temporary, progressive, and permanent illness or disability

	Transition from health to illness	*Stage of accepted illness*	*Convalescence*
Temporary illness	Signs and symptoms relatively easily recognized and validated in reference group relationships; assumption of sick role uncomplicated	Deviance from wellness known to be temporary; adaptation transient; change in self-concept minor; usually no stigma; impact of hospitalization limited	No residual physical or behavioral aberration; sick role leave taking facilitated by overt progress toward higher level of wellness; recovery in literal meaning: regaining of premorbid functions
Progressive disability	Signs and symptoms may be vague, ambiguous and insidious; transition may be prolonged and traumatic; assumption of sick role difficult; transition may be repeated with each progression of the disability	May be postponed due to vague transition period; this stage vacillating and unpredictable, especially if there are remissions and exacerbations; adaptation is to marked and continuous changes; sick role has vicissitudes; self-concept is in transition and the sick role becomes a marginal life role; impact of hospitalization is severe and often repeated; stigma may be covert	Virtually none, although remissions may be "convalescences"; no return to premorbid levels of function; some residual aberration that is constantly progressing
Permanent disability	Signs and symptoms may be sudden and abrupt or may occur after long progression; in either case, disability is usually overt and consensual validation regarding transition from health to illness is immediate	Sick role becomes a major life role that is verified in reference group relationships; grieving over loss of body part or function may occur in this stage; impact of hospitalization severe and prolonged; stigma usually overt; adaptation is in relation to permanent, significant change	Marked residual aberration; rehabilitation—physical, emotional, and social incorporation of the disability, reassessment and reorganization of environment, self-concept, and significant relationships; no return to premorbid levels of function related to the disability

fined as ill, how they adopt the sick role, and how they emerge from it.

This chapter explores some aspects of adaptation to illness in relationship to the sick role and to different types of illness, such as temporary illness and progressive and permanent disability. The latter classification, with its ramifications, is superimposed on models that define stages of adaptation to illness from a psychosocial frame of reference. The emerging framework allows exploration of some abstractions regarding the illness experience as they differ in type, stage, and implication for nursing. Related concepts of self, norms, reference groups, deviance, and interaction are explored as an integral part of this framework (Table 8).

References

1. Parsons, Talcott: Definitions of health and illness in the light of American values and

social structure. In Jaco, E. G., editor: Patients, physicians and illness, New York, 1958, The Free Press.

2. Faulkner, William: As I lay dying, New York, 1930, Random House, Inc.

3. Mechanic, David: Medical sociology, New York, 1968, The Free Press.

4. Martin, Nancy: Nursing in rehabilitation. In Beland, Irene, editor: Clinical nursing: pathophysiological and psychosocial aproaches, New York, 1970, The MacMillan Co.

5. Goffman, Erving: Stigma, Englewood Cliffs, N. J., 1963, Prentice-Hall, Inc.

6. Mechanic, David: The concept of illness behavior, J. Chron. Dis. **15:**189-194, 1962.

7. Kasl, S. V., and Coff, S.: Health behavior, illness behavior, and sick-role behavior, Arch. Environ. Health **12:**531-540, 1966.

8. Lederer, Henry D.: How the sick view their world, J. Soc. Issues **8:**4-15, 1952.

9. Suchman, Edward A.: Stages of illness and medical care, J. Health Soc. Behav. **6:**114-128, 1965.

10. Freidson, Eliot: Patients' views of medical practice, New York, 1961, Russell Sage Foundation.

11. Hadley, Betty Jo: Becoming well: a study in role change, unpublished doctoral dissertation, University of California, Los Angeles, Jan., 1966.

12. Eridson, Kai T.: Patient role and social uncertainty: a dilemma of the mentally ill. In Milton, Ohmer, editor: Behavior disorders: perspectives and trends, New York, 1965, J. B. Lippincott Co.

13. Norris, Catherine M.: The work of getting well, Amer. J. Nurs. **69:**2118-2121, Oct., 1969.

14. Goffman, Erving: Asylums, Chicago, 1961, Aldine Publishing Co.

15. Coe, Rodney M.: Sociology of medicine, New York, 1970, McGraw-Hill Book Co.

16. Crate, Marjorie: Nursing functions in adaptation to chronic illness, Amer. J. Nurs. **65:**72-76, Oct., 1965.

17. Kübler-Ross, Elisabeth: Lectures at the Seventh Kramer Foundation Educational Institute in the series, Toward Therapeutic Long Term Care, University of Chicago Continuing Education Center, Chicago, Jan. 16-17, 1970.

18. Holsclaw, Pamela: Nursing in high emotional risk areas, Nurs. Forum **4:**36-45, 1965.

19. Wright, Beatrice A.: Physical disability: a psychological approach, New York, 1960, Harper & Row, Publishers.

20. Frankl, Viktor E.: The doctor and the soul, New York, 1965, Alfred A. Knopf, Inc.

21. Bettelheim, Bruno: To nurse and to nurture, Nurs. Forum, **1:**60-76, 1962.

Chapter 30

Anxiety: a concept in the care of the heart surgery patient

Judy Haselhorst

The concept of anxiety is not formally included in preoperative evaluation protocols for most patients undergoing surgery. Nevertheless, surgeons and anesthesiologists often cancel or postpone surgery for patients who seem highly anxious or emotionally upset, and nurses become quite concerned about such patients.

Anxiety in a patient is frequently considered a negative or potentially hazardous experience. However, Basowitz and associates[1] claim that anxiety is a precursor of defensive or adjustive processes as well as a possible consequence of their breakdown. Thus anxiety can stimulate adaptive processes, a factor that is generally considered to be positive and beneficial. Several studies have demonstrated the increased ability to learn and the increased perception that accompany low levels of anxiety.[2,3] On the other hand, anxiety can result in negative or harmful situations; overuse of defensive processes and coping mechanisms can lead to behavior problems and maladaptation that affect the person's social relationships and psychological ability to deal with additional stress.

Physiological manifestations of anxiety (changes in blood pressure, pulse and respiration, and cardiac rhythmicity) can be life threatening for a cardiac surgery patient who is already in physical disequilibrium. If the goal of health care is to help a patient attain an optimal state of health and prevent complications and if the goal for achieving the optimal state of health in a cardiac surgery patient is to decrease energy needs of the body and therefore the burden on the heart, then during particular phases of a patient's surgical experience it may be crucial to help control this patient's anxiety, thereby decreasing his energy requirements to avoid life-threatening complications. However, anxiety may be desirable at less dangerous points during a patient's hospitalization. Decisions as to the most desirable course of action must await empirical investigation.

This chapter focuses on the concept of anxiety, methods of measurement, some applicable research findings, and use of the concept in caring for the heart surgery patient.

The concept of anxiety

*Anxiety is the state in which a being
is aware of its possible non-being.*

Paul Tillich[4]

Major surgery can be regarded as a profound threat to a person due to confrontation with several types of imminent danger—acute pain, bodily damage, helplessness, and the possibility of death. Such threats to one's being evoke anxiety or fear. These two states often co-exist and may be highly related to each other. Anxiety is most commonly defined as a disturbed mental state regarding some future or uncertain event that elicits painful or disturbing feelings of uneasiness or suspense.[5] In addition, the anxious individual usually cannot precisely identify the cause of his apprehension.[6] However, fear is usually evoked by an identifiable threat; it is accompanied by a desire to avoid or escape that which is threatening. May[7] defines anxiety as "the apprehension cued off by a threat to some value which the individual holds essential to his existence as a personality."* In a similar vein, Cattell and Scheier[8] define anxiety as a "phenomenon that manifests itself in immediate experience as an unpleasant emotional feeling with a characteristic anticipatory character—the expectation of impending danger."†

The process of heart surgery (that is, the patient's entire course, pre- and postoperatively) can be long and involved. The patient meets numerous health professionals and is faced with many crucial decisions and situations. Phases a patient goes through in the heart surgery experience include the following: referral by the family physician, the diagnostic phase involving both medical and surgical aspects, the operative phase involving mainly surgical aspects, the convalescent phase involving short- and long-term contact with medical and surgical aspects, and return to the family physician.[9] Throughout these phases the patient is necessarily in a stressful situation. The variety of physically stressful diagnostic and evaluative procedures and the uncertainty concerning the future can lead to a feeling of uneasiness or anxiety.

Various factors contributing to anxiety have been identified. Cattell lists conflict, repression, somatic illness, uncertainty, insufficient education, and isolation from the community as being threatening.[8] Titchener and Levine[10] are more general in stating that the anxiety which one finds in surgical patients "is not related as much to the object of their fear as it is to personality structure, unconscious motivation, imagination, fantasy, early history, and the form of adaptation characteristic for the individual."* That is, two people confronted with the same surgical procedure having the same past physical history and probability for survival after surgery may react differently due to (1) the meaning the individual attaches to his illness and surgery and (2) the individual's previous adaptive patterns. It is also conceivable that one of these patients might survive and the other not. Titchener also states that the objects of fear in the surgical experience are loss of life, loss of body part, fear of castration, and fear of separation.[10] Levitt[3] is more general in stating that anxiety occurs as a result of restriction on one's behavior in gratifying his needs, desires, and impulses.

Several studies support these factors as causes of anxiety associated with surgery. Cassaday and Altrocchi[11] interviewed forty

---

*From May, Rollo: The meaning of anxiety, New York, 1950, The Ronald Press Co.

†Cattell, R. B., and Scheier, I. H.: The nature of anxiety: a review of thirteen multivariate analyses comprising 814 variables, Psychol. Rep. 4:351-388, 1958.

*From Titchener, J. L., and Levine, M.: Surgery as a human experience: the psychodynamics of surgical practice, New York, 1960, Oxford University Press, Inc.

patients to elicit their concerns regarding surgery. They found that the most important concerns of almost half the patients were related to diagnosis and death. The other most important concerns, in order of their frequency, were physical discomfort, socioeconomic problems, a feeling of helplessness, and fear of disability. Robbins[12] found that pain, duration and curability of the illness, treatment, changes in ability to function, social devaluation, financial loss, separation from family, and death were definite causes of anxiety. In a rather extensive study of surgical patients, Janis[2] found that many patients feared loss of control such as incontinence as well as fear of death. Janis contends that there are events in the surgical experience such as unfamiliar organic sensations, restriction of body functions, and enforced hygienic routines that convey information that "all is not going well."[2] These events are stimuli for the development of anxiety.

A major question to be asked is, how does anxiety affect the heart surgery patient? If it can be agreed that surgery presents a threat to a person's being, it can be assumed that heart surgery patients will experience some anxiety during the surgical experience. There have been several studies regarding psychological disturbances occurring in patients with heart surgery. Egerton and Kay[13] noted postoperative delirium (motor restlessness, disordered thinking, and sensory disturbances) in 41% of the sixty adult patients in their study. They cite as possible precipitating factors sleep deprivation, drugs, abnormal sensory input, and dehydration. Predisposing factors included a significant incidence of mental illness in the patients who experienced delirium, brain damage, and current pressing personal problems not related to hospitalization. Could the abnormal sensory input have led to increased anxiety with delirium as a defense mechanism? Kornfeld and associates[14] studied 119 adult patients having either open or closed heart surgery. They found overall incidence of delirium to be 38%. Of the patients having repair of a congenital cardiac defect, closed mitral commissurotomy, and aortic valve replacement, the incidence of delirium was 30% in each of these procedures; in mitral valve replacements, 40%, and in double valve replacements, 78%. There was no significant relationship between delirium and age, sex, marital status, duration of surgery, bypass time, or hypothermia time.[14] Most of Kornfeld's patients looked back on the experience as disturbing due to the frightening atmosphere, unusual sounds, a sense of being chained, and lack of sleep. It is interesting to note that the delirium occurred after a lucid period of three to four days, which suggests that postoperative factors or unresolved preoperative concerns may be operative in these psychological reactions. Kornfeld suggests that the onset of these reactions resembles the psychoses of sleep and sensory deprivation. However, other factors also need to be considered, such as sensory overstimulation and social deprivation. Krauss and Ruiz[15] investigated anxiety and time perspective and found that highly anxious individuals perceive time events more in the past than in terms of present or future. This may occur when the patient attempts to lower his anxiety by avoiding consideration of present or future unknowns or threatening situations.

Studies indicate that some researchers believe anxiety can be detrimental to a patient's course, whereas other researchers believe anxiety can be advantageous. A question requiring further investigation is, what is the effect of anxiety on the patient's postoperative course? Kennedy and Bakst[16] studied the influence of emotions on the outcome of cardiac surgery. They claim that anxiety relates directly to survival. The sample of 136 patients was divided into six groups according to their preoperative emotional state and desire to have surgery. The researchers found the death rate lowest in the group best motivated for surgery. There was a higher incidence of medical and psychological complications in the groups with higher anxiety and ambivalence toward surgery.[16] Janis found that patients with high- or low-preoperative fear exhibited behavioral and psychological disturbances after surgery, whereas patients with moderate amounts of preoperative fear had a more normal recovery.[2]

From these and other studies[17] it is evident that psychological disturbances often occur after heart surgery and that a patient's anxiety level affects his surgical experience.

It is helpful to consider Spielberger's conceptual framework in understanding types of anxiety.[18] The first step in identifying a type of anxiety is cognitive appraisal of the external stimuli (stresses). This appraisal is affected by internal stimuli (for example, thoughts, feelings, or biological needs) and by A-Trait (anxiety proneness). A situation may be perceived as threatening or nonthreatening. If it is nonthreatening, a behavioral sequence occurs in direct response to the situation. If the situation is threatening, one of two reactions occur. There may be feelings of apprehension (A-State) and activation of the autonomic nervous system, or defense mechanisms may be initiated that alter cognitive appraisal. With occurrence of anxiety state or use of defense mechanisms, a behavioral response is initiated to avoid or cope with the situation.

Measurement of anxiety

> *Whatever exists, exists in some quantity and can in principle be measured.*
>
> R. B. Cattell[19]

Anxiety may be manifested behaviorally or physiologically. Cattell ranks the following physiological variables according to their degree of association with anxiety:

(1) increases in systolic pulse pressure, heart rate, respiration rate, and basal metabolic rate; (2) a decrease in electrical skin resistance; (3) increases in urine acidity and ketosteroid excretion; and (4) decreases in alkalinity of saliva and serum cholinesterase.[20] Deane and Zeaman[21] found the heart rate accelerated in normal persons in anxious anticipation of an electrical shock; after the shock there was marked cardiac deceleration. Magendantz and Shortsleeve[22] found S-T segment and T-wave changes in the electrocardiographic patterns of patients without cardiovascular disease who exhibited anxiety. These physiological variables, mostly autonomic nervous system reactions, can be used to monitor state anxiety. Changes in these variables can indicate an increase or decrease in anxiety level, although other factors may enter into the change, for example, diurnal variation. The fact that these physiological variables are readily observable and are not voluntarily controlled is a definite advantage for their use as an aid for identifying the presence of state anxiety. On the other hand, Levitt[3] states that physiological measures are seldom related to each other, to psychological indexes, or to intensity of stress, and that patterns of physiological reactivity to anxiety are idiosyncratic. In addition, physiological measures are often highly variable between individuals as well as in any one individual, expensive when obtained over a prolonged period of time, and primarily limited to measuring the state aspect of anxiety. Thus the use of physiological indexes to measure anxiety is highly controversial.

Along with physiological measures, there are numerous psychological tools to measure anxiety. The following is a noninclusive sample of the major tools used. Levitt classifies as most important the projective techniques (for example, ink blots) in which the person builds structure around vague stimuli, thereby revealing his personality. This is one method of measuring covert anxiety, although a major disadvantage of this technique is the skill and training required for interpretation of results.[3] The most popular technique is the inventory or questionnaire in which the person responds to a series of items according to what he thinks he feels. The resulting score is considered a quantitative account of the person's anxiety level.[3] Although this instrument requires only a short period of time and is easy to administer and score, subjects may repeatedly choose the same response category or select the category that is socially desirable rather than the one expressing their true feelings. These disadvantages can be minimized in the test construction. One of the first anxiety inventories developed was the Taylor manifest anxiety

SELF-ANALYSIS QUESTIONNAIRE

A. State anxiety form

	Not at all	Somewhat so	Moderately so	Very much
1. I feel calm	1	2	3	4
3. I am tense	1	2	3	4
9. I feel anxious	1	2	3	4
20. I feel pleasant	1	2	3	4

B. Trait anxiety form

	Almost never	Sometimes	Often	Almost always
21. I feel pleasant	1	2	3	4
23. I feel like crying	1	2	3	4
27. I am "calm, cool, and collected"	1	2	3	4
31. I am inclined to take things hard	1	2	3	4

Fig. 13

Statements from Spielberger's "Self-Analysis Questionnaire" illustrating the state, **A**, and trait, **B**, forms of the instrument. (Reproduced by special permission from Spielberger, C. D.: The state-trait anxiety, 1969, Consulting Psychologists Press Inc.)

scale (MAS). This inventory consisted of a number of items taken from the Minnesota multiphasic personality inventory (MMPI). This scale (MAS) measures a predisposition to anxiety rather than anxiety in immediate state.[3] The IPAT anxiety scale (developed by R. B. Cattell and his co-workers at the Institute for Personality and Ability Testing through factor analysis and identification of sixteen personality traits) seems to measure anxiety proneness. The items do not refer to a momentary state but rather a continuing situation—the trait factor. However, the instrument is well developed and extensively used.[8, 21, 23, 24] A third inventory is the state-trait anxiety inventory (STAI) developed by C. D. Spielberger.[25] This inventory incorporates both state and trait measures using a different form for each (Fig. 13). Levitt states, "The STAI is the most carefully developed instrument, from both theoretical and methodological standpoints."[3] It is easily and rapidly administered, scored, and readily understood by subjects.

Two factors important to consider when measuring an individual's state and level of anxiety are (1) the individual's awareness of his anxiety and (2) the fluctuation of anxiety levels. It is also important to distinguish between overt and covert anxiety. Overt anxiety involves a recognition of the feeling state; the individual is often aware of his anxiety and frequently is willing to discuss his concern.[19] Covert anxiety is concealed anxiety or anxiety that is not readily apparent to the individual or to others.[19] In addition, covert anxiety involves the state and trait types of anxiety. State anxiety is a condition of the moment, "a transitory emotional state or condition that varies in intensity and fluctuates over time."[25] State anxiety (A-State) can be measured with self-report questionnaires or physiological measures such as heart rate, blood pressure, or galvanic skin response. Trait anxiety (A-Trait) "refers to relatively stable individual differences in anxiety proneness, that is, to differences in the disposition or tendency to respond with elevation in A-State in situations that are perceived as threatening."[25] It is necessary to distinguish between state and trait anxiety, since specific stresses (for example, surgery) may produce different characteristic levels of anxiety in different individuals.

In summary, researchers list many behavioral disturbances and heightened defense mechanisms that result from anxiety. Investigations that include heart surgery patients have shown the occurrence of delirium and other behavioral disturbances in the postoperative and convalescent periods. Physical concomitants of anxiety show biochemical and physiological changes that could influence the physical convalescence of the heart surgery patient. Uncertainty, isolation from the community, and unusual somatic sensations can cause anxiety in any person, particularly a surgical patient. Increased death rates and increased rates of psychological and medical complications have been found in patients with high anxiety levels.

If the goal of the health team is to promote the highest state of mental and physical health possible, then it is necessary to systematically evaluate the outcome of the surgical process as it relates to the patient's pre- and postoperative physical and mental status, the medical therapy, and the nursing intervention.

Additional aspects of pre- and postoperative anxiety

Using the definition of anxiety presented in this chapter, it can be assumed that most hospitalized patients will experience some degree of anxiety. As previously stated, high levels of anxiety are related to increased morbidity and mortality after heart surgery and to psychological disturbances. Also present in anxiety states are autonomic nervous system responses, including increases in blood pressure, pulse, respiration, and metabolism. Briefly stated, anxiety states consume energy. It is often necessary to help the heart surgery patient decrease his energy requirements, thereby increasing the possibility of cardiac compensation. However, anxiety has been shown to be useful in preparing a person for future events, and therefore it is probable that some anxiety is quite necessary for a heart surgery patient. Nevertheless, it is frequently of greater importance to decrease or cope with a patient's anxiety level than to stimulate anxiety.

As soon as a tentative diagnosis of heart disease is made by a patient's private physician, it becomes a stimulus for anxiety. There may be a feeling of helplessness from inability to control the situation and insecurity about what will happen next. But most of all there may be a threat to the self-image. Depending on the degree of cardiac damage (assuming acquired heart disease), the patient may have been relatively well, at least in his own estimation. Now his role is threatened, be it breadwinner, housewife, or student. Referral to a cardiac team is made and a thorough physical evaluation begins. This evaluation most often includes cardiac catheterization and pulmonary function and hematology studies. These procedures are physically as well as psychologically threatening, and, in addition, the patient encounters a variety of health personnel who are for the most part unfamiliar to him. He may feel helpless when subjected to stringent hospital routines and multiple tests without opportunity to manipulate the situations. Although the patient receives some information regarding what to expect during a scheduled test (for example, cardiac catheterization) from the nurse, doctor, or other patients, if he has never undergone the test be-

fore, he develops fantasies (or as Janis puts it, he goes through the work of worrying) to prepare himself to cope with any eventuality. Development of anxiety depends on the degree of reality of the fantasies. If the patient has been told what he will experience and what he will see, and thus what he can realistically expect, high-anxiety levels will probably be avoided in the evaluation and diagnostic phases. Another factor causing anxiety is isolation from a familiar social setting and from significant others. Absence from family and friends who give predictable responses to one's behavior and provide needed support during periods of stress is anxiety producing.

Once the decision to operate has been made, new anxiety-producing stimuli occur. These may include fear of the anesthetic, uncertainty concerning the success of surgery, and fear of death. There may be anxiety about the function of a new valve, whether it will be heard by others or become ineffective or malfunctioning. Surgery is frequently delayed to allow time for the patient to rest and hopefully achieve some degree of cardiac compensation. This time seems long and unnecessary to the patient who may complain that the doctors are just putting him off, that his case is worse than they thought, that they really do not know what is wrong with him, and that he cannot rest with all those tests. Anxiety levels may increase at this time. It is also during this time that a clinical nurse specialist visits the patient to teach him about his surgery. For some patients, knowing that they will have tubes, intravenous feedings, and monitors makes it easier for them to adjust in the postoperative period. However, for other patients this information is either not heard or is used for exaggerated worrying, thereby causing increased levels of anxiety. These and other situations can act as stimuli for anxiety in the preoperative phase.

The first forty-eight hours are often

crucial for the heart surgery patient. He is surrounded by equipment, personnel, and often by other critical or acutely ill patients. There may be environmental stimuli such as words or expressions by personnel or unusual functioning of equipment that the patient interprets as threatening. In some cases the endotracheal tube remains in place for twenty-four hours during which the patient may be unable to summon the attention of a nurse, since intensive care units are often devoid of signal lights. Theoretically, there is someone in attendance in an intensive care area at all times. However, there are short periods of time when the nurse or attendant is out of the room, and if the patient feels he needs help and is unable to summon anyone, he may panic. As previously stated this expenditure of energy does not facilitate cardiac compensation. DeMeyer's study[26] indicates that patients (1) felt tied down by electrocardiograph leads and unable to escape the environment; (2) were disturbed by the noise around them and the number of persons checking on them; (3) lost their sense of time because of perpetual light; (4) were disturbed when people talked about them without including them; and (5) felt a sense of urgency in the environment. As convalescence proceeds, anxiety-provoking stimuli decrease, except for the patient whose heart disease and limitations fulfilled dependency needs.[27] In this patient, relief from the physical limitations of heart disease tends to produce anxiety.

Although the preceding information has been related to the heart surgery patient, it can be applied to most hospitalized patients with modifications for the individual patient, his disease process, and his hospital course.

Recognizing and coping with anxiety

Once one accepts that anxiety is usually present in patients and that high levels of anxiety are undesirable, it is necessary to be able to recognize anxiety states in order to cope with them. McReynolds[28] lists numerous behaviors that are descriptive of anxiety including trembling, moist hands, nervous mannerisms (for example, tapping feet or rubbing chin), pacing, headaches, tremulous or quivering voice, sighing, flushed or pale face, digestive disturbances, sleep disturbances, crying, and biting nails. One can also assess the level of anxiety by the ability of the patient to perceive the situation around him. In mild anxiety one is alert and perceptive. With moderate anxiety there is decreased ability to perceive and concentrate, and muscular tension usually develops. And in severe anxiety only details are perceived, time and events become distorted, and there is obvious physical and emotional discomfort.

Once recognized, anxiety must be dealt with, and nurses serve an important function when they assist patients to cope with their anxiety. A nurse, observing behavioral manifestations of anxiety and commenting, "you seem upset," may stimulate a torrent of complaints, crying, or withdrawal. All too often the encounter ends here with both nurse and patient feeling uncomfortable. Titchener suggests that the most effective way of dealing with anxiety is to provide the patient with opportunity to perceive the anxiety, assimilate it, and discharge his feelings.[10] This would entail continuing the encounter with the patient and helping him recognize the connection between the anxiety and his behavior. This could be done by asking him what he does when he is nervous or upset. The next step involves helping the patient formulate the cause of the anxiety. The following is an example of a situation that often occurs in the hospital. A nurse passing noon medications encounters a patient who is obviously upset. He is flipping the pages of a book without reading them, and the ashtray is full of the remains of smoked cigarettes. The nurse might greet the patient, give him his medication, ask him how the book is, and leave. Or she might greet him and mention that he appears distressed.

Patient: Oh, this book isn't any good. I don't know why my wife brought me such junk. She knows I don't like this kind of story. It makes me nervous.
Nurse: You are upset then?
Patient: Of course!
Nurse: What do you do when you are nervous?
Patient: Oh, I smoke and pace.
Nurse: When did this nervousness start?
Patient: Early this morning.
Nurse: Do you remember what happened before it started?
Patient: Nope! . . . Oh, I guess my roommate's doctors came in. Say, when is my doctor coming? He said he was going to have a conference with my other doctors this morning and decide about surgery. Is the conference still going on?
Nurse: Your doctor hasn't been in yet?
Patient: No.
Nurse: You expected him and he didn't come?
Patient: Yes! And it's driving me crazy.
Nurse: So maybe it isn't the book that makes you nervous, but the fact that your doctor hasn't come yet.

In this situation the nurse took definite steps to reduce the patient's anxiety first by helping him to recognize his anxiety and then by assisting him to uncover the apparent cause. Stimuli for this patient's anxiety seemed to be the physician's delayed visit and concern over the results of the doctors' conference about the patient's future.

It has been stated, frequently without research basis, and glibly accepted that preoperative teaching is important for the patient. If he knows what is going to happen and what will be required of him, he will know what to expect, his anxiety will be decreased, and he will be able to participate in his therapy. DeMeyer[26] states that how a patient perceives and reacts to the intensive care unit is altered by the preparation for the experience. Healy[29] suggested that if preoperative teaching did benefit the patient in his postoperative period, it would be manifest in faster recuperation, minimal use of drugs, and

fewer complications. In her study the majority of 181 major surgery cases who had received preoperative instruction went home sooner than was expected and were off all narcotics by the sixth postoperative day. A study by Varvaro[30] indicated that patients who were taught preoperatively showed interest, felt like individuals, perceived the staff as being interested in them, and were observed to be more relaxed and calm and more willing to cooperate in essential postoperative procedures of coughing, deep breathing, and turning.

Weiler[31] interviewed 100 postoperative open heart surgery patients to determine what information patients considered essential and most meaningful and what information was not helpful. She found that the most important areas of instruction were (1) deep breathing and coughing, (2) information about pain, oxygen, and chest tubes, (3) description of intensive care, (4) information regarding seeing a minister, rabbi, or priest, (5) visiting hours, and (6) communication of information to relatives.[31] Janis[2] suggests that "the arousal of some degree of anticipatory fear may be one of the necessary conditions for developing inner defenses of the type that can function effectively when the external dangers materialize."* He adds that probably "the most effective preparatory communications would be those which gave a detailed factual account of the outstanding perceptual experiences that will most likely occur, concentrating on the vague ambiguous events which will most likely be misinterpreted."* Janis' main thesis is that once one accomplishes the "work of worrying," one is able to adjust more adequately to a painful reality situation.

During preoperative teaching sessions the nurse is often in a position that per-

---

*From Janis, I. L.: Psychological stress: psychoanalytical and behavioral studies of surgical patients, New York, 1958, John Wiley & Sons, Inc.

mits her to detect and alleviate a patient's anxiety. Answering questions the patient has about surgery will do much to decrease anxiety. If the anxiety level of the patient is low or moderate so as not to interfere severely with his attention and perception, it would be advisable to plan preoperative teaching according to the advice of Janis; that is, "the most effective preparatory communications would be those which gave a detailed factual account of the outstanding perceptual experiences that will most likely occur."[2] It is also conceivable that there are some patients with high anxiety levels who should not receive preoperative instruction due to their decreased perceptual field and their tendency to select out details without relating them to the situation. It is possible for these patients to develop even higher levels of anxiety by worrying about an insignificant or minor facet included in preoperative instructions. It is, therefore, important for the nurse to be flexible and perceptive in the timing, methods, and content of preoperative teaching.

Another factor applicable to dealing with anxiety in the preoperative period is mentioned by Kennedy.[32] She suggests that since the preoperative heart patient is "up and about," he is often assigned to staff least knowledgeable about dealing with anxiety or to staff who have many other patients "since he only needs his bed made." This situation does not help the anxious patient cope with his anxiety very effectively.

State and trait anxiety in heart surgery patients

This author investigated state and trait anxiety in thirty-five white adult patients admitted to a large private metropolitan hospital for corrective (open or closed) heart surgery. The purpose of the study was to determine when heart surgery patients tend to be most anxious, if a relationship exists between anxiety levels and postoperative morbidity, the periods of

greatest fluctuation in anxiety levels, and the relationship between trait and state anxiety levels in heart surgery patients.

Subjects consisted of seventeen female and eighteen male patients ranging in age from 26 to 69 years. None of the subjects had previously been diagnosed as having a psychological disturbance. On admission, the state anxiety form was administered followed by the trait anxiety form. Thereafter, the state anxiety form was readministered three times: the afternoon or evening before surgery after preoperative instruction; about forty-eight hours after surgery while the patient was still in the intensive care unit and able and willing to respond; and after the patient was transferred to the general surgical ward for convalescence. During the latter convalescent phase, data were obtained from the subjects concerning what they were told to expect postoperatively and whether or not specific items (for example, chest tubes) were included in preoperative instruction. In addition, subjects were asked the following questions: (1) Was there any time during your hospitalization that was more disturbing than others? (2) When do you think you were most anxious or scared? These data were used to determine how the patient's perception of his experience compared with his measured anxiety levels.

Data obtained from the surgeons for determining presurgical physical state and for measuring surgical outcome included the surgical risk to the patient, evaluation of the patient's postsurgical state, and the complications experienced by the patient postoperatively. Demographic data were obtained from the chart and the patient to determine the relationship between these data and the patient anxiety levels.

Although Spielberger found a significant decrease in anxiety levels postoperatively in general surgery patients,[33] this investigator found a peak in anxiety levels in the immediate postoperative period for heart surgery patients.[34] Periods of significant state anxiety fluctuations ($p \leq$ .05) were found between the admission and the postoperative levels of anxiety, between the preoperative and the postoperative anxiety levels, and between the postoperative and the convalescent anxiety levels. Admission, preoperative, and convalescent anxiety levels were lower than were those found in the postoperative period. This may indicate more effective use of defenses in the preoperative and convalescent phases, whereas in the postoperative period there is a breakdown in defenses with the patient consciously aware of his discomfort and anxiety. The postoperative period is highly stressful and threatening to a patient. Often he is in pain, other patients around him go into and out of crises and often die, there are unusual machines and routines, and there is a high concentration of personnel. If the personnel are highly anxious, this is frequently conveyed to the patient.

Although it was found that the level of anxiety varies significantly during a patient's hospital course and peaks in the postoperative period, no relationship was found between the levels of anxiety and the outcome of surgery. There also was no significant relationship between preoperative anxiety levels and previous surgery. However, a significant ($p \leq$ .05) relationship was found between postoperative anxiety and previous surgery; a greater number of patients who had previous surgery had lower anxiety levels postoperatively. This finding might indicate that the most effective type of preoperative teaching would be that which simulated the experiences of the postoperative period. However, in this study preoperative instruction had little effect on anxiety levels.[34]

Significant correlations ($p \leq$ .05) were found between trait anxiety and the admission anxiety levels and between trait and the postoperative anxiety levels. Spielberger[25] states that there is higher correlation between trait and state in conditions of threat to self-esteem, whereas the correlation is lower in situations of physical danger. It would appear, then, that the admission and postoperative periods present threats to a person's self-esteem, whereas the preoperative period may be more characterized by consciousness of physical danger. The low correlation coefficient in the convalescent period between trait and state anxiety may similarly reflect the awareness of physical danger. With preparations under way for discharge, the patient is aware that he is or will soon be testing the physical success of the surgery. It is interesting to note that this study did not show that persons with high anxiety trait respond with elevations in state anxiety more frequently and with greater intensity than persons with low trait anxiety.

Seventy-four percent of the patients in this study stated that their most disturbing time occurred postoperatively, and 69.5% stated that this was also their most anxious period. These findings are consistent with test results. Again it cannot be said that these feelings adversely affected the patient's course, but it can be concluded that the postoperative period is the most psychologically uncomfortable period in a cardiac surgery patient's hospital experience.

Conclusion

At the present time there are inconclusive research results regarding the desirability of anxiety states or their effect on the surgical patient's hospitalization experience. Thus additional research is very important. Measurements of anxiety levels at various times during hospitalization and during residence in the community prior to and after hospitalization to establish patterns of anxiety of patients and to compare these patterns with the patient's postsurgical course (including length of hospital stay, success of surgery, complications, need for pain medication, and behavioral disturbances) are needed.

Findings from these studies can help determine more effective methods of health care.

References

1. Basowitz, Harold, Persky, H., Korshin, S., J., and Grinker, R. R.: Anxiety and stress, New York, 1955, McGraw-Hill Book Co., Inc.
2. Janis, I. L.: Psychological stress: psychoanalytical and behavioral studies of surgical patients, New York, 1958, John Wiley & Sons, Inc.
3. Levitt, Eugene E.: The psychology of anxiety, New York, 1967, The Bobbs-Merrill Co., Inc.
4. Tillich, Paul: The courage to be, New Haven, 1952, Yale University Press.
5. Murray, J. A. H.: A new English dictionary on historical principles, Oxford, 1888, Clarendon Press.
6. English, Horace, and English, Ava: A comprehensive dictionary of psychological and psychoanalytical terms, New York, 1958, Longmans, Green & Co., Inc.
7. May, Rollo: The meaning of anxiety, New York, 1950, The Ronald Press Co.
8. Cattell, R. B., and Scheier, I. H.: The nature of anxiety: a review of thirteen multivariate analyses comprising 814 variables, Psychol. Rep. 4:351-388, 1958.
9. Norman, J. C.: Cardiac surgery, New York, 1967, Appleton-Century-Crofts.
10. Titchener, J. L., and Levine, M.: Surgery as a human experience: the psychodynamics of surgical practice, New York, 1960, Oxford University Press, Inc.
11. Cassaday, John, and Altrocchi, June: Patient concerns about surgery, Nurs. Res. 9:219-221, 1960.
12. Robbins, P. R.: Some explorations into the nature of anxieties relating to illness, Genet. Psychol. Monogr. 66:91-141, 1962.
13. Egerton, N., and Kay, J. H.: Psychological disturbances with open heart surgery, Brit. J. Psychiat. 110:433-439, 1964.
14. Kornfeld, D. S., Zimberg, S., and Malm, J. R.: Psychiatric complications of open heart surgery, New Eng. J. Med. 273:287-292, 1965.
15. Krauss, Herbert, and Ruiz, Rene A.: Anxiety and temporal perspective, J. Clin. Psychol. 23:340-342, 1967.
16. Kennedy, Janet A., and Bakst, Hyman: The influence of emotions on the outcome of cardiac surgery: a predictive study, Bull. N. Y. Acad. Med. 42:809-845, 1966.
17. Fox, Henry, Rizzo, N. D., and Gifford, S.: Psychological observations of patients undergoing mitral surgery: a study of stress, Psychosom. Med. 16:186-208, 1954.
18. Spielberger, C. D., editor: Anxiety and behavior, New York, 1966, Academic Press, Inc.
19. Cattell, R. B.: The scientific analysis of personality, Baltimore, 1965, Penguin Books, Inc.
20. Cattell, R. B.: Anxiety and motivation: theory and crucial experiments. In Spielberger, C. D., editor: Anxiety and behavior, New York, 1966, Academic Press, Inc.
21. Deane, George, and Zeaman, D.: Human heart rate during anxiety, Percept. Motor Skills 8:103-106, 1958.
22. Magendantz, H., and Shortsleeve, J.: Electrocardiographic abnormalities in patients exhibiting anxiety, Amer. Heart J. 42:849-857, 1951.
23. Levitt, E., and Persky, H.: Experimental evidence for the validity of the IPAT anxiety scale, J. Clin. Psychol. 18:458-461, 1962.
24. Rankin, R. J., and Balfrey, W. R.: Impact of delayed auditory feedback on the IPAT 8-parallel-form anxiety scales, Psychol. Rep. 18:583-586, 1966.
25. Spielberger, C. D., Gorsuch, R. L., and Lushene, R. E.: The state-trait anxiety inventory: preliminary test manual for form X, Tallahassee, 1968, Department of Psychology, Florida State University.
26. DeMeyer, JoAnna: The environment of the intensive care unit, Nurs. Forum 6:262-272, 1967.
27. Fordham, Mary: Cardiovascular surgical nursing, New York, 1962, The Macmillan Co.
28. McReynolds, Paul: On assessment of anxiety: I. By a behavior checklist, Psychol. Rep. 16:805-808, 1965.
29. Healy, K. M.: Does preoperative instruction make a difference? Amer. J. Nurs. 68:62-67, 1968.
30. Varvaro, F. F.: Teaching the patient about open heart surgery, Amer. J. Nurs. 65:111-115, 1965.
31. Weiler, Sister M. C.: Postoperative patients evaluate preoperative instruction, Amer. J. Nurs. 68:1465-1467, 1968.
32. Kennedy, M. J.: Coping with emotional stress in the patient awaiting heart surgery, Nurs. Clin. N. Amer. 1:3, 1966.
33. Spielberger, C. D.: Personal communication, 1970.
34. Haselhorst, J. A.: State-trait anxiety and the

outcome of heart surgery, unpublished masters thesis, University of Illinois at the Medical Center, Chicago, 1970.

Bibliography

Abdellah, Faye G.: Criterion measures in nursing, Nurs. Res. 10:21-26, 1961.

American Psychiatric Association: Diagnostic and statistical manual: mental disorders, Washington, D. C., 1952, American Psychiatric Association.

Anxiety: Recognition and intervention, programmed instruction, Amer. J. Nurs. 65:129-152, 1965.

Beland, Irene L.: Clinical nursing: pathophysiological and psychosocial approaches, New York, 1965, The Macmillan Co.

Bendig, A. W.: Age-related changes in covert and overt anxiety, J. Gen. Psychol. 62:159-163, 1960.

Bosselman, Beulah: Neurosis and psychosis, Springfield, Ill., 1964, Charles C Thomas, Publisher.

Braimbridge, M. V.: Post-operative cardiac care, Oxford, 1965, Blackwell Scientific Publications Ltd.

Bronzo, Anthony, and Powers, Gerald: Relationship of anxiety with pain threshold, J. Psychol. 66:181, 1967.

Coston, Harriet: Myocardial infarction: stages of recovery and nursing care, Nurs. Res. 9:178, 1960.

Fenz, Walter: Specificity in somatic responses to anxiety, Percept. Motor Skills 24:1183-1190, 1967.

Fine, B. J., and Gaydos, H. F.: Relationship between individual personality variables and body temperature response patterns in the cold, Psychol. Rep. 5:71-78, 1959.

Fox, D. S.: Fundamentals of research in nursing, New York, 1966, Appleton-Century-Crofts.

Goldman, Mervin: Principles of clinical electrocardiography, Los Altos, Calif., 1967, Lange Medical Publications.

Graffam, Shirley: Care of the surgical patient, New York, 1960, McGraw-Hill Book Co., Inc.

Hiltner, Seward, and Menninger, Karl: Constructive aspects of anxiety, Nashville, 1963, Abingdon Press.

Hodges, William F.: Effects of ego threat and threat of pain on state anxiety, J. Personality Soc. Psychol. 8:364-372, 1968.

Johnson, D. T.: Effects of interview stress on measures of state and trait anxiety, J. Abnorm. Psychol. 73:245-251, 1968.

Kelly, D. H. W.: Measurement of anxiety by forearm blood flow, Brit. J. Psychiat. 112:789-798, 1966.

King, S. H.: Perceptions of illness and medical practice, New York, 1962, Russell Sage Foundation.

Kittle, C. F., et al: Factors influencing risk in cardiac surgical patients: cooperative study, presented at the American Heart Association Meeting, Miami, Fla., Nov., 1968.

Lazarus, Richard S.: Psychological stress and the coping process, New York, 1966, McGraw-Hill Book Co., Inc.

Mainzer, H., and Krause, M.: The influence of fear on the electrocardiogram, Brit. Heart J. 2:221-230, 1940.

Megargee, Edwin I.: Research in clinical assessment, New York, 1966, Harper & Row, Publishers.

Mendels, Joe: Stress polycythemia, Amer. J. Psychiat. 123:1570-1572, 1967.

Meyer, B. C.: Psychiatry in surgical practice, AORN J. 5:49-50, 1967.

Moss, C. S., and Waters, T. J.: Intensive longitudinal investigation of anxiety in hospitalized juvenile patients, Psychol. Rep. 7:379-380, 1960.

Peddie, G., and Bruch, F.: Cardiovascular surgery: a manual for nurses, New York, 1961, G. P. Putnam's Sons.

Peitahinis, J.: Psychological care of patient important to surgery's outcome, Hosp. Top. 43:113-119, 1965.

Quint, Jeanne C.: Delineation of qualitative aspects of nursing care, Nurs. Res. 11:204-206, 1962.

Rodale, Jerome I., editor: The synonym finder, Emmaus, Pa., 1961, Rodale Books, Inc.

Schlotfeldt, Rozella: Problems in the development of adequate criteria, Nurs. Res. 11:211-213, 1962.

Smith, S. L.: An exploratory study to identify stressors producing myocardial ischemia in the pre- and postoperative periods of patients having open heart surgery, unpublished masters thesis, University of Washington, Seattle, 1965.

Taufic, Marjorie R.: Nursing care of the cardiovascular surgery patient, Nurs. World 130:10-13, 1956.

Tepperman, J.: Metabolic and endocrine physiology, Chicago, 1968, Year Book Medical Publishers, Inc.

Wadeson, R. W.: Anxiety in the dreams of a neurosurgical patient, Arch. Gen. Psychiat. 14:249-252, 1966.

White, M. E.: An outline guide for the care of the post-operative cardiac patient, Springfield, Ill., 1961, Charles C Thomas, Publisher.

Whyman, A., and Moos, R. H.: Time perception and anxiety, Percept. Motor Skills 24:567-570, 1967.

Chapter 31

Current status of cardiac valvular replacement and the professional nurse

Doreen M. Harris

Since Hufnagel first implanted a prosthetic valve in the descending aorta of a patient in 1952, significant advancements have been made in the replacement of diseased cardiac valves. The development of effective means of extracorporeal circulation, modification of the design and materials of the prosthesis, and continuing experience in the selection and clinical management of the patient have contributed to the acceptance of surgical replacement as an important alternative in the treatment of patients with valvular deformity. A major manufacturer of valvular prostheses reports that between 1960 and 1970 approximately 60,000 of their prostheses were implanted, with usage over the last few years increasing about 15% every year compounded yearly.[1] This estimate illustrates the significance of this type of surgery for practicing nurses. Valvular replacement is no longer confined to the university medical centers involved in clinical research. Nurses in smaller hospitals throughout the country are caring for these patients at some time during their illness experience. To plan and deliver nursing care to these patients intelligently, the professional nurse must have a basic understanding of how the prosthesis and its design affect the patient physiologically and psychologically. This chapter seeks to review the current knowledge concerning prosthetic valve design and to examine the nursing care specifically related to the design of the valve and to the effects of valvular replacement. The effects of other aspects of the surgery, such as extracorporeal circulation, are not included.

To understand the function and clinical complications of valvular replacement, it is helpful to review briefly the anatomy and function of the normal valve. Anatomically, a valve consists of pliable leaflets attached to a circular ring at commissures. The leaflets of the atrioventricular (tricuspid and mitral) valves are anchored to the papillary muscles of the ventricles by strings of endothelially covered collagen (chordae tendineae) to prevent eversion during ventricular systole.

Valve function has been most carefully studied in the mitral and aortic valves. In the mitral valve leaflet motion is believed to be passive and dependent on changes in the direction of the pressure differential across the valve.[2] Opening results from a decrease in ventricular pressure below that of the atrium due to rapid ventricular diastolic relaxation. Closure of the mitral valve is believed to be due to atrial relaxation, resulting in its pressure becoming less than ventricular pressure. Recent electron microscopy studies revealing the presence of a neuromuscular apparatus within the mitral valve leaflet may modify this theory of valve function into a more active one.[3] Additional research is required.

Acquired or congenital lesions may interfere with normal valve function by restricting outflow through stenosis or by allowing regurgitant backflow through incompetent valve closure. Valvular deformity may be asymptomatic or cause minimal discomfort or physical restriction. If, however, the individual's exertional ability becomes severely restricted (functional class III or IV, New York Heart Association classification), surgical repair or replacement of the diseased valve may be necessary. An exception to this is the asymptomatic patient with severe aortic stenosis. His valve may be replaced to prevent sudden death.

Valve prostheses—problems and modifications

The problem of how to replace these delicate valves continues to confront cardiac surgeons and biomedical engineers. The ideal criteria for judging the suitability of a prosthesis are based on early laboratory and clinical experience with prosthetic models. Although no prosthesis available meets most, let alone all, of these criteria, they are as follows:

1. Ease of implantation to minimize length of extracorporeal circulation and its adverse effects
2. Rapid and secure healing
3. Absence of thrombus formation
4. Insignificant physiological valvular gradient
5. No regurgitation
6. Lack of significant injury to blood cells
7. Long-term durability[4]

The Starr-Edwards caged-ball prosthesis, one of the earliest designs, was tested clinically in 1960. Initial problems including endocarditis, thromboembolism, stenosis, leakage, decreased cardiac output from obstruction of the aortic outflow tract after mitral replacement, septal irritation, and ball variance have led to modifications of the ball-valve design and of prosthetic materials and to the development of new designs.

The Starr-Edwards model has been modified in several ways. The orifice-external ratio has been increased to reduce stenotic tendencies. The sewing margin is flanged to decrease perivalvular leak; in addition, silicone foam padding has been added to the sewing ring, affording some compressability and coaptation to the irregular tissue surface. The silicone ball has been replaced with a smaller one made of hollow Stellite 21, since ball variance was significant in the former due to impurities and lipid absorption.[5]

Thromboembolism has been a major cause of late mortality after prosthesis implantation despite long-term anticoagulation. To solve this problem investigators sought to eliminate the prosthesis-tissue interface where it was believed thrombus formation originated. The nonmoving metal parts were covered with a thin fabric lattice of Dacron that allowed an ingrowth of autogenous tissue histologically similar to endothelium.[6] Although this cloth has decreased the incidence of thromboemboli, it has renewed the problem of stenosis, since the cloth and the tissue ingrowth encroach on the orifice area.[7] In addition the cloth has presented the question of long-term durability, particularly on the cage legs and the seat of the orifice that are subject to wear from the moving ball. To meet the problem at the orifice, recent Starr-Edwards models (6310 and

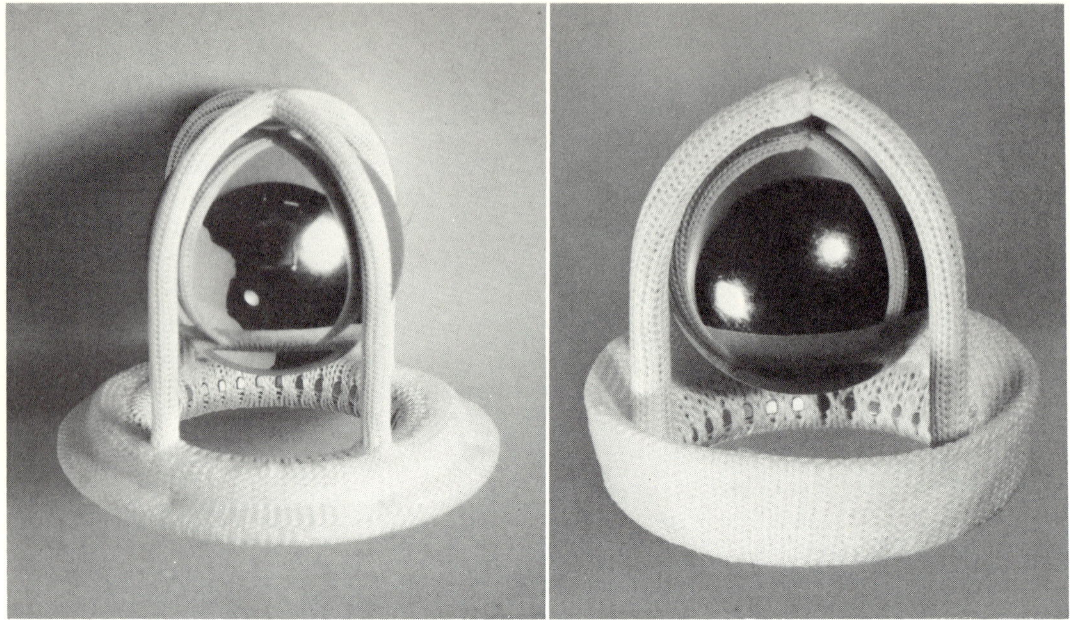

Fig. 14

Starr-Edwards caged-ball valves. **A,** Model 6310 mitral valve prosthesis. **B,** Model 2310 aortic valve prosthesis. (Courtesy of Edwards Laboratories, Santa Ana, Calif.)

2310) incorporate exposed metallic supports in the orifice to reinforce the strength of the seat against which the ball closes and to allow the orifice area to be increased without concern for cloth durability (Fig. 14). A serendipitous effect of the cloth covering of the cage legs has been a decrease in the noise level produced by ball motion, an effect that may decrease the patient's subjective awareness of and possible anxiety over the presence of the prosthesis.[8]

Pharmacological control of thromboembolic complications is also being researched. Based on the theory that platelet aggregation is the initiating event in thrombus formation in an area of rapid blood flow investigations have been conducted to determine therapy to prevent this phenomenon. Dipyridamole (Persantine) has been found to increase the concentration of adenosine and adenosine triphosphate, both of which cause coronary vasodilation. However, adenosine triphosphate also acts as an important high-energy source. This may foster healing of injured tissue, a factor in platelet aggregation and thromboembolic formation. Results of one study, in which administration of dipyridamole was begun ten to fourteen days after prosthetic replacement in conjunction with anticoagulation therapy, demonstrated absence of thromboemboli or hemorrhage when this combined therapy was continued for at least one year.[9]

A third line of investigation to make prostheses thromboresistant involves the use of a surface possessing high negativity. It is believed that a negatively charged surface repels the formation of a clot.[10]

Although opening and closure of the ball-valve prosthesis is similar to the normal valve, the onset is slightly delayed due to the force necessary to overcome the ball's inertia.[11] Of note is the slight, fixed regurgitation of blood through the

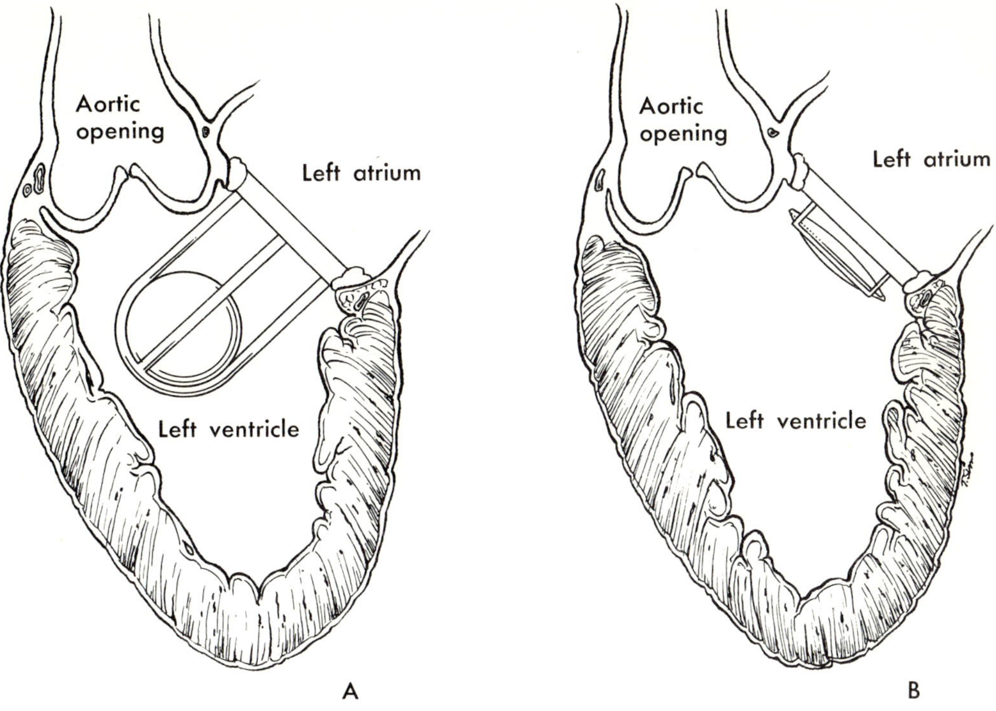

Fig. 15

A, Protrusion of caged-ball valve into the left ventricle. **B,** Low profile valve in the mitral position. (Modified from Brewer, Lyman A., editor: Prosthetic heart valves, Springfield, Ill., 1969, Charles C Thomas, Publisher.)

valve as a result of this delay. This regurgitation becomes proportionally more significant at heart rates greater than 100/ minute. Likewise the transvalvular energy loss (the cost of achieving blood flow in terms of pressure expended) increases with an increased heart rate. Tachycardia must be avoided postoperatively, therefore, since both the volume and energy load on the heart would be increased.

The presence of the caged-ball prosthesis in the mitral position protruding into the ventricle has produced two complications, particularly in patients with small ventricles. (1) During ventricular systole the cage may obstruct aortic outflow, thus reducing cardiac output. (2) The cage may strike the interventricular septum during systole. This may injure the myocardium, may initiate irritable ventricular

foci, and cause a resultant arrhythmia (Fig. 15). In response to these problems, low profile mitral prostheses have been developed with minimal protrusion into the ventricle. Designs include use of a lens or disc within a cage or a single or double hinge.

An example of the caged lens valve is the Cross-Jones valve. Advantages of this design are (1) its low profile, (2) less delay in opening and closing because of its lighter weight, and (3) decreased force of closure of the lens on the orifice seat. Disadvantages also exist. The lens may become cocked open, presenting severe stenosis and regurgitation. If the blood flow through the valve is oblique, the lens may tilt, which results in turbulent blood flow that fosters thromboembolism.[12] The question of durability is raised with the use of cloth-covered cage legs. The material of the lens must not wear the cloth and vice versa. The search for this material continues.[13]

The hinged-double leaflet valve such as the Gott-Daggett also offers low profile and rapid response to blood flow. The chief disadvantages of this design are (1) the large area of stasis distally between the leaflets and (2) turbulence from the free edges of the leaflets.[14]

Because blood stasis and turbulence are

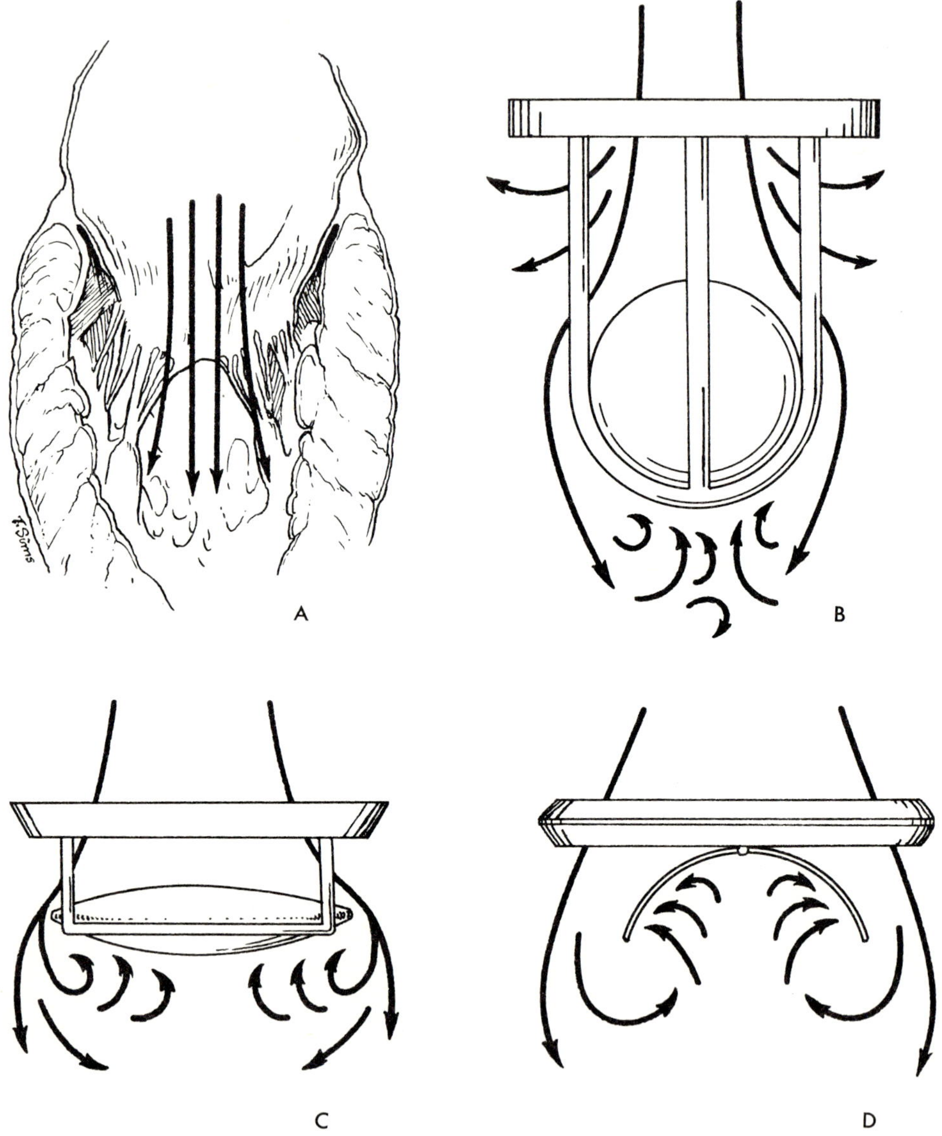

Fig. 16

Blood flow characteristics. **A,** Normal mitral valve with central blood flow. **B,** Starr-Edwards ball valve. **C,** Disc-type low profile valve. **D,** Gott-Daggett hinged-double leaflet valve. (**B, C,** and **D** from Brewer, Lyman A., editor: Prosthetic heart valves, Spingfield, Ill., 1969, Charles C Thomas, Publisher.)

believed to predispose to thrombus formation, prosthetic designs have recently been subjected to intensive investigation of their blood flow characteristics (Fig. 16). The conclusion seems to be that central flow as provided by the normal valve is ideal. Prostheses designed to open as leaflets have had limited success because of their lack of flexibility and stenotic outflow. The sinus of the valve that ensures optimum opening with efficient closure is absent. Hufnagel[34] has developed a low profile trileaflet valve covered with Hepacone, an antithrombogenic substance, with which he has had satisfactory hemodynamic results. Research continues on many designs to modify the shape of the valve and its closure device to provide minimal turbulence and stasis.

Speed of insertion may be particularly critical in older, more debilitated patients, or in patients requiring multiple valvular replacements. In response to this need, Magovern developed a sutureless aortic ball valve that is held in place by two rows of opposing metal teeth. It must not be attached to friable tissue due to danger of disruption. Possible dislodgement, perivalvular leak, and injury to the myocardial conduction system are among the disadvantages of the sutureless valve.

Research has brought about modifications in valvular prostheses, and current models more closely meet the ideal criteria. However, the nurse may still care for a patient in some setting who has a functioning prosthesis of an older design. It is her responsibility to learn what type of prosthesis the patient has and plan her observations and interventions accordingly. For example, a patient whose prosthesis has a silicone ball may develop ball variance several years after surgery; this may occur abruptly. This phenomenon can be detected through auscultatory changes, particularly absence of the opening click, and by symptoms of outflow obstruction. Although the cardiac monitor may indicate normal sinus rhythm, the nurse may detect an irregular pulse on palpation. Asynchronous prosthetic valve sounds may be heard as the ball moves with difficulty within the cage.[5]

Complications

Although improvements in valve design and materials have been made, postoperative complications still exist. Intimately involved in the care of these patients, the nurse must anticipate potential complications through purposeful observations for early signs and take prompt action if any develop. As a member of the health team involved in the continuing clinical research concerning optimal prosthetic design, she must report any deviations from the expected course of recovery.

The chief prosthesis-related complication after valvular replacement continues to be thromboembolism. Symptoms depend on the operative site and actual site of embolization. The most severe adverse effect is complete occlusion of the prosthesis, resulting in a rapid diminution of cardiac output and death. Smaller emboli may travel to the coronary, cerebral, or systemic arteries from the left side of the heart or to the lungs from the right side. In addition to design modification previously discussed, anticoagulation with a coumarin drug continues to be an important means of preventing this complication. After insertion of a cloth-covered prosthesis, anticoagulants may be prescribed only until tissue ingrowth is complete, experimentally determined to be about six months.[6] If the prosthesis is not completely cloth covered, anticoagulation is continued indefinitely.

Coumarin therapy requires a precise balance to avoid bleeding while maintaining therapeutic levels of anticoagulation. The patient and the health team must be aware of factors that may influence this balance. Coumarin derivatives compete with vitamin K for binding sites with the enzyme necessary for the production of prothrombin and factors VII, IX, and X in the liver.[15] A change in vitamin K intake, therefore, will alter coumarin activity. Vitamin K is fat soluble, available in the diet, and manufactured by normal intestinal flora. A decrease in fat intake or a decrease in intestinal flora due to ingestion of broad-spectrum oral antibiotics will decrease available vitamin K, thereby increasing coumarin activity. Coumarin derivatives are metabolized in the liver; liver dysfunction slows this degradation, causing accumulation and prolonged activity of the anticoagulant. Drug interactions have been observed in patients taking other drugs concurrently with coumarin anticoagulants. Such interactions result from several mechanisms. Coumarin activity is increased by the following:

1. Decreased degradation of coumarins; for example, concurrent administration of phenylbutazone (Butazolidin), diethylstilbestrol (stilbestrol), or phenyramidol (Analexin).
2. Displacement of coumarin from plasma protein-binding sites thereby increasing concentration of free coumarin; for example, concurrent administration of phenylbutazone, clofibrate (Atromid-S), sulfonamides, or salicylates.

Coumarin activity is decreased when there is increased metabolic degradation of coumarins. This occurs with the use of the following drugs: barbiturates, chloral hydrate, glutethimide (Doriden), meprobamate (Equanil and Miltown), and griseofulvin (Fulvicin and Grifulvin).[16]

Coumarin derivatives in turn may potentiate the effects of other drugs by inhibiting their metabolic degradation in the liver. This occurs when coumarin compounds are used with diphenylhydantoin (Dilantin) and tolbutamide (Orinase).

During initiation or termination of anticoagulation therapy or administration of a drug affecting coumarin activity, careful monitoring of the patient's rate of thrombin formation becomes important. Modification of the coumarin dosage schedule may be necessary. A patient must be cautioned against self-medication without his physician's approval, since salicylates and other over-the-counter drugs are frequently considered harmless by the uninformed individual. The nurse can also teach the patient to observe for symptoms of excessive anticoagulation, such as hematuria, bleeding gums, or bruising tendencies. While increasing his awareness of possible complications of anticoagulant therapy, try not to also increase his anxiety over his recovery and prognosis. Although complications exist, they are rarely life threatening, as is so often true of thrombus formation.

The second significant complication of valvular replacement is endocarditis, with a reported mortality of 2% to 4%.[17] It is more frequent after aortic valve replacement and is usually manifested within the first year after surgery.[17] Origin of the microorganism is probably operative contamination or seeding of the prosthesis from bacteremia that results from infection of the respiratory tract, urinary tract, or cutdown site. Symptoms of infected prostheses and endocarditis may not occur until late in the disease process.[18] These symptoms usually include a chronic or recurrent low-grade fever of obscure etiology as well as symptoms of mechanical dysfunction of the prosthesis from vegetative overgrowth or from disruption of the suture line. These infections are frequently refractory to antibiotic therapy. Valvular surgery patients are subject to certain factors predisposing them to endocarditis:

1. Preoperative debilitation
2. Implantation of foreign materials, including sutures, that provide a nidus for vegetative growth
3. Change in host resistance after mechanical injury to white blood cells and protein from extracorporeal circulation

To minimize the possibility of endocarditis, strict intraoperative asepsis is sought and broad-spectrum antibiotics (methicillin, oxacillin, or cephalothin) are given prophylactically before, during and after surgery.[17] The latter therapy may create a fourth factor predisposing the patient to the development of infection by altering his autogenous flora, thereby allowing multiplication of resistant strains.

Nursing actions related to prevention of endocarditis include attention to possible sources of infection. Respiratory infection can be avoided by aseptic suctioning and effective respiratory toilet. Aseptic technique in the insertion and care of the urinary catheter and prevention of urinary stasis in the bladder and tubing can help prevent urinary tract infection. Cutdown sites should be dressed daily with an antibiotic ointment and the nurse should observe the patient for signs of phlebitis. Since nursing care is provided for the hospitalized patient around the clock, the nurse may be the first to recognize signs of endocarditis. Auscultation is an important tool in detecting possible mechanical dysfunction from impaired ball motion or dislodgment of the valve; this will be discussed in more detail later. Before discharge the patient should be instructed to report any unexplained chronic or recurrent low-grade fever to his physician.

Although one study reported slight hemolysis with all ball-valve prostheses,[19] most patients with valve replacements have red blood cell survival rates that approach normal or are significantly longer than are those of patients with unrepaired valves.[20] Red blood cell survival may be reduced due to occult bleeding from anticoagulation. Low-grade hemolysis is compensated by increased bone marrow production to prevent anemia.

The extent of hemolysis may be influenced by the following factors:

1. Increased cardiac output that may increase hemolysis
2. Increased hemolysis in aortic prostheses due to increased flow velocity
3. Lipemia that increases susceptibility of red blood cells to mechanical disruption
4. Men more susceptible than women
5. Presence of endothelium on the sewing ring that may decrease hemolysis[18]

It must be emphasized that the degree of hemolysis considered here is asymptomatic. Severe hemolysis associated with anemia and fatigability results from mechanical dysfunction. If this occurs within the first few postoperative months, it is usually related to a perivalvular leak; after several years, however, the development of hemolytic anemia usually indicates ball variance, requiring immediate surgery.[21]

Despite prosthetic modification, dysrhythmias may be seen after valvular replacement. In the aortic position, inadequate perfusion of the coronaries during extracorporeal circulation with myocardial anoxia may cause ventricular dysrhythmias; injury to the conduction system during implantation may cause partial or complete heart block. A ball-valve in the mitral position may obstruct aortic outflow or cause myocardial septal irritation with ectopic ventricular foci. The nurse should be able to identify these dysrhythmias and report their occurrence and frequency.

Selected nursing care aspects

Several aspects of the nursing care of patients after valvular replacement are specifically related to the presence of the prosthesis. Prevention of and observation and intervention for possible complications have been discussed. It is important to stress the need for professional nurses to develop skill in using the stethoscope if they are to function optimally in the care of patients with valvular prostheses.

Certain auscultatory changes are obvious after surgery. The opening click is most prominent. The mitral valve can be heard best at the apex of the heart, the aortic valve at the left sternal border or the second right intercostal space, and the tricuspid valve in the region of the xiphoid.[22] The opening click is usually slightly delayed due to ball inertia.

The nurse should not only listen for the apical beat after prosthesis insertion, but also for the presence or development of cardiac murmurs. Low-grade murmurs may be normal. An early diastolic grade I murmur after aortic replacement with a Starr-Edwards valve usually results from slight aortic regurgitation due to ball inertia. This murmur is low pitched and can be heard by placing the bell of the stethoscope lightly on the chest wall. Too much pressure may obscure the sound. A grade I to II systolic ejection murmur is common after a Starr-Edwards aortic replacement.[23] It is high pitched and may therefore be heard best with the diaphragm of the stethoscope.

It is obvious that to detect a murmur the professional nurse should listen in the appropriate anatomic location with both the bell and the diaphragm of her stethoscope. Grade I and II murmurs are quite difficult to hear and require an experienced ear. Recordings are available to aid the nurse in listening to heart sounds.* If she is inexperienced, however, a murmur that she may identify in one of the anatomic locations listed above is more likely to be a louder grade (III to VI) and, therefore, more significant. This is particularly true if it appears suddenly. Phonocardiography is frequently used to aid in the diagnosis of murmurs that may be a sign of endocarditis, perivalvular leak, valve disruption or incompetence, or ball variance. All murmurs should be recorded and reported.

The patient may exhibit different reactions to the sound of the prosthesis. The amount of sound perceived by the patient

---

*Available from Merck Sharp & Dohme, West Point, Pa.

seems to vary with the following factors:

1. Anxiety concerning his heart or his surgery
2. Postoperative interval—increased myocardial activity during the first six months
3. Thickness of the chest wall
4. Size of the heart

The patient may be reassured by the opening click, the regularity of which may be interpreted as a sign of recovery. To others the noise may be unnerving, particularly when the patient lies down, since the heart rests against the chest wall and rib cage that serve as sounding boards. If dysrhythmias are present, it is more likely to be upsetting. Patients should be encouraged to accept the sound as a normal result of exchange of their diseased valve for an efficient replacement. If the patient initially seems bothered by the noise, the nurse can suggest that he avoid lying on his left side or use a foam rubber pillow to muffle the sound.[24] He will probably become accustomed to it as time passes. If he continues to worry, the nurse should consider the possibility that this complaint may be a manifestation of a deeper anxiety over his prognosis or modified life-style, and she should consult with the physician.

In the event of cardiac arrest the nurse should distinguish between ventricular asystole and fibrillation as the cause to avoid unnecessary external cardiac massage. Rare cases of dislodgment of the unyielding prosthesis[25] or rupture of a coronary artery[26] have been reported. Although resuscitative measures are essential, they should be definitive. Defibrillation is the choice of treatment for ventricular fibrillation and, some authors suggest, initially when the cause of the arrest is not known.[26] If massage is necessary, the patient should be monitored for possible consequences.

Cardiac valve transplants

In the search for the valvular replacement that would meet the ideal criteria and have central flow, investigators have begun to look beyond prostheses to autogenous, homologous, and even heterogenous tissues. Homograft valves present the advantages of (1) central blood flow, (2) absence of thromboemboli even without anticoagulation, (3) low incidence of endocarditis, and (4) possibility of late degeneration.[27] Currently fresh homografts removed under sterile conditions and stored for up to two weeks in an antibiotic solution at 4° C. seem to be preferred because of the structural changes resulting from sterilization and storage techniques.[28, 29] In addition, valves from young female donors are preferred, for these tissues are less likely to exhibit thickening and degeneration of the collagen fibers. Rejection of the homograft does not seem to be a problem, since the primary antigen is in the cells and the normal valve becomes both acellular and avascular with age.[23]

To facilitate insertion of the homograft and to determine valve competence before implantation, several investigators sew the homograft to a cloth-covered support prior to insertion.[28, 30] This support presents several of the same disadvantages associated with a prosthesis: (1) the presence of an unyielding metal ring; (2) the danger of thromboemboli until ingrowth occurs; and (3) prongs that protrude into the ventricle from the atrioventricular position.

To utilize living, autogenous tissue that they believe will exhibit less late degeneration, some researchers have turned to the fascia lata that is readily available, shows good tensile strength, and is relatively easy to suture.[31] The fascia lata may be fashioned into a semilunar or trileaflet valve on a cloth-covered support. To prevent thrombus formation while the cloth endothelializes, the patient may be anticoagulated for six weeks. Even without anticoagulation, a one-year follow-up of these patients revealed no thromboemboli.[23, 32]

Early experimental research has been conducted on the use of heterograft valves because of their availability in a variety of sizes. Calf and pig valves seem most appropriate according to criteria of size, leaflet characteristics, tensile strength, and durability.[33] Although no emboli have been observed, evidence of early or late immunological rejection is inconclusive. Anatomic variations in the valve structure have caused problems of late degeneration.[23]

The nurse who is aware of the type of valve inserted in her patient can plan her patient's care more knowledgeably. Tissue grafts have a decreased incidence of thromboembolism and endocarditis and may not require anticoagulation. Auscultatory changes will not be as apparent; the development of a systolic murmur after mitral replacement or a diastolic murmur after aortic replacement may indicate leaflet incompetence and should be recorded as well as reported to the physician. The tissue graft without a support is easily compressed so external cardiac massage can be done safely. Lastly, the patient will not be able to hear the tissue valve open or close, eliminating the need to adjust to the noise of a prosthesis.

Conclusion

Comparisons of clinical results from various prosthetic and tissue valve replacements are difficult. Each team of physicians not only have different experiences, they also employ different techniques of insertion as well as different criteria for patient selection. In addition there is wide variation in preoperative and postoperative management. If the professional nurse keeps in mind, however, the design of the prosthesis or tissue graft her patient has received, she should be able to develop a pertinent and individualized plan of care for him.

References

1. Edwards Laboratories: Personal communication, 1970.
2. Brockman, S. K., Collins, H. A., and Snyder,

H. E.: The normal mode of action of the mitral valve and its alteration following replacement by a prosthetic ball valve, J. Thorac. Cardiovasc. Surg. 50:820-825, 1965.

3. Cooper, T., Sonnenblick, E. H., Priola, D. V., Napolitano, L. M., and Dempsey, P. J.: An intrinsic neuromuscular basis for mitral valve motion. In Brewer, L. A., editor: Prosthetic heart valves, Springfield, Ill., 1969, Charles C Thomas, Publisher.

4. Sauvage, L. R., Berger, K., Wood, S. J., Viggers, R. F., and Robel, S. B.: In vivo testing of prosthetic heart valves and criteria for specimen evaluation. In Brewer, L. A., editor: Prosthetic heart valves, Springfield, Ill., 1969, Charles C Thomas, Publisher.

5. Leatherman, L. L., Leachman, R. D., McConn, R. G., Hallman, G. L., and Cooley, D. A.: Malfunction of mitral ball-valve prostheses due to swollen poppet, J. Thorac. Cardiovasc. Surg. 57:160-163, 1969.

6. Bull, B., Fuchs, J. C. A., and Braunwald, N. S.: Mechanism of formation of tissue layers on the fabric lattice covering intravascular prosthetic devices, Surgery 65:640-648, 1969.

7. Reis, R. L., Glancy, D. L., O'Brien, K., Epstein, S. E., and Morrow, A. G.: Clinical and hemodynamic assessments of fabric-covered Starr-Edwards prosthetic valves, J. Thorac. Cardiovasc. Surg. 59:84-91, 1970.

8. Koorajian, S., Keller, D. P., Pierie, W. R., Starr, A., and Herr, R.: Criteria and systems for testing artificial heart valves in vitro. In Brewer, L. A., editor: Prosthetic heart valves, Springfield, Ill., 1969, Charles C Thomas, Publisher.

9. Sullivan, J. M., Harken, D. E., and Gorlin, R.: Pharmacologic control of thromboembolic complications of cardiac valve replacement, New Eng. J. Med. 279:576-580, 1968.

10. Sawyer, P. N., Srinivasan, S., Lee, M. E., Martin, J. G., Murakami, T., and Stanczewski, B.: The influence of the metal interface charge on longe-term function of prosthetic heart valves. In Brewer, L. A., editor: Prosthetic heart valves, Springfield, Ill., 1969, Charles C Thomas, Publisher.

11. Nolan, S. T., Stewart, S., Fogarty, T. J., Dixon, S. H., and Morrow, A. G.: In vivo studies of instantaneous blood flow across mitral ball-valve prostheses: effects of cardiac output and heart rate on transvalvular energy loss, Ann. Surg. 169:551-559, 1969.

12. Cross, F. S., Akao, M., and Jones, R. D.: Comparison of ball and lens heart valve prostheses, Surgery 62:797-806, 1967.

13. Cross, F. S., Akao, M., and Jones, R. D.: The evaluation of experimental mitral valve prostheses in the dog, Surgery 65:89-97, 1969.

14. Smeloff, E. A., Davey, T. B., and Kaufman, B.: Patterns of blood flow through artificial valves. In Brewer, L. A., editor: Prosthetic heart valves, Springfield, Ill., 1969, Charles C Thomas, Publisher.

15. Gadboys, H. L., Litwak, R. S., Niemetz, J., and Wisch, N.: Role of anticoagulants in preventing embolization from prosthetic heart valves, J. A. M. A. 202:282-286, 1967.

16. Interactions of oral anticoagulants with other drugs, Med. Lett. Drugs Ther. 9:97, 1967.

17. Killen, D. A., Collins, H. A., Koenig, M. G., and Goodman, J. S.: Prosthetic cardiac valves and bacterial endocarditis, Ann. Thorac. Surg. 9:238-247, 1970.

18. Hairston, P., and Lee, W. L.: Management of infected prosthetic heart valves, Ann. Thorac. Surg. 9:229-237, 1970.

19. O'Connell, T. J., Geiger, J. P., and Aronstam, E.: Accelerated hemolysis following mitral valve replacement with the Davila prosthesis, Ann. Thorac. Surg. 9:44-50, 1970.

20. Brodeur, M. T. H., Koler, R. D., Starr, A., and Griswold, H. E.: RBC survival in patients with mitral valvular disease and mitral valve prostheses, Circulation 33 (suppl.):140-151, 1966.

21. Starr, A.: Panel discussion: current clinical problems in prosthetic heart valves. In Brewer, L. A., editor: Prosthetic heart valves, Springfield, Ill., 1969, Charles C Thomas, Publisher.

22. Najmi, M., and Segal, B.: Auscultatory and phonocardiographic findings in patients with prosthetic ball valves, Amer. J. Cardiol. 16:794-799, 1965.

23. Gonzalez-Lavin, Lorenzo: Personal communication, 1970.

24. Farrell, K. M.: Telltale hearts, Amer. J. Nurs. 67:1239-1240, 1967.

25. Wilcox, B. R.: Disruption of a mitral-valve prosthesis: post external cardiac massage, J. A. M. A. 194:93-94, 1965.

26. Burnside, J., Daggett, W. M., and Austen, W. G.: Coronary artery rupture by a mitral valve prosthesis after closed chest massage, Ann. Thorac. Surg. 9:267-271, 1970.

27. Ross, D., and Yacoub, M. H.: Homograft replacement of the aortic valve: a critical review, Progr. Cardiovasc. Dis. 11:275-293, 1969.

28. Angell, W. W., and Shumway, N. E.: The homograft prosthesis. In Brewer, L. A.,

editor: Prosthetic heart valves, Springfield, Ill., 1969, Charles C Thomas, Publisher.

29. Barratt-Boyes, B. G., Roche, A. H. G., Brandt, P. W. T., Smith, J. C., and Lowe, J. B.: Aortic homograft valve replacement: a long-term follow-up of an initial series of 101 patients, Circulation **40**:763-775, 1969.

30. Sugie, S., Watanabe, M., Aoki, T., Murakami, T., Tanabe, T., Takagi, M., Kubo, Y., Ohta, S., Misaka, K., Tomiyama, M., and Sugiyama, M.: Clinical experience with supported homograft heart valve for mitral and aortic valve replacement, J. Thorac. Cardiovasc. Surg. **57**:455-463, 1969.

31. Myers, W. O., and Miller, D. R.: Autogenous fascial aortic valves in dogs, J. Thorac. Cardiovasc. Surg. **57**:805-811, 1969.

32. Ionescu, M. I., Ross, D. N., Deac, R., Grimshaw, V. A., Taylor, S. H., Whitaker, W., and Wooler, G. H.: Autologous fascia lata for heart valve replacement, Thorax **25**:46-56, 1970.

33. Harris, P. D., Kowalik, A. T. W., Beach, P. M., Parodi, E., Castanay, R., Bowman, F. O., and Malm, J. R.: A comparative study of selected physical properties of aortic homografts and heterografts, J. Thorac. Cardiovasc. Surg. **57**:830-833, 1969.

34. Hufnagel, C. A., Conrad, P. W., Gillespie, J. F., Pifarre, R., and Ilano, A.: A new method for the prevention of thrombus formation in valvular prosthesis, Amer. Coll. Cardiol., abst., Feb., 1966.

Bibliography

Carpentier, A., Lemaigre, G., Robert, L., Carpentier, S., and Dubost, C.: Biologic factors affecting long-term results of valvular heterografts, J. Thorac. Cardiovasc. Surg. **58**:467-483, 1969.

Hufnagel, C. A., and Conrad, P. W.: A new approach to aortic valve replacement, Ann. Surg. **167**:791-795, 1968.

Starr, A., Herr, R. H., and Wood, J. A.: Mitral replacement review of 6 years experience, J. Thorac. Cardiovasc. Surg. **54**:333-358, 1967.

Chapter *32*

An evaluation of visiting policies for intensive and coronary care units

Joan E. Zetterlund

One of the most significant advances in the improvement of care of the seriously ill has been the establishment of intensive and coronary care units. Segregation of patients into a specialized area with highly technical machinery and experienced personnel to detect and treat potentially fatal complications has substantially reduced mortality. In the coronary care unit, for example, constant monitoring of cardiac activity, availability of defibrillators, pacemakers, and antiarrhythmic drugs, and alert nursing and medical personnel who recognize beginning arrhythmias and initiate proper treatment constitute a combination of factors that provide maximum opportunity for recovery.

Ultimate recovery and rehabilitation after a critical illness, however, depend not only on physical care, but also on consideration of psychological, emotional, and social reactions to illness. As nurses increase their awareness of the importance of these reactions, recovery of the "whole person" is accelerated.

Patients and their families are understandably appreciative and grateful for the care provided in intensive and coronary care units. One policy of many units that has been of concern to some patients and families, however, is the restriction of visiting periods to 5 minutes every hour. This policy was first recommended for intensive care units by the United States Public Health Service,[1] together with the suggestion that a family room be located on or near the unit to permit relatives to be near the patient without "interfering" with his treatments. Recommendations by the United States Public Health Service in relation to visiting policies in coronary care units are essentially the same, but these recommendations state that the number and length of visits should be kept at a level consistent with the patient's condition and with the effective operation of the unit.[2] In some units, because visits are brief and space is limited, chairs are not provided, which requires the visitor to stand at the patient's bedside during the entire visit.

Evaluation of the therapeutic value of such a policy has been limited and is absent from current literature. It is the purpose of this chapter to present the results of such an evaluative study within the context of discussion of the emotional, psychological, and social factors influencing recovery from serious illness. The myocardial infarction patient has been chosen as an example of the seriously ill patient. Much of the discussion, however, is relevant to patients with other types of serious or critical illness.

Psychological and emotional reactions to myocardial infarction

The most common reaction to myocardial infarction is anxiety, which may be severe. Rosen and Bibring[3] define anxiety as an individual's response to perceived danger. The degree of anxiety a person experiences is determined by his assessment of the danger and his ability to overcome the threat. Anxiety is greatest when the nature of the threat is uncertain and when the ways of conquering it are not known.

Anxiety from fear of death

Uncertainty, to be sure, is the hallmark of coronary-artery disease and myocardial infarction. Immediately after infarction there is a sense of uncertainty regarding life itself; the patient, doctor, or nurse cannot be assured that an irreversible arrhythmia, cardiogenic shock, or cardiac rupture will not occur and prove fatal. Thus fear of death and the fear of living with the thought of impending death are common reactions that produce anxiety after a myocardial infarction.[4, 5] Factors contributing to a patient's fear of death include not only the pain and difficulty in breathing caused by the illness, but also the measures initiated by the doctor or nurse as soon as the patient enters the hospital or unit—a "beeping" monitor is attached to his chest, an intravenous solution is started in his arm, an injection is given to relieve his pain, oxygen may be administered, and he is told to lie as quietly as possible. Accelerated activity in both the emergency room and intensive or coronary care unit may also compound this fear of death.

In discussing the meaning of death, Feifel[6] states, "It has been said that we may *learn* looking backward—we *live* looking forward." Man is essentially future oriented, and his sense of feeling alive is closely related to the idea of moving toward a future with purposes and goals.[7] To be alive, however, is to face at some time the inevitable reality of death. Despite this fact, our society generally considers death a taboo subject, and little time is spent discussing the meaning and implications of death. As a result, fear of death is a common phenomenon among both the sick and those who are in good health. Zilboorg[8] believes that no one is free from the fear of death because of its threat to the instinct of self-preservation present in every man. He states that fear of death is normally repressed but emerges to our level of consciousness whenever our life is threatened. The object of this fear may be death itself or the process of dying. This process pertains to a sense of imminent disintegration or collapse of one's total personality.[9] Also involved in a person's fear of death or of the process of dying may be a sense of guilt regarding opportunities that have been lost or wasted, tasks that remain unfinished, or wrongs that have been done.[6]

Anxiety from change in self-image

A second source of anxiety after myocardial infarction is change in self-image. After infarction, the patient must integrate the awareness of the lesion into his concept of himself, his interpersonal relationships, and his total pattern of living.[10] The resultant change in self-image will depend in part on the patient's basic personality characteristics, his perception of himself, and the meaning of illness to him. Studies by Cleveland and Johnson[11] reveal that the postinfarct patient perceives himself as a "fragile object" and feels he must be extremely cautious with his life. He feels inadequate and inferior because of failure to live up to ego ideals and because of his decreased ability to achieve his desired goals in his business, family, and social situations.

Change in body image is an important part of the patient's new image of himself. Impaired heart function is a threat to his physical integrity, especially if he has always taken pride in his physical strength and abilities. He may regard his body as damaged because of anticipation of physical disability. Physical inactivity after infarction may also be a serious threat to self-image if activity has been an integral part of the patient's life.[4]

An additional "blow" to the postinfarct patient's self-image is his impaired self-sufficiency. He is forced to change his independent role to one of dependency. As a result, he may feel guilty about burdening others with tasks he has always done prior to his illness, and his helplessness may make him question the willingness of nurses and other health team members to tolerate the inconvenience of caring for him.[7]

Factors influencing reactions to myocardial infarction
Age

Age may be an important factor influencing a patient's reaction to myocardial infarction; change in self-image is especially affected. Rosen and Bibring[3] did a study comparing the reactions of 30-year-old and 50-year-old men to myocardial infarction. According to these researchers, men 50 years of age are already in conflict over their changing role from activity and health of youth to passivity, bodily decline, decreased social and economic achievement, and dependency of later years. After myocardial infarction this conflict is accentuated, resulting in increased anxiety and depression. In this study, patients in their fifties were described by nurses as withdrawn, depressed, hard to get to know, agitated, or rude. Observation of

30-year-old patients revealed that the diagnosis of myocardial infarction and its resulting helpless, dependent role are so unusual for a young patient that it may take him a longer time to accept and integrate the seriousness of his illness and that he may initially deny his illness. Patients in their thirties were described as overly cheerful, jovial, and flirtatious, and their behavior revealed emphasis on masculine strength and independence.

Miller[12] also carried out a study to evaluate the relationship of age to anxiety, depression, and achievement motivation in patients with coronary-artery disease. Although specific ages were not stated in the study, results revealed that younger patients had more psychological disturbances than did older patients, with greater increase in pessimism about success and achievement in life. Sex was not a significant variable in this study.

Personality

One of the most influential factors in determining reactions to myocardial infarction is the patient's personality prior to his illness.[13] If the person is immature and emotionally unstable, with little tolerance of frustration, his capacity to cope with his illness will be impaired. In essence, the patient's pattern of response to stress prior to illness will directly influence his response to myocardial infarction.

In an attempt to improve understanding of psychological factors related to coronary-artery disease, a number of studies have been done to determine personality characteristics of patients with this illness. Although there is disagreement regarding the validity of results, there are similarities in data obtained. The "typical" coronary disease patient has been described as a man of high standards—a "pillar of society" who is concerned about future achievements. He has great control over his behavior, drives, and impulses, and his activities are guided rationally rather than emotionally. He is hard driving and goal directed.[14-16]

Socioeconomic background

The relationship between socioeconomic background and reactions to an initial myocardial infarction was observed by Rosen and Bibring.[3] The blue collar worker was primarily concerned with the effect of illness on his work; if he was assured of returning to employment of equal status and pay, his anxiety was reduced. He also appeared to accept the authority of his doctor and did not question the treatment or care he received. The white collar worker, however, was concerned primarily with his illness, and feared the future course of his illness could not be controlled. It is interesting to note that patients with advanced academic degrees experienced a higher level of anxiety.

Severity of illness

Severity of illness would also seem to affect a person's reaction to myocardial infarction. Dovenmuehle and Verwoerdt,[17] however, have concluded from their studies that a mild illness does not differ from a severe one in its potential to cause serious depression within the first three years of illness. Frequent hospitalization, even in mild cardiac illness, does result in increased depression.

Mechanisms of coping with anxiety

After myocardial infarction, patients may cope with their anxiety in several ways. The defense mechanisms most commonly observed are denial and regression.

Denial

Dovenmuehle and Verwoerdt[17] describe denial as "an avoidance mechanism by means of which the very existence of a phenomenon is repudiated." A patient may deny the illness itself, the associated concerns and problems, or the emotional reac-

tions to the illness. Denial is a frequent complication of coronary-artery disease in active, aggressive men.[10] An aggressive man ordinarily will react to external threats with anger and hostility. If the threat is internal, as is myocardial infarction, the patient cannot remove the threat or escape from it. As a result, he frequently denies the seriousness of his illness, suppresses concern about it, and overcompensates by increasing his physical activity to prove his intactness.

Browne and Hackett[18] observed the mechanism of denial in a group of myocardial infarction patients. Evaluation of reactions of patients to constant cardiac monitoring revealed that eighteen of the nineteen patients in the study reacted to both the monitor and their illness with the same denial of fear, apprehension, or depression. Patients expressed denial in various ways, but two distinct patterns were observed, differentiated by the degree of rigidity with which denial was maintained. The authors called these patterns major denial and partial denial. Twelve of the nineteen patients were described as those using major denial to cope with the anxiety of their illness; six patients were classified as partial deniers. Major deniers considered fear as weakness, and many emphasized courage, indifference to fear, and manly endurance as important attributes. They stated they experienced no anxiety because of either illness or monitor. Partial deniers, on the other hand, initially denied being frightened by their illness or the monitor, but eventually admitted their fear.

Thoughts and fears about death differed in the two groups. Major deniers considered death an abstract and impersonal concept and could not elaborate on their concept of personal death, whereas partial deniers eventually began to admit fear of death and concern for their future. In both groups underlying anxiety was indirectly evidenced by slips of the tongue, inconsistent comments, and frightening dreams. Studies by Cleveland and Johnson[11] also reveal inconsistencies between a postinfarct patient's conscious and subconscious perceptions of himself and his illness.

Regression

A second coping mechanism that may be observed after myocardial infarction is regression to childhood patterns of behavior. A patient with a dependent personality is especially prone to regress; he may assume a state of helplessness and want others to take complete care of him. This coping mechanism may be of temporary advantage in the critical stage of illness, but if prolonged, chronic invalidism may result. Thus the patient may use his illness to escape from responsibilities or problems of everyday life.[4, 10, 15]

The role of the family

Preceding discussion has been related primarily to differences within the individual patient that may affect his reactions to myocardial infarction. To limit our concern to the patient would be incorrect, for each patient interprets his illness in relation to others as well as himself. No person exists in a vacuum. As Westman[19] states, "Each individual is deeply imbedded in a matrix of complicated and vitally important relationships with other people." Thus understanding a patient's reaction to serious illness cannot be achieved without consideration of the group of which he is a member and his position in that group.

The group in which a patient is most intimately involved is his family. The family is the basic unit of society—the unit of growth and experience and of fulfillment and failure.[20] Interrelationships within the family substantially influence the identity and self-image of a person, whether he is in a state of good health or illness.[7] In addition, family relationships provide an individual with the roles he will have in

life. Koos[21] defines a role as "the specific way of behaving expected of the individual in a certain situation by the group." Each member of the family has one or more roles to perform to enable the group to function. For example, in the American family the father is usually the breadwinner and disciplinarian. In most families there is also a pattern of dominance; for cultural, personality, or other reasons, one person is usually the "boss" in the family, with other members being subservient, in varying degrees, to the dominant person and to each other. Roles within the family are not static, however. Each member must continually adjust both to normal stages every family experiences and to unexpected periods of stress, such as illness.[21]

After myocardial infarction, a person's role in the family is changed as he is forced to assume a new role of "patient." This role is unique because it frees the individual from both privileges and responsibilities of other social and family roles.[19] If the patient is father, breadwinner, and disciplinarian in the family, as is frequently true of patients with myocardial infarction, someone else has to assume his role if balance is to be maintained within the family unit. Other family members may resent this reversal of roles.

Family members also react to the uncertainty associated with myocardial infarction. When an individual is admitted to a coronary care unit, the threat to the patient's life and survival brings about a threat to the structure and survival of the family. The resulting anxiety of family members is readily communicated to the patient and contributes to his response to illness.[22, 23] Therefore a patient's psychological and emotional reactions to myocardial infarction cannot be fully evaluated without considering the reactions of the family group of which he is a member. Moreover, the importance of patient-family interrelationships in the recovery and rehabilitation of patients with myocardial infarction must be given proper concern.

During hospitalization on a coronary care unit the primary opportunity for continuing patient-family relationships is during visiting periods. Because of the recognition of the importance of these periods, together with an awareness of the occasional unfavorable comments from both patients and families regarding the restriction of visiting periods, a study was carried out to evaluate the therapeutic value of restricted family visits. Myocardial infarction patients and their families were interviewed to determine their opinions of visiting privileges on the coronary care unit. In addition, physiological reactions of patients to visits were determined by observing changes in cardiac rate and rhythm during family visits.

Visiting privileges

Patients participating in the study were in the coronary care units of two hospitals. The written policy of both units stated that one member of the patient's family may visit for 5 minutes every hour. Patients and families were informed of the policy by nurses of these units. In one hospital, length of visiting periods was not generally enforced by nurses. Length of observed visits varied from 5 to 40 minutes. At the other hospital, visits began every hour on the hour. After 5 minutes, the ward secretary went from room to room announcing the end of the visiting period. Because of the secretary's other responsibilities, the time of her announcement sometimes was delayed; also, some visitors were reluctant to leave until spoken to more than once. As a result, length of visits ranged from 5 to 23 minutes, although most were between 5 and 10 minutes.

Reactions of patients

Five of the seventeen patients interviewed stated they preferred visits limited to 5 minutes every hour. Reasons for their opinions included the following: "patients on coronary care units are very sick, and need rest, and it's easier to rest when there are no visitors"; "when my sons visit, my heart goes 'thump, thump,' so I just like to see their faces and know they're all right." Another patient stated longer visiting periods would interfere with his personal needs, such as using the urinal or commode. This patient was in a semiprivate room and had become embarrassed one afternoon when he was using the commode and his roommate's wife came to visit.

Eleven patients stated that 5 minutes were too brief. Five of these patients suggested that 10- or 15-minute visits would be adequate in most situations. Two male patients commented that a patient in their situation has "family business" to discuss, and that 5 minutes is not long enough to do so satisfactorily. Another patient stated he would frequently think of his family having to wait 55 minutes just to visit 5 minutes. He said he felt more relaxed when visits were longer. An additional comment was that being in the coronary care unit was "like being in jail; the visitor comes in, and the 'policeman' is right there to ask her to leave." Three patients clarified their statements by saying that each patient's condition and "how he feels" should affect visiting privileges. A male patient said he did not want any visitors when he was critically ill and receiving frequent intravenous doses of antiarrhythmic drugs, but during the remainder of his stay in the unit, "when the pain went, it didn't matter how long people stayed."

Only one patient was noncommittal in his opinion of visiting privileges. He stated, "I don't say much during visits, anyway, so it really doesn't make any difference to me if it's 5 minutes or longer."

Reactions of families

Only one of the nine family members interviewed agreed with the advisability of 5-minute visits. The wife of one patient "generally" agreed with the policy, but said she wanted to stay longer and "just sit with my husband when he was very sick."

The remaining seven visitors preferred longer visits. Four stated there should be some restriction, but that the amount of time spent with the patient should depend on the severity of his illness. One visitor commented that the head nurse should determine the length of visits for each patient, and that "one rule should not apply to all patients."

Cardiac changes

Another aspect of the study sought to determine if patients' stress levels would differ if the length of visits were controlled by hospital personnel in contrast to control by the patient and his family. Measurement of stress was indicated by changes in cardiac rate and rhythm during visits as compared with rate and rhythm while the patient was resting, with no visitors. Strips of electrocardiograph monitor recordings were obtained during thirty-five visits to the seventeen patients involved in the study.

As stated previously, although both units had a written policy limiting visits to 5 minutes every hour, nurses in one unit generally did not enforce the policy. As a result, length of visits was controlled essentially by the patient and his family. Observation of heart rates of patients in this unit showed a mean increase of 10% at the beginning of the visits, but mean cardiac rates decreased to the mean resting rate at the termination of visits. This decrease in rate suggests that levels of stress may be decreased at this time if length of visits are controlled by the patient and his family.

In contrast, observation of patients in the unit in which the visiting policy was enforced revealed that mean cardiac rate remained increased between 6% and 7% above mean resting rate throughout the entire visit. This observation seems to support comments by two patients in this unit that 5 minutes is not time enough to resolve family problems or other concerns the patient wishes to discuss with a member of the family.

Changes in cardiac rhythm were noted during visits in four instances. One patient experienced slight temporary irregularity of heart rate at the beginning of the visit. The other three patients experienced temporary changes in rhythm at the termination of a visit. When interviewed, two of these latter three patients stated they preferred visits restricted to 5 minutes. However, the two visits that precipitated arrhythmias were 23 and 40 minutes in length. These observations suggest that visits longer than the period of time desired by the patient may result in increased stress, as reflected in cardiac changes.

Implications for nursing

The study presented in this chapter is limited both by the relatively small number of patients and families involved and by the fact that consideration of emotional, psychological, and social reactions of the seriously ill patient was centered specifically on the patient with myocardial infarction. However, since many of the reactions a patient experiences after an acute cardiac illness are similar to those of other seriously ill patients, implications can be derived that will be important for nurses in both intensive and coronary care units.

It is understood that because of the serious and complex nature of their health problems, patients in intensive and coronary care units require care by nurses who are highly competent in recognizing and dealing with physical crises that threaten recovery. Nurses are becoming increasingly aware that recovery may also be influenced by the effects of anxiety from fear of death or of the unknown, change in self-image, and isolation from a familiar environment, family, and friends. Some of this anxiety can be relieved by the nurse as she anticipates manifestations of anxiety in her patients and evaluates each patient's ability to cope with his reactions to serious illness. By recognizing that each patient's behavior is influenced by many factors unique to himself and by responding to each patient as an individual human being, the nurse can also help prevent the potentially impersonal environment induced by modern technology and automation. A former patient in an intensive care unit has said, "In contrast to the cold steel of my respirator or transparent glass of my suction jar, I wanted the touch of a warm, human hand."[24]

Of utmost importance for the nurse is consideration of the patient's family in recovery and rehabilitation after serious illness. Some nurses and health team members tend to look on the patient's family as a burden. This is especially true in intensive and coronary care units where the demands for complex physical care are so great. In addition, increased anxiety and concern of family members may lead to their seemingly endless questions and pleas for reassurance from nursing personnel. Since attitudes and feelings of family members contribute to the patient's response to his illness, it would seem important that the nurse become more aware of the role of the patient's family. It cannot be denied that some visitors may upset patients and interfere with promotion of rest, for preexisting family problems and conflicts follow the patient to the hospital. The nurse should observe for manifestations of such stress-producing situations and seek solutions to them. She should also recognize that new conflicts and tensions may result from reversal of roles and insecurity precipitated by serious illness. Thus the nurse's attitude toward the family should be as understanding as that toward the patient. Effective communica-

tion should be established with both patient and family so the uniqueness of each patient-family relationship may be realized.

The right of the family to be with the patient during the critical stages of his illness must also be recognized. Before intensive and coronary care units existed, members of the family usually stayed at the bedside of a seriously ill relative. Perhaps nurses felt more secure knowing that someone was with the patient when they did not have the time to observe him as often as they would have desired. But nurses now are able to observe patients closely on intensive and coronary care units, and the amount of time for patients and families to be together has been rigidly restricted in some units. Do such restrictions conflict with the right of the patient and family to be with each other at this important time? Is this right a moral or legal one? Perhaps this latter question is one that nurses may have to answer in the near future as increased emphasis is placed on the legal aspects of human rights.

Evaluation of the results of the study presented in this chapter reveals that patients on coronary care units desire periods of time to renew and clarify relationships with their family and discuss family concerns. Comments about the length and frequency of visits vary considerably, influenced by the unique response of each individual patient and family member to serious illness. However, most patients and family members agreed that one policy should not apply to all patients, but that visiting privileges should be determined by each patient's condition.

If length and frequency of family visits to patients in intensive and coronary care units were determined on an individual basis, several questions would have to be answered:

1. Who would be responsible for evaluating each patient's condition?

2. When a patient's condition becomes

more critical, should length and frequency of visits be increased or decreased?

3. Who would evaluate the patient's response to visitors? If this is the nurse's responsibility, how would she observe family visits without interfering with patient-family interaction?

4. What criteria determine a favorable or unfavorable response to visitors?

5. How does the nurse reply to a patient who asks her why her roommate is allowed visitors for a longer period of time than she?

6. If the intensive or coronary care unit is one large room with several patients, what effects do visitors of one patient have on other patients?

These are only some of the questions that indicate the complexity of the problem of determining visiting policies for intensive and coronary care units. Perhaps the easiest solution would seem to be to effect a uniform policy for all patients. However, as nurses become more aware of the importance of the family in the recovery of seriously ill patients, it seems desirable if not essential to allow some flexibility in visiting policies and to seek new ways to integrate family visits into the care plan for individual patients. For example, in units that do not provide a chair for visitors, visits may be more relaxed and meaningful if the family member could sit by the patient's bedside rather than stand hovering over him. If patients were asked their preferences regarding family visits, they may have at least some feeling of control over what happens to them in their new and strange environment, and anxiety may be reduced. The presence and reassuring touch of a family member may also help a seriously ill patient adapt to his unfamiliar hospital environment and reduce confusion.

Nurses in each intensive and coronary care unit have the final responsibility in identifying other ways that families may contribute to the recovery of seriously ill

patients and in determining the degree of flexibility in visiting policies for their unit. However, if additional studies of the role of the family and family visits were carried out, more reliable guidelines or criteria for determining visiting policies would be available to all nurses interested in the care of the seriously ill.

References

1. United States Department of Health, Education and Welfare, Public Health Service: Elements of progressive patient care, no. 930-C-1, Washington, D. C., 1962, Government Printing Office.
2. United States Department of Health, Education and Welfare, Public Health Service: A facility designed for coronary care, no. 930-D-19, Washington, D. C., 1965, Government Printing Office.
3. Rosen, J., and Bibring, G.: Psychological reactions of hospitalized male patients to a heart attack, Psychosom. Med. **28**:808-821, 1966.
4. Braceland, F. J.: Coronary spectrum: psychiatric aspects, J. Rehab. **32**:53-55, 1966.
5. Kinlein, M. L.: Nursing the coronary patient, J. Rehab. **32**:39-41, 1966.
6. Feifel, H.: Attitudes toward death in some normal and mentally ill populations. In Feifel, H., editor: The meaning of death, New York, 1959, McGraw-Hill Book Co., Inc.
7. Verwoerdt, A.: Communication with the fatally ill, Springfield, Ill., 1966, Charles C Thomas, Publisher.
8. Zilboorg, G.: Fear of death, Psychoanal. Quart. **12**:465-475, 1943.
9. Weisman, A. D., and Hackett, T. P.: Predilection to death, Psychosom. Med. **23**:232-256, 1961.
10. Reiser, M. F.: Emotional aspects of cardiac disease, Amer. J. Psychiat. **107**:781-785, 1951.
11. Cleveland, S. E., and Johnson, D. L.: Personality patterns in young males with coronary disease, Psychosom. Med. **24**:600-610, 1962.
12. Miller, C. K.: Psychological correlates of coronary artery disease, Psychosom. Med. **27**:257-265, 1965.
13. Likoff, W.: Coronary spectrum: the attack, J. Rehab. **32**:25-26, 1966.
14. Cady, L. D., Gertler, M. M., Gottsch, L. G., and Woodbury, M. A.: The factor structure

of variables concerned with coronary artery disease, Behav. Sci. **6:**37-41, 1961.

15. Heal, F. C.: Recent advances in the psychosomatic aspects of cardiac disease, Psychosomatics **3:**365-370, 1962.

16. Minc, S.: Psychological factors in coronary heart disease, Geriatrics **20:**747-755, 1965.

17. Dovenmuehle, R. H., and Verwoerdt, A.: Physical illness and depressive symptomatology: factors of length and severity of illness and frequency of hospitalization, J. Geront. **18:**260-266, 1963.

18. Browne, I. W., and Hackett, T. P.: Emotional reactions to the threat of impending death: a study of patients on the monitor cardiac pacemaker, Irish J. Med. Sci. **6:**177-187, 1967.

19. Westman, J. C.: The patient's family, Univ. Mich. Med. Cent. J. **30:**147-150, 1964.

20. Ackerman, N. W.: The family in crisis, Bull. N. Y. Acad. Med. **40:**171-187, 1964.

21. Koos, E. L.: The sociology of the patient, New York, 1959, McGraw-Hill Book Co., Inc.

22. Kübler-Ross, E.: On death and dying, New York, 1969, The Macmillan Co.

23. Lambertsen, E. C.: Coronary care unit therapy must include support for the patient's family, Mod. Hosp. **110:**128, 1968.

24. Carlson, D.: The unbroken vigil, Richmond, 1968, John Knox, Press.

Bibliography

Duff, R. S., and Hollinshead, A. B.: Sickness and society, New York, 1968, Harper & Row Publishers.

Fisher, S. H.: Psychological factors and heart disease, Circulation **27:**113-117, 1963.

Fitzwater, J.: Planning an intensive care unit, Amer. J. Nurs. **67:**310-314, 1967.

George, J.: Monitoring the myocardial infarction patient: emotional reactions of nurse and patient, Nurs. Clin. N. Amer. **1:**549-557, 1966.

Glaser, B. G., and Strauss, A. L.: Awareness of dying, Chicago, 1966, Aldine Publishing Co.

Kinlein, M. L.: Myocardial infarction: the crucial hours, Amer. J. Nurs. **64:**C-10-13, Nov., 1964.

Kornfeld, D. S., Maxwell, T., and Momrow, D.: Psychological hazards of the intensive care unit. nursing care aspects, Nurs. Clin. N. Amer. **3:**41-51, 1968.

Lambertsen, E. C.: The nature and objectives of intensive care nursing, Nurs. Clin. N. Amer. **3:**3-6, 1968.

Meltzer, L. E., Pinneo, R., and Kitchell, J. R.: Intensive coronary care—a manual for nurses, Philadelphia, 1965, CCU Fund, Presbyterian Hospital.

Powers, M., and Storlie, F.: The apprehensive patient, Amer. J. Nurs. **67:**58-63, 1967.

Roberts, S. L.: The patient's adaptation to the coronary care unit, Nurs. Forum **9:**56-63, 1970.

Strauss, A. L.: The intensive care unit: its characteristics and social relationships, Nurs. Clin. N. Amer. **3:**7-15, 1968.

United States Department of Health, Education and Welfare, Public Health Service: Coronary care units, No. 1250, Washington, D. C., 1965, Government Printing Office.

Yu, P. N., Imboden, C. A., Fox, S. M., and Killip, T.: Coronary care unit, Mod. Conc. Cardiovasc. Dis. **34:**23-30, 1965.

Chapter 33

Medication information: patient knowledge and nursing responsibility

Joy L. Brown

Although the use of medicinal agents in the treatment of illness can be traced back to ancient times, it has only been recently that drugs have figured decisively in health care. They have contributed significantly to increased life expectancy by decreasing mortality from acute illnesses and have provided a means for treatment of chronic conditions such as diabetes mellitus and hypertension, which were previously fatal. Today, drugs have become a major means of attaining and maintaining physical and mental well being. However, none of the drugs in use today is without hazard to the patient. An increasing number of problems have arisen due to adverse drug response and incorrect administration.

The effective and safe use of drugs is dependent on the patients' acquisition and retention of essential information about their medication. However, such instruction is rarely provided the patient in a systematic, carefully planned manner. Patients' attempts to obtain medication information from nurses on patient care units meet with varying degrees of success. Some nurses discourage such time-con-suming activity with curt replies, whereas others avoid teaching obligations with statements such as "I can't give you that information, you'll have to ask your doctor." Frequently the hospitalized patient receives medication information on the day of discharge when his anxiety level is high and a variety of concerns and activities divert his attention. In one study, of one hundred and eight patients interviewed, 65% received no instructions in any aspect of their care and only 17% reported receiving more than 5 minutes of instruction.[1] The out-patient fares no better in the busy physician's office or clinic where he often receives a handful of prescriptions and a few hurried sentences of instruction. Pharmacists dispensing the medications are rarely of assistance to the patient. Labeling of prescription drugs is frequently restricted to the dosage and administration schedule with the name, strength, or purpose of the medication stated only if the physician has specifically requested that they be included. Thus the patient frequently finds himself confronted by a confusing array of drugs that he is expected to take correctly with little or no guidance.

Instances of incorrect administration of medications due to misinterpretation of directions or inadequate information are not uncommon. The need for greater clarity and more detailed information is illustrated by the following examples.

Miss M, who previously had taken two tablets of digoxin daily, was instructed to alternate one tablet of digoxin with two tablets daily. One week after this change in her medication schedule she called her physician complaining of nausea and vomiting. Upon questioning, it was discovered that she was taking three tablets of digoxin every day. In this instance the directions for taking the medication had not been clearly stated and were misunderstood by the patient.

Mrs. Z, a cardiac patient with a history of angina, was discharged from the hospital with prescriptions for several medications, including Prednisone that was to be taken once a day. Although she was given this drug in the hospital for her chest pain, she was not told what it was or how it acted. However, she had taken nitroglycerin previously for her chest pain and assuming the new medication to be similar in its action, she took a tablet whenever she experienced episodes of chest pain. This patient was not given enough information about the purpose and action of her new medication to ensure its correct administration.

Mr. B, for whom long-term anticoagulant therapy was prescribed for treatment of thrombophlebitis and pulmonary embolus, took his medication exactly as prescribed. However, recent blood tests indicated an unexpected increase in coagulation time. Upon investigation it was found that his bursitis was acting up and he was treating it with 15 grains of aspirin every four hours. Mr. B was unaware that aspirin should not be taken by persons on anticoagulants because of its synergistic effect. He had not been informed of this medication restriction.

Concern about medication errors made by patients at home has led several investigators to study the scope of the problem and identify contributory factors. In a study of 178 elderly patients taking medication at home, Schwartz[2] found that 105 were making medication errors. Neely and Patrick[3] report that thirty of fifty patients they surveyed made errors; of these 48% were errors of omission and 34% were attributed to inaccurate knowledge of the drugs. The number of medications a patient was taking was found to be related to medication errors. Curtis[4] reports that fifteen of sixteen patients who made errors were taking three or more drugs. Neely and Patrick[3] found similar results. Lack of understanding of a drug's purpose may also affect patient's adherence to prescribed regimen. In a study of 245 patients for whom a seven-day course of penicillin was prescribed, eighty-four admitted to not taking the full amount of the drug; when patient instruction was revised to include an explanation of the necessity of completing the full course, compliance increased from 60% to 70%.[5]

Nursing and pharmacology texts stress the importance of administering the right drug in the right dosage at the right time. This applies to patients at home as well as nurses on patient care units. In addition, information regarding precautions and symptoms of adverse reactions must be provided if patients are to safely administer their drugs. Schimmel reports that of hospitalized patients who had serious reactions to therapy, 51% were the result of drug therapy.[6] Patients taking medication at home are not under constant observation by the physician or nurse and must be taught to recognize and report significant symptoms.

There are other instances in which a patient's knowledge of his medications is useful. With today's system of health care a patient may be under treatment by several specialists at the same time for separate problems. The patient who is knowledgeable about his medications is able to give an accurate drug history. He can assist the people responsible for his care in developing a more complete picture of the patient's health status and enable them to formulate a better plan of care. Possible duplication of drugs, incompatibilities, antagonism, or potentiation might thus be avoided. Patients in need of emergency medical care or hospitalization who are taking medications in which blood levels must be maintained, such as steroids, insulin, or anticoagulants, could provide this information so that the medication could be continued or the dosage changed as needed.

To provide adequate instruction, it is necessary to identify those areas in which information is lacking. The following study was conducted to investigate the extent of patients' knowledge of their prescription medications and identify related factors.

Study design

The information presented is derived from a study of fifty patients attending the general medicine clinic at a large public teaching hospital. All these individuals had been taking at least one oral prescription medication on a regular basis for two weeks prior to the study.

Semistructured interviews were conducted in which the subjects were asked to identify the name, purpose, dosage, and administration schedule of all prescription medications. They were also asked if any additional instructions or information had been given regarding the medications. The information obtained was compared to that found in the medical records to determine existing discrepancies. Medication scores were obtained on the basis of number of correct responses.

Results

The fifty patients interviewed were taking a total of 134 drugs; the number of

Table 9. Number and percentage of correct responses in all medication information categories for 134 medications prescribed

Category	Number	Percentage
Name	59	44.0
Purpose	75	56.0
Dosage	118	88.1
Schedule of administration	107	79.9
Additional information	6	4.5

medications per patient ranged from 1 to 6. For only 29 of the 134 drugs was all necessary information (name, purpose, dosage, and administration schedule) correctly given by the subjects. As can be seen from Table 9, the name of the medication was known for 59 of the drugs. The correct purpose was stated seventy-five times. Correct dosage was reported for 118 of the medications, whereas administration schedule was correctly cited in 107 instances.

These findings suggest that in patient teaching the dosage and time of administration are stressed, whereas the name and purpose of medications are given less attention, or, possibly, the former information has greater meaning for the patients. The hospital pharmacy where most of the prescriptions were filled does include the name of the drug on the label; thus this information can be readily obtained if the patient so desires.

Despite the high percentage of correct responses for dosage and administration schedule, in a total of forty-three separate instances drugs were apparently being taken incorrectly. Of these, fourteen instances would have resulted in serious underdosage and nine in overdosage. Although no one dosage or schedule appeared to have a great number of incorrect responses, of three patients with complicated schedules, all gave incorrect responses. For example, one patient who was supposed to be alternating one tablet once

Table 10. Age of subjects as related to number of medications taken, education level, and medication information scores

Age and number of subjects	Number of prescribed medications			Education level		Medication information scores	
	1	*2-3*	*4+*	*≤ 8*	*> 8*	*low*	*high*
21 - 44 (N = 13)	6	5	2	4	9	6	7
45 - 64 (N = 22)	1	15	6	10	12	5	17
65 + (N = 15)	2	10	3	11	4	13	2
Total (N = 50)	9	30	11	25	25	24	26

a day with one tablet twice daily indicated the instructions were one tablet three times a day.

Additional information such as precautions and side effects were reported for only six medications. In three instances patients on anticoagulants cited reporting of bleeding to the physician as important. Two patients taking potassium depleting diuretics remembered being instructed to drink orange juice. The failure of patients to be cognizant of side effects, signs of toxicity, and other precautions is of significance. Of the drugs included in the study, 65.7% were cardiovascular drugs such as digitalis, antihypertensives, and diuretics. None of the patients taking antihypertensive medications indicated awareness of orthostatic hypotension as a side effect with which to be concerned, although some reported episodes of dizziness. None of the patients on digitalis preparations mentioned anorexia, nausea, vomiting, or change in heart rhythm as important signs to report, even though some of them had previously been hospitalized for digitalis toxicity.

The results of this study indicate that while patients receive instruction in how to take their medications and perhaps general information related to purpose, few either receive or retain information about the name, therapeutic effect, or symptoms of adverse reactions. Whether unintentional or purposely avoided for fear of alarming patients, failure to provide them with information necessary for the safe administration of drugs appears to be a serious omission in patient education.

In addition to the above findings, the data were analyzed in an attempt to identify significant variables affecting patients' drug information. Although neither the number of medications nor the length of time on medication appeared significant, age was a significant factor. Table 10 shows that fewer drugs were prescribed for patients below the age of 45 than for those 45 or older. This could be due to severity of illness; older patients had chronic or degenerative diseases affecting multiple organ systems (for example, atherosclerosis), whereas younger patients were more likely to have a single organ dysfunction (for example, hypothyroidism).

The elderly were also less knowledgeable about drugs they were taking than was true for younger persons; thirteen of the elderly had low medication information scores. Educational level was significant. Eleven of the fifteen patients 65 or older had less than an eighth grade education; in general, persons with less than eight years of formal education knew less about their medications than those with more schooling. Race, sex, marital status, occupation, and religion were not found to be significant.

Conclusion

The results of this study indicate a need for patient education. Lack of adequate instruction is detrimental to health care. With the current emphasis on self-care, the patient must have that information which will enable him to carry out therapy effectively and safely. It is the responsibility of the health professions to provide this information.

Nursing implications

As the role of the professional nurse has expanded, her responsibilities for educating the patient in various aspects of his care have increased. Whether in the hospital, clinic, or physician's office, functioning as a primary health agent or in a more traditional role, the nurse is involved with helping the patient adjust to his illness and to care for himself. Providing drug information is an integral part of nursing care.

For the outpatient whose contact with the physician and nurse is limited, special effort must be made to provide time for instruction. In the hospital, educating the patient may take place over a longer time period as he becomes aware of and indicates readiness to assume responsibility for various aspects of his care. A patient in an intensive care unit may only want to know that the medication being administered will relieve his pain, whereas a convalescing patient nearing discharge is more interested in specific information about his drugs.

A nursing history is a useful tool in planning for patient teaching. Exploration of the patient's attitudes toward illness and the use of drugs, and his trust in those involved in his care have bearing on patient instruction and may indicate reluctance or resistance on the part of the patient to comply with therapy. For example, a person who does not like to take medication may tend to disregard an increase in a drug dosage. Specific information about the patient's home routine, difficulty in taking particular dosage forms, poor eyesight, or unsteadiness is helpful in in-

dividualizing teaching and in planning a workable medication routine. An arthritic patient may have difficulty opening the new childproof medication containers. Accuracy in pouring liquids may be a problem for persons with hand tremor. For the busy housewife with children to get off to school, breakfast is not a convenient time to take her medication. The elderly patient who becomes confused easily must be helped to develop a system that will ensure correct medication administration. Once such a patient assessment is obtained, a personalized plan can be developed and instituted that, along with providing specific drug information, adapts the therapy to the patient.

Patient education need not nor should it be provided solely in planned formal teaching sessions. Impromptu questions should be answered fully. Such inquiries are indicative of the patient's readiness and willingness to learn, and the opportunity for patient teaching should be utilized.

However, this does not imply that instructing the patient about his medications should be dependent on chance encounters. A well-formulated plan incorporating all necessary information should be utilized to ensure that the patient receives adequate instruction well before his discharge date. When possible any family members involved in the patient's care should be included in formal teaching sessions. Patient instruction should be carried out in a relaxed, friendly atmosphere and adequate time should be provided for questions and discussion of the information provided. In some settings, group sessions may be useful in exploring common problems and attitudes toward drug therapy.

After completion of medication instruction, an assessment of the patient's ability to safely administer his medications should be made. If additional instruction and supervision are thought advisable and referral to a community health agency is made, information about the patient, the teaching program employed, and assessment of the patient's knowledge should be provided. For all patients, follow-up evaluation is necessary to identify areas of knowledge in need of reinforcement and to determine the success of the teaching methods employed.

In teaching the patient about his medications, the nurse has the opportunity to apply knowledge from various areas. She must know the therapeutic and adverse effects of drugs. She must recognize individual psychosocial factors of significance and apply knowledge of educational psychology in evolving and instituting a teaching plan. To be effective, the nurse must recognize the importance of medication instruction and accept her responsibility for such patient education. Familiarization with recent advances and development in drug therapy, and the implementation, evaluation, and revision of teaching methods is demanding and time consuming. But by so doing, the nurse, in ensuring that the patient can administer his medications effectively and safely, makes a significant contribution to patient care.

References

1. Spiegel, Allen D.: Questions of hospital patients—unasked and unanswered, Postgrad. Med. 43:215-218, 1968.
2. Schwartz, Doris: Medication errors made by aged patients, Amer. J. Nurs. 62:51-53, 1962.
3. Neely, Elizabeth, and Patrick, Maxine.: Problems of aged persons taking medications at home, Nurs. Res. 17:52-55, 1968.
4. Curtis, Elizabeth B.: Medication errors made by patients, Nurs. Outlook 9:290-291, 1961.
5. Mohler, Daniel N., Wallin David G., and Dreyfus, Edward G.: Studies in the home treatment of streptococcal disease, New Eng. J. Med. 252:1116-1118, 1955.
6. Schimmel, Elihu M.: The physician as a pathogen, J. Chron. Dis. 16:1-4, 1963.

Bibliography

Brown, Joy L.: Patients information about their prescription medications, unpublished master's thesis, University of Illinois at the Medical Center, Chicago, Ill., 1969.
Redman, Barbara Klug: The process of patient teaching in nursing, St. Louis, 1968, The C. V. Mosby Co.

Index